LIPPINCOTT
MANUAL *of*
NURSING
PRACTICE
POCKET
GUIDES

Pediatric Nursing

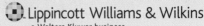 Lippincott Williams & Wilkins
a Wolters Kluwer business
Philadelphia · Baltimore · New York · London
Buenos Aires · Hong Kong · Sydney · Tokyo

STAFF

Executive Publisher
Judith A. Schilling McCann,
RN, MSN

Editorial Director
H. Nancy Holmes

Clinical Director
Joan Robinson, RN, MSN

Senior Art Director
Arlene Putterman

Editorial Project Manager
Jennifer Lynn Kowalak

Clinical Project Manager
Beverly Ann Tscheschlog,
RN, BS

Editors
Naina D. Chohan,
Julie Munden

Clinical Editor
Kathryn Henry, RN, BSN

Copy Editors
Kimberly Bilotta (supervisor),
Dorothy P. Terry,
Pamela Wingrod

Designers
Linda Jovinelly Franklin
(project manager),
Matie Anne Patterson

Cover Design
PubTech, LLC

Digital Composition Services
Diane Paluba (manager),
Joyce Rossi Biletz,
Donna S. Morris

Manufacturing
Beth J. Welsh

Editorial Assistants
Megan L. Aldinger,
Karen J. Kirk, Linda K. Ruhf

Design Assistant
Georg W. Purvis IV

Indexer
Barbara Hodgson

Library of Congress
Cataloging-in-Publication Data

Pediatric nursing.
     p. ; cm.—(Lippincott manual of nursing
practice pocket guides)
  Includes bibliographical references and index.
  1. Pediatric nursing—Handbooks, manuals,
etc. I. Lippincott Williams & Wilkins. II. Title.
III. Series.
  [DNLM: 1. Pediatric Nursing—Handbooks.
WY 49 P3705 2007]
RJ245.P43 2007
618.92'00231—dc22
ISBN 1-58255-585-0 (alk. paper)
                                        2006001207

Contents

Contributors
and consultants

Brandy Andrew, ARNP, MSN
Assistant Nursing Professor, Pediatric Nurse
    Practitioner
Northern Kentucky University
Highland Heights

Peggy D. Baikie, RN, MS, CNNP, CPNP
Clinical Coordinator/Nurse Practitioner
St. Anthony Hospitals
Denver
Adjunct Professor
Metropolitan State College of Denver

Stephanie C. Butkus, RN, MSN, CPNP, IBCLC
Assistant Professor
Kettering (Ohio) College of Medical Arts

Kim Cooper, RN, MSN
Nursing Department Program Chair
Ivy Tech Community College
Terre Haute, Ind.

Patricia L. Eells, RN, MS, CPNP
Pediatric Nurse Practitioner
Pediatric Heart Lung Center, The Children's
    Hospital
Denver

Diane M. Elmore, RN, MSN, APN, FNP-C
Nursing Faculty
Great Basin College
Elko, Nev.
Family Nurse Practitioner
Northeastern Nevada Regional Hospital
Elko

Dana M. Etzel-Hardman, RN, BSN, CPN
Training & Educational Specialist
Children's Hospital of Pittsburgh
Duquesne University

Karla Lamley, RN, MSN, CFNP
Registered Nurse
Mesa (Ariz.) General Hospital

Deborah Mayo, ARNP/CPNP, MSN
Pediatric Nurse Practitioner
Oklahoma State Department of Health
Guthrie

Noel C. Piano, RN, MS
Instructor
Lafayette School of Practical Nursing
Williamsburg, Va.

Janet Somlyay, RN, MSN, CNS, CPNP
Maternal-Child Clinical Nurse Specialist
United Medical Center
Cheyenne, Wyo.

Trinidad Villaruel, RN, MSN
Clinical Nurse Specialist
Children's Hospital of New York (New York
    Presbyterian)

Lynette M. Wachholz, ARNP, MN, IBCLC
Pediatric Nurse Practitioner, Lactation
    Consultant
The Everett Clinic – Harbour Pointe
Mukilteo, Wash.

Julee Waldrop, RN, MSN, FNP, PNP
Clinical Associate Professor
The University of North Carolina
Chapel Hill

Robin R. Wilkerson, RN, PhD
Associate Professor of Nursing
University of Mississippi
Jackson

Part one

Disorders

Acquired immunodeficiency syndrome

DESCRIPTION

- Results from the human immunodeficiency virus (HIV) attacking helper T cells
- Three main groups of children infected with HIV
  - Infants of HIV-infected mothers, acquiring the infection either during pregnancy, birth, or via breast-feeding
  - Adolescents acquiring the infection through sexual contact or I.V. drug abuse
  - Infants, children, and adolescents acquiring the virus via contaminated blood products
- Not spread by casual contact with an infected child; spread only by an exchange of body fluids, including breast milk, blood, semen, or vaginal fluids
- Incubation period for HIV infection much shorter in children than in adults
  - In teenagers and young adults: incubation period may last 10 or more years
  - Children acquiring virus by placental transmission: usually become HIV-positive by age 6 months and develop clinical signs by age 3
- Passive antibody transmission: accounts for all infants born to HIV-infected mothers testing positive for antibodies to the virus up to about age 18 months; during this time, detection of the HIV antigen confirms diagnosis
- Also called *AIDS*

PATHOPHYSIOLOGY

- HIV strikes helper T cells bearing the CD4 antigen.
- Antigen serves as a receptor for the retrovirus and allows it to enter the cell.
- After invading a cell, HIV replicates, leading to cell death, or becomes latent.

■ HIV infection leads to acute disease either directly, through destruction of CD4+ cells, other immune cells, and neuroglial cells; or indirectly, through the secondary effects of CD4+ T-cell dysfunction and resultant immunosuppression.

CAUSES

■ Contaminated blood products
■ Infected mother (during pregnancy, birth, or breast-feeding)
■ I.V. drug abuse
■ Sexual contact with infected partner

ASSESSMENT FINDINGS

■ Failure to thrive
■ Lymphadenopathy
■ Mononucleosis-like prodromal symptoms
■ Neurologic impairment, such as loss of motor milestones and behavioral changes
■ Night sweats
■ Recurring opportunistic infections, such as *Pneumocystis carinii* pneumonia (PCP)
■ Recurring diarrhea
■ Weight loss
■ Hepatosplenomegaly
■ Repeated fungal infections (thrush)
■ Multiple bacterial infections

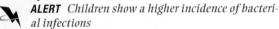 ***ALERT*** *Children show a higher incidence of bacterial infections*

TEST RESULTS

■ CD4+ T cell count measures the severity of immunosuppression.
■ Culture and sensitivity tests reveal infection with opportunistic organisms.

■ Enzyme-linked immunosorbent assay and Western blot
are positive for HIV antibody.
■ Viral culture or p24 antigen test reveals the presence of
the virus in children younger than age 18 months.

TREATMENT

▶ **COLLABORATION** *The patient requires the skill of an
immunologist specializing in HIV infection. He may
also need the assistance of pulmonary specialists, if his
respiratory system is compromised and nutritional therapy to optimize his condition. Supportive therapy (for pain
relief and psychological support) promotes patient com-
fort. The patient (and his family) may also benefit from re-
ferrals to AIDS societies and support programs.*
■ Blood administration, if necessary
■ Follow-up laboratory studies
■ High-calorie diet provided in small, frequent meals
■ I.V. fluids to maintain hydration
■ Nutritional supplements, if necessary
■ Parenteral nutrition, if necessary
■ Antibiotic therapy according to the sensitivity of the in-
fecting opportunistic organism
■ Antiviral agents: zidovudine
■ Protease inhibitors
■ Non-nucleoside reverse transcriptase inhibitors
■ Monthly gamma globulin administration
■ Prophylactic antibiotic therapy with co-trimoxazole to
prevent PCP
■ Routine immunizations (but varicella vaccine isn't rec-
ommended for HIV-infected children)

KEY PATIENT OUTCOMES

The patient (or his family) will:
■ achieve management of symptoms
■ demonstrate use of protective measures, including energy conservation, maintenance of well-balanced diet, and
getting adequate rest

PREVENTING HIV TRANSMISSION

■ Use precautions in all situations that risk exposure to blood, body fluids, and secretions. Diligently practicing standard precautions can prevent the inadvertent transmission of human immunodeficiency virus (HIV), hepatitis B, and other infectious diseases that are transmitted by similar routes.
■ Teach the parents, family, and friends about disease transmission and prevention of extending the disease to others.
■ Tell the patient not to donate blood, blood products, organs, tissue, or sperm.
■ If the patient uses I.V. drugs, caution him not to share needles.
■ Inform the patient that high-risk sexual practices for HIV transmission are those that exchange body fluids, such as vaginal or anal intercourse without a condom.
■ Discuss safe sexual practices, such as hugging, petting, mutual masturbation, and protected sexual intercourse. Abstinence is the most effective method to prevent transmission.
■ Advise the female patient of childbearing age to avoid pregnancy. Explain that an infant may become infected during pregnancy, birth, or breast-feeding.

■ utilize available support systems to assist with coping
■ voice feelings about changes in sexual identity and social response to disease
■ develop no illness complications
■ comply with the treatment regimen. (See *Preventing HIV transmission.*)

NURSING INTERVENTIONS

■ Monitor the patient's developmental progress at regular intervals and adapt activity program as needed.
■ Provide appropriate play activities.
■ Encourage fluid intake.
■ Assess respiratory and neurologic status.
■ Maintain standard precautions.
■ Administer medications, as ordered.
■ Instruct the child and his parents about infection control measures in the home.

- Because an AIDS diagnosis is devastating for the child and his family, provide psychosocial support.
- Assess the child's support system, and provide referrals as necessary.

PATIENT TEACHING

Be sure to cover:
- hand-washing procedures
- how and when to use protective equipment, such as gloves, gowns, and masks
- household and laundry cleaning measures
- spill clean-up
- disposal of contaminated equipment and supplies
- trash disposal.

Allergic rhinitis

DESCRIPTION

- Immune response of the upper airways triggered by inhaled airborne allergens
- Seasonal allergic rhinitis — an immunoglobulin (Ig) E-mediated type I hypersensitivity response to an environmental antigen (allergen) in a genetically susceptible person
- Perennial rhinitis — inhaled allergens provoke antigen responses, producing signs and symptoms year-round
- Affects more than 20 million Americans
- Most prevalent in young children and adolescents

PATHOPHYSIOLOGY

- The body's immune system overresponds to common allergens in the nose.
- Antibodies attach to mast cells, which release several chemicals, including histamine, and cause dilation of blood vessels, skin redness, swollen membranes in the nose, and mucous production.

CAUSES

Perennial allergic rhinitis
- Animal dander
- House dust and dust mites
- Molds
- Processed materials or industrial chemicals
- Tobacco smoke

Seasonal allergic rhinitis
- Grass and weed pollens (in summer)
- Mold spores (occasionally, in summer and fall)
- Tree pollens (in spring)
- Weed pollens (in fall)

ASSESSMENT FINDINGS

Perennial allergic rhinitis
- Nasal polyps
- Dark circles under the eyes (allergic shiners)

Seasonal allergic rhinitis
- Pale, cyanotic, edematous nasal mucosa
- Red and edematous eyelids and conjunctivae
- Excessive lacrimation

TEST RESULTS

- Sputum and nasal secretions reveal a high number of eosinophils.
- IgE levels are normal or elevated; this may be linked to seasonal overproduction of interleukin-4 and -5 (involved in the allergic inflammatory process).
- Allergy testing (skin prick tests, intracutaneous tests, or in vitro radioallergosorbent testing) is positive for specific allergens.

TREATMENT

- Elimination of environmental antigens, if possible

- Increased fluid intake to loosen secretions
- Restrict activities in areas of allergen exposure
- Antihistamines
- Leukotriene receptor antagonists
- Intranasal corticosteroids
- Nasal decongestants
- Immunotherapy

KEY PATIENT OUTCOMES

The patient (or his family) will:
- maintain current health status
- verbalize feelings and concerns
- express feelings of increased comfort.

NURSING INTERVENTIONS

- Implement measures to relieve signs and symptoms and increase the patient's comfort.
- Encourage increased fluid intake.
- Elevate the head of the bed and provide humidification.

  ALERT *Before initiating immunotherapy using desensitization injections, assess the patient's symptoms. After giving the injection, observe him for 30 minutes to detect adverse reactions, including anaphylaxis and severe localized erythema. Make sure that epinephrine and emergency resuscitation equipment are available.*

- Monitor the patient's compliance with the prescribed drug regimen.
- Monitor changes in control of signs and symptoms.
- Monitor for indications of drug misuse.

PATIENT TEACHING

Be sure to cover:
- importance of calling the physician if the patient experiences a delayed reaction to immunotherapy (desensitizing injections)

- reduction of environmental exposure to airborne aller-gens
- possible lifestyle changes, such as relocation to a pollen-free area either seasonally or year-round, in severe and re-sistant allergic rhinitis
- medication dosage, administration, and adverse effects.

Anemia, iron deficiency

DESCRIPTION

- Decreased total iron body content, leading to diminished erythropoiesis
- Produces smaller (microcytic) cells with less color on staining (hypochromia)
- Most common form of anemia

PATHOPHYSIOLOGY

- Body stores of iron, including plasma iron, decrease.
- Transferrin, which binds with and transports iron, in-creases.
- Insufficient body stores of iron leads to a depleted red blood cell (RBC) mass and to a decreased hemoglobin (Hb) concentration.
- Oxygen-carrying capacity of the blood is, ultimately, de-creased. (See *Iron absorption and storage*, page 10.)

CAUSES

- Blood loss secondary to drug-induced GI bleeding or due to heavy menses or hemorrhage from trauma, GI ulcers, or malignant tumors
- Can be related to lead poisoning
- Inadequate dietary intake of iron
- Intravascular hemolysis-induced hemoglobinuria or paroxysmal nocturnal hemoglobinuria
- Iron malabsorption

IRON ABSORPTION AND STORAGE

Found in abundance throughout the body, iron is needed for erythro-poiesis. Two-thirds of total-body iron is found in hemoglobin (Hb); the other third, mostly in the reticuloendothelial system (liver, spleen, and bone marrow), with small amounts in muscle, serum, and body cells.

Adequate iron in the diet and recirculation of iron released from dis-integrating red blood cells maintain iron supplies. The duodenum and upper part of the small intestine absorb dietary iron. Such absorption depends on gastric acid content, the amount of reducing substances (ascorbic acid, for example) present in the alimentary canal, and amount of iron intake. If iron intake is deficient, the body gradually depletes its iron stores, causing decreased Hb levels and, eventually, signs and symptoms of iron deficiency anemia.

ASSESSMENT FINDINGS

- Red, swollen, smooth, shiny, and tender tongue (glossitis)
- Corners of the mouth may be eroded, tender, and swollen (angular stomatitis)
- Spoon-shaped, brittle nails
- Tachycardia
- Decreased appetite
- Fatigue
- Weakness
- Irritability

TEST RESULTS

- Serum Hb is decreased (males, less than 13 g/dl; females, less than 12 g/dl); in severe anemia, mean corpuscular Hb is decreased.
- Serum hematocrit is decreased (males, less than 37%; females, less than 36%).
- Serum iron levels with high total iron binding capacity are decreased.
- Serum ferritin levels are decreased.

- With microcytic and hypochromic cells, serum RBC count is decreased (in early stages, RBC count may be normal, except in infants and children).
- Bone marrow studies reveal depleted or absent iron stores (done by staining) as well as normoblastic hyperplasia.
- GI studies, such as guaiac stool tests, barium swallow and enema, endoscopy, and sigmoidoscopy, rule out or confirm the diagnosis of bleeding causing the iron deficiency.

TREATMENT

- Underlying cause must first be determined
- Nutritious, nonirritating foods
- Iron-rich diet
- Planned rest periods during activity
- Oral preparation of iron or a combination of iron and ascorbic acid
- I.M. iron in rare cases

KEY PATIENT OUTCOMES

The patient will:
- maintain weight
- maintain vital signs within prescribed limits during activity
- express feelings of increased energy
- express feelings of increased comfort.

NURSING INTERVENTIONS

- Note the patient's signs or symptoms of decreased perfusion to vital organs.
- Provide oxygen therapy, as necessary.
- Assess the family's dietary habits for iron intake, noting the influence of childhood eating patterns, cultural food preferences, and family income on adequate nutrition.
- Ask the dietitian to give the patient nonirritating foods.
- Give prescribed analgesics for headache and other discomfort.

RECOGNIZING IRON OVERDOSE

Excessive iron replacement may produce such signs and symptoms as diarrhea, fever, severe stomach pain, nausea, and vomiting.

When these signs and symptoms occur, notify the physician and give prescribed treatment, which may include chelation therapy, vigorous I.V. fluid replacement, gastric lavage, whole-bowel irrigation, and supplemental oxygen.

- Evaluate the patient's drug history. Certain drugs, such as pancreatic enzymes and vitamin E, can interfere with iron metabolism and absorption; aspirin, steroids, and other drugs can cause GI bleeding.
- Provide frequent rest periods.
- If the patient receives iron I.V., monitor the infusion rate carefully and observe for an allergic reaction.
- Use the Z-track injection method when administering iron I.M.
- Provide good nutrition and meticulous care of I.V. sites.
- Monitor the patient's vital signs.
- Monitor the patient's compliance with prescribed iron supplement therapy.
- Be alert for signs of iron replacement overdose. (See *Recognizing iron overdose*.)

PATIENT TEACHING

Be sure to cover:
- the disorder and its diagnosis and treatment
- dangers of lead poisoning, especially if the patient reports pica
- importance of continuing therapy, even after the patient begins to feel better
- absorption interference of iron supplementation with milk or antacid
- increased absorption with vitamin C
- avoidance of staining teeth by drinking liquid supplemental iron through a straw
- when to report adverse effects of iron therapy

- basics of a nutritionally balanced diet
- importance of avoiding infection and when to report signs of infection
- need for regular checkups
- compliance with prescribed treatment.

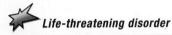 *Life-threatening disorder*

Anemia, sickle cell

DESCRIPTION

- Congenital hemolytic disease that results from a defective hemoglobin (Hb) molecule (HbS), causing red blood cells (RBCs) to become sickle shaped
- Sickle-shaped cells impairing circulation, resulting in chronic ill health (fatigue, dyspnea on exertion, swollen joints), periodic crises, long-term complications, and premature death
- Autosomal recessive disorder
- No universal cure (Bone marrow transplantation offers a cure; however, the procedure is risky, few patients have matched donors, and it's costly.)
- Most common in tropical Africans and in people of African descent
- Abnormal gene present in about 1 in 12 blacks; if two such carriers have offspring, each child has 1-in-4 chance of developing disease
- Occurs in 1 in every 500 blacks in the United States alone
- Also occurs in Puerto Rico, Turkey, India, the Middle East, and the Mediterranean area

PATHOPHYSIOLOGY

- Abnormal HbS found in the patient's RBCs becomes insoluble whenever hypoxia occurs.
- RBCs become rigid, rough, and elongated, forming a crescent or sickle shape.

- Sickling may produce hemolysis (cell destruction).
- Altered cells accumulate in capillaries and smaller blood vessels, making the blood more viscous.
- Normal circulation is impaired, causing pain, tissue infarctions, and swelling.

CAUSES

- Homozygous inheritance of the HbS-producing gene (defective Hb gene from each parent)

ASSESSMENT FINDINGS

- Signs and symptoms usually not developing until after age 6 months
- History of chronic fatigue, unexplained dyspnea, or dyspnea on exertion
- Joint swelling
- Aching bones
- Chest pain
- Ischemic leg ulcers
- Increased susceptibility to infection
- Pulmonary infarctions and cardiomegaly
- Jaundice or pallor
- May appear small in stature for age
- Delayed growth and puberty
- Spiderlike body build (narrow shoulders and hips, long extremities, curved spine, and barrel chest) in adult
- Tachycardia
- Hepatomegaly and, in children, splenomegaly
- Systolic and diastolic murmurs
- Sleepiness with difficulty awakening
- Hematuria
- Pale lips, tongue, palms, and nail beds
- Body temperature over 104° F (40° C) or a temperature of 100° F (37.8° C) persisting for 2 or more days

In painful crisis

■ Most common crisis and the hallmark of the disease, usually appearing periodically after age 5, characterized by severe abdominal, thoracic, muscle, or bone pain and, possibly, increased jaundice, dark urine, and a low-grade fever

■ Painful swelling of the fingers and toes in infants and children younger than age 3 may be the first symptom

In aplastic crisis

■ Pallor, lethargy, sleepiness, dyspnea, possible coma, markedly decreased bone marrow activity, and RBC hemolysis

In acute sequestration crisis

■ Occurring in infants between ages 8 months and 2 years, causes lethargy and pallor and, if untreated, progresses to hypovolemic shock and death

In hemolytic crisis

■ Liver congestion and hepatomegaly

TEST RESULTS

■ Stained blood smear shows sickle cells, and Hb electrophoresis shows HbS. (Electrophoresis should be done on umbilical cord blood samples at birth to provide sickle cell disease screening for all neonates at risk.)

■ RBC count is decreased, white blood cell and platelet counts are elevated, erythrocyte sedimentation rate is decreased, and serum iron level is increased.

■ RBC survival and reticulocytosis are decreased; Hb level is normal or low.

■ Serum potassium, serum creatinine, and bilirubin are elevated.

■ Lateral chest X-ray detects the characteristic "Lincoln log" deformity. (This spinal abnormality develops in many adults and some adolescents with sickle cell anemia, leaving the vertebrae resembling logs that form the corner of a cabin.)

■ Ophthalmoscopic examination reveals corkscrew or comma-shaped vessels in the conjunctivae.

TREATMENT

▶ **COLLABORATION** *Sickle cell anemia requires a multidisciplinary approach to care. Specialists in hematology, cardiology, and immunology may be involved, depending on the patient's status and whether the patient is experiencing a sickle cell crisis. A pain management specialist may assist with pain control during an acute crisis. A dietitian may assist with meal planning and measures to ensure adequate hydration.*

■ Avoidance of extreme temperatures, high altitudes, and nonpressurized air travel
■ Avoidance of stress
■ Well-balanced diet
■ Adequate amounts of folic acid-rich foods
■ Adequate fluid intake
■ Bed rest with crises
■ Activity, as tolerated
■ Vaccines, such as polyvalent pneumococcal vaccine and *Haemophilus influenzae* B vaccine
■ Prompt treatment of infections
■ Analgesics
■ Iron supplements
■ Penicillin for children starting at age 2 to 4 months, continuing until age 5, or beyond if the child has had a splenectomy
■ Transfusion of packed RBCs, if Hb level decreases suddenly or if condition deteriorates rapidly
■ Sedation and administration of analgesics, blood transfusion, oxygen therapy, and large amounts of oral or I.V. fluids, in an acute sequestration crisis
■ Genetic counseling for all carriers of the disease

KEY PATIENT OUTCOMES

The patient will:
- demonstrate age-appropriate skills and behaviors to the extent possible
- exhibit adequate ventilation
- maintain collateral circulation
- maintain balanced fluid volume where input will equal output
- express feelings of increased comfort and decreased pain
- maintain normal peripheral pulses
- maintain normal skin color and temperature
- consider wearing a MedicAlert bracelet.

NURSING INTERVENTIONS

- Encourage the patient to talk about his fears and concerns.
- Encourage the male patient to seek care for priapism.
- Make sure that the patient receives adequate amounts of folic acid-rich foods such as green leafy vegetables.
- Encourage adequate fluid intake.
- Apply warm compresses, warmed thermal blankets, and warming pads or mattresses to painful areas of the patient's body, unless he has neuropathy.
- Administer analgesics and antipyretics, as necessary.
- When cultures demonstrate the presence of infection, give prescribed antibiotics.
- Give the patient prescribed prophylactic antibiotics.
- Use strict sterile technique when performing treatments.
- Encourage bed rest with the head of the bed elevated.
- Administer oxygen as needed.
- Administer blood transfusions.
- If the patient requires general anesthesia for surgery, help ensure that he receives adequate ventilation.
- Monitor the patient's vital signs, intake and output, and complete blood count and other laboratory study results.

PATIENT TEACHING

Be sure to cover:
- avoidance of tight clothing that restricts circulation
- conditions that provoke hypoxia, such as strenuous exercise, vasoconstricting medications, cold temperatures, unpressurized aircraft, and high altitude
- importance of normal childhood immunizations, meticulous wound care, good oral hygiene, regular dental checkups, and a balanced diet as safeguards against infection
- need for prompt treatment of infection
- need to increase fluid intake to prevent dehydration, which can cause increased blood viscosity
- symptoms of vaso-occlusive crisis
- need for hospitalization in a vaso-occlusive crisis in which I.V. fluids, parenteral analgesics, oxygen therapy, and blood transfusions may be necessary
- need to inform all health care providers that the patient has this disease before undergoing any treatment, especially major surgery
- pregnancy and the disease
- balanced diet, including folic acid supplements during pregnancy
- need to inform school personnel of illness, treatment, and emergency measures.

Aortic stenosis

DESCRIPTION

- Narrowing of the aortic valve, affecting blood flow in the heart
- Classified as congenital, acquired, or rheumatic
- With congenital heart disease, symptoms possibly absent until adulthood, even though stenosis has been present since childhood
- About 80% of patients male

PATHOPHYSIOLOGY

- Stenosis of the aortic valve results in impeded blood flow.
- The left ventricle requires greater pressure to open the aortic valve.
- This added workload increases myocardial oxygen demands.
- Diminished cardiac output reduces coronary artery blood flow.
- Left ventricular hypertrophy and failure results.

CAUSES

- Congenital aortic bicuspid valve
- Idiopathic fibrosis and calcification
- Rheumatic fever

ASSESSMENT FINDINGS

- May be asymptomatic
- History possibly including dyspnea on exertion, dizziness, angina, exertional syncope, fatigue, palpitations, and paroxysmal nocturnal dyspnea
- Small, sustained arterial pulses slowly rising
- Distinct lagging between carotid artery pulse and apical pulse
- Orthopnea
- Prominent jugular vein A waves
- Peripheral edema
- Diminishing carotid pulses with delayed upstroke
- Apex of the heart possibly displaced inferiorly and laterally
- Suprasternal thrill
- Blood pressure may be normal

ALERT An early systolic ejection murmur may be present in children and adolescents who have non-calcified valves. The murmur is low-pitched, rough, and rasping and is loudest at the base in the second intercostal space.

IDENTIFYING THE MURMUR OF AORTIC STENOSIS

A low-pitched, harsh crescendo-decrescendo murmur that radiates from the aortic valve area to the carotid artery characterizes aortic stenosis.

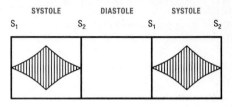

- Paradoxical splitting of the second heart sound developing as stenosis becomes more severe
- Prominent S_4
- Harsh, rasping, mid- to late-peaking systolic murmur that's best heard at the base and commonly radiates to carotids and apex (see *Identifying the murmur of aortic stenosis*)

TEST RESULTS

- Chest X-ray may show valvular calcification, dilation of the aorta, left ventricular enlargement, pulmonary vein congestion and, in later stages, left atrial, pulmonary artery, right atrial, and right ventricular enlargement.
- Echocardiography shows decreased valve area, increased gradient, and increased left ventricular wall thickness.
- Cardiac catheterization shows increased pressure gradient across the aortic valve, increased left ventricular pressures, and presence of coronary artery disease.
- Electrocardiography may show left ventricular hypertrophy, atrial fibrillation, or other arrhythmia.

TREATMENT

- Periodic noninvasive evaluation of the severity of valve narrowing, even mild stenosis may worsen over time
- Lifelong treatment and management of congenital aortic stenosis
- Low-sodium, low-fat, low-cholesterol diet
- Modified activity according to severity of disease
- Cardiac glycosides
- Antibiotic infective endocarditis prophylaxis

> **ALERT** *The use of diuretics and vasodilators may lead to hypotension and inadequate stroke volume.*

- Percutaneous balloon aortic valvuloplasty (usually limited to children)
- In children without calcified valves, simple commissurotomy under direct visualization
- Ross procedure may be performed in patients younger than age 5

KEY PATIENT OUTCOMES

The patient will:
- perform activities of daily living without excess fatigue or exhaustion
- avoid complications
- maintain cardiac output
- demonstrate hemodynamic stability
- maintain balanced fluid status
- maintain joint mobility and range of motion
- develop and demonstrate adequate coping skills.

NURSING INTERVENTIONS

- Give the patient prescribed drugs.
- Maintain a low-sodium diet. Consult with a dietitian.
- If the patient requires bed rest, stress its importance. Provide a bedside commode.
- Alternate periods of activity and rest.

- Allow the patient to voice concerns about the effects of activity restrictions.
- Keep the patient's legs elevated while he sits in a chair.
- Place the patient in an upright position and administer oxygen, as needed.
- Allow the patient to express his fears and concerns.
- Monitor the patient's vital signs, intake and output, daily weight, and respiratory status.
- If the patient has surgery, monitor for signs and symptoms of thrombus formation, hemodynamics, arterial blood gas results, blood chemistry results, and chest X-ray results.

PATIENT TEACHING

Be sure to cover:
- the disorder and its diagnosis and treatment
- medications and potential adverse reactions
- when to notify the physician
- periodic rest in the patient's daily routine
- leg elevation whenever the patient sits
- dietary and fluid restrictions
- importance of consistent follow-up care
- signs and symptoms of heart failure
- infective endocarditis prophylaxis
- pulse rate and rhythm
- monitoring for atrial fibrillation and other arrhythmias.

 Life-threatening disorder

Asthma

DESCRIPTION

- Chronic reactive airway disorder that involves episodic, reversible airway obstruction, resulting from bronchospasm, increased mucus secretions, and mucosal edema
- Signs and symptoms ranging from mild wheezing and dyspnea to life-threatening respiratory failure

- Signs and symptoms of bronchial airway obstruction possibly persisting between acute episodes
- May occur at any age; about 50% of all patients with asthma under age 10, affecting twice as many boys as girls
- In about one-third of patients, onset between ages 10 and 30
- Disease shared with at least one immediate family member in about one-third of cases
- Intrinsic and extrinsic asthma possibly coexisting in many asthmatics

PATHOPHYSIOLOGY

- Tracheal and bronchial linings overreact to various stimuli, causing episodic smooth-muscle spasms that severely constrict the airways.
- Mucosal edema and thickened secretions further block the airways.
- Immunoglobulin (Ig) E antibodies, attached to histamine-containing mast cells and receptors on cell membranes, initiate intrinsic asthma attacks.
- When exposed to an antigen such as pollen, the IgE antibody combines with the antigen. (On subsequent exposure to the antigen, mast cells degranulate and release mediators.)
- Mediators cause bronchoconstriction and edema of an asthma attack.
- During an asthma attack, expiratory airflow decreases, trapping gas in the airways and causing alveolar hyperinflation.
- Atelectasis may develop in some lung regions.
- Increased airway resistance initiates labored breathing. (See *What happens in status asthmaticus*, page 24.)

CAUSES

- Sensitivity to specific external allergens or from internal, nonallergenic factors

FOCUS IN

WHAT HAPPENS IN STATUS ASTHMATICUS

A potentially fatal complication, status asthmaticus arises when impaired gas exchange and heightened airway resistance increase the work of breathing. This flowchart shows the stages of status asthmaticus.

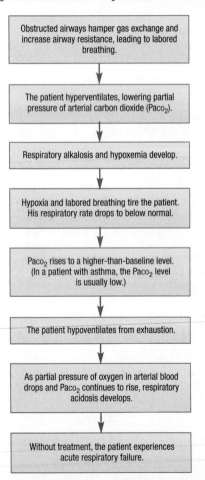

Obstructed airways hamper gas exchange and increase airway resistance, leading to labored breathing.

↓

The patient hyperventilates, lowering partial pressure of arterial carbon dioxide ($Paco_2$).

↓

Respiratory alkalosis and hypoxemia develop.

↓

Hypoxia and labored breathing tire the patient. His respiratory rate drops to below normal.

↓

$Paco_2$ rises to a higher-than-baseline level. (In a patient with asthma, the $Paco_2$ level is usually low.)

↓

The patient hypoventilates from exhaustion.

↓

As partial pressure of oxygen in arterial blood drops and $Paco_2$ continues to rise, respiratory acidosis develops.

↓

Without treatment, the patient experiences acute respiratory failure.

Bronchoconstriction
- Cold air
- Drugs, such as aspirin, beta-adrenergic blockers, and non-steroidal anti-inflammatory drugs
- Exercise
- Hereditary predisposition
- Psychological stress
- Sensitivity to allergens or irritants such as pollutants
- Tartrazine (a food additive with conflicting evidence regarding effects on asthma)
- Viral infections

Extrinsic asthma (atopic asthma)
- Animal dander
- Food additives containing sulfites and any other sensitizing substance
- House dust or mold
- Kapok or feather pillows
- Pollen

Intrinsic asthma (nonatopic asthma)
- Emotional stress
- Genetic factors

ASSESSMENT FINDINGS

- Intrinsic asthma often preceded by severe respiratory tract infections, especially in adults
- Irritants, emotional stress, fatigue, endocrine changes, temperature and humidity variations, and exposure to cigarette smoke and noxious fumes possibly aggravating intrinsic asthma attacks
- Asthma attack possibly beginning dramatically, with simultaneous onset of severe, multiple symptoms, or insidiously, with gradually increasing respiratory distress
- Exposure to a particular allergen followed by a sudden onset of dyspnea and wheezing and by tightness in the chest accompanied by a cough that produces thick, clear, or yellow sputum

- Visibly dyspneic
- Ability to speak only a few words before pausing for breath
- Use of accessory respiratory muscles
- Diaphoresis
- Increased anteroposterior thoracic diameter
- Hyperresonance
- Tachycardia, tachypnea, mild systolic hypertension
- Inspiratory and expiratory wheezes
- Prolonged expiratory phase of respiration
- Diminished breath sounds
- Cyanosis, confusion, and lethargy indicate the onset of life-threatening status asthmaticus and respiratory failure

TEST RESULTS

- Arterial blood gas (ABG) analysis reveals hypoxemia.
- Serum IgE levels are increased (from an allergic reaction).
- Complete blood count with differential shows increased eosinophil count.
- Chest X-ray may show hyperinflation with areas of focal atelectasis.
- Pulmonary function studies may show decreased peak flows and forced expiratory volume in 1 second, low-normal or decreased vital capacity, and increased total lung and residual capacities.
- Serial peak flow measures are decreased (as reported by the patient).
- Skin testing may identify specific allergens.
- Bronchial challenge testing shows the clinical significance of the allergens identified by skin testing.
- Pulse oximetry measurements may show decreased oxygen saturation.

TREATMENT

- Identification and avoidance of precipitating factors
- Desensitization to specific antigens

- Establishment and maintenance of patent airway
- Fluid replacement
- Activity as tolerated
- Bronchodilators
- Corticosteroids (inhaled or systemic)
- Histamine antagonists
- Leukotriene antagonists
- Anticholinergic bronchodilators
- Low-flow oxygen
- Antibiotics
- Heliox trial (before intubation), if available
- I.V. magnesium sulfate (controversial)

ALERT *The patient with increasingly severe asthma that doesn't respond to drug therapy is usually admitted for treatment with corticosteroids, epinephrine, and sympathomimetic aerosol sprays. He may require endotracheal intubation and mechanical ventilation.*

KEY PATIENT OUTCOMES

The patient will:
- maintain adequate ventilation
- maintain a patent airway
- maintain normal activity levels
- use effective coping strategies
- report feelings of comfort
- effectively monitor peak flow readings
- maintain skin integrity.

NURSING INTERVENTIONS

- Give the patient prescribed drugs.
- Place the patient in high Fowler's position.
- Encourage pursed-lip and diaphragmatic breathing.
- Administer prescribed humidified oxygen.
- Adjust oxygen according to the patient's vital signs and ABG values.
- Assist with intubation and mechanical ventilation, if appropriate.

- Perform postural drainage and chest percussion, if tolerated.
- Suction an intubated patient as needed.
- Treat the patient's dehydration with I.V. or oral fluids, as tolerated.
- Anticipate bronchoscopy or bronchial lavage.
- Keep the room temperature comfortable.
- Use an air conditioner or a fan in hot, humid weather.
- Monitor the patient's vital signs, intake and output, response to treatment, signs and symptoms of theophylline toxicity, breath sounds, ABG results, pulmonary function test results, pulse oximetry, complications of corticosteroids, and anxiety level.

PATIENT TEACHING

Be sure to cover:
- the disorder and its diagnosis and treatment
- medications and potential adverse reactions
- when to notify the physician
- avoidance of known allergens and irritants
- metered-dose inhaler or dry powder inhaler use
- pursed-lip and diaphragmatic breathing
- use of peak flow meter
- effective coughing techniques
- maintaining adequate hydration
- importance of communicating with school and caregivers regarding health needs
- referral to a local asthma support group.

Atopic dermatitis

DESCRIPTION

- Chronic, noncontagious skin disorder characterized by superficial skin inflammation and intense itching
- Marked by exacerbations and remissions

- May appear at any age but typically begins during infancy or early childhood (may then subside spontaneously, followed by exacerbations in late childhood, adolescence, or early adulthood)
- In approximately 75% of affected children, development of hay fever or asthma

PATHOPHYSIOLOGY

- Allergic mechanism of hypersensitivity results in a release of inflammatory mediators through sensitized antibodies of the immunoglobulin (Ig) E class.
- Histamine and other cytokines induce acute inflammation.
- Abnormally dry skin and a decreased threshold for itching set up the "itch-scratch-itch" cycle, eventually causing lesions (excoriations, lichenification).

CAUSES

- Exact cause unknown (combination of genetic and environmental factors likely)
- Possible contributing factors:
  – Chemical irritants
  – Extremes of temperature and humidity
  – Food allergy
  – Infection
  – Psychological stress or strong emotions

  ALERT *About 10% of juvenile cases of atopic dermatitis are caused by allergic reactions to certain foods, especially eggs, peanuts, milk, and wheat.*

ASSESSMENT FINDINGS

- Atopy, such as asthma, hay fever, or urticaria (or similar family history) (see *Factors contributing to atopy,* page 30)
- History of exposure to allergen

FACTORS CONTRIBUTING TO ATOPY

- Changes associated with industrialization, such as exposure to new chemicals like diesel fumes, have proven to increase the antigenicity of common pollens.
- Increased exposure to antigens, such as dust mites (in wall-to-wall-carpets), especially at an early age, contributes to a predisposition to developing allergies.
- Dietary changes, such as increased fat intake and an earlier weaning from human breast milk, may be contributing factors.
- Vaccination may cause a shift in T-cell function away from the normal helper T-cell (Th1) response to the Th2 allergic response by limiting early bacterial and viral infections.
- Lack of exposure to intestinal parasites may contribute to a similar shift in T-cell functioning.
- Frequent use of antibiotics, especially in early childhood, may decrease normal intestinal flora and further contribute to the shift.

- Dry, itchy skin and rashes on the face, inside the elbows, behind the knees, and on the hands and feet
- Erythematous, weeping lesions
- Pink pigmentation and swelling of the upper eyelid and a double fold under the lower lid (Morgan's line or Dennie's sign) (see *Signs of atopic dermatitis*)

TEST RESULTS

- Blood studies reveal eosinophilia.
- Serum IgE levels are elevated.
- Physical examination findings are positive.
- Skin testing is positive.

TREATMENT

- Meticulous skin care
- Environmental control of offending allergens
- Nonirritating topical lubricants
- Corticosteroids (topical or systemic)
- Antipruritics

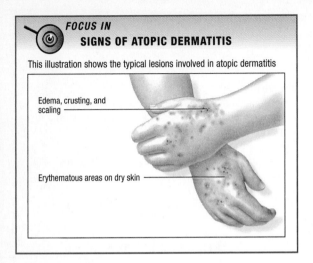

FOCUS IN
SIGNS OF ATOPIC DERMATITIS

This illustration shows the typical lesions involved in atopic dermatitis

Edema, crusting, and scaling

Erythematous areas on dry skin

- Antihistamines
- Antibiotics if secondary infection develops
- Immunomodulators to control inflammation and reduce immune system reactions

KEY PATIENT OUTCOMES

The patient will:
- express relief from itching and pain
- demonstrate improved skin condition
- remain free from infection
- effectively implement environmental control measures
- identify potential adverse effects of prescribed medications.

NURSING INTERVENTIONS

- Offer support.
- Dissuade the patient from scratching during urticaria.
- Apply prescribed topical medications.

■ Monitor the patient's compliance with drug therapy and nutritional status.

PATIENT TEACHING

Be sure to cover:
■ when and how to apply topical corticosteroids
■ importance of regular personal hygiene using only luke-warm water and mild soap
■ signs and symptoms of secondary infection
■ avoidance of laundry additives, such as fragrances and dyes
■ avoidance of allergens
■ distraction strategies to avoid scratching.

Atrial septal defect

DESCRIPTION

■ Acyanotic congenital heart defect that features an open-ing between the left and right atria, which allows blood to flow from left to right, resulting in ineffective pumping of the heart, thus increasing the risk of heart failure
■ Three types:
  – Ostium secundum defect (the most common type): oc-curs in the region of the fossa ovalis and, occasionally, extends inferiorly, close to the vena cava
  – Sinus venosus defect: occurs in the superior-posterior portion of the atrial septum, sometimes extending into the vena cava, and almost always associated with ab-normal drainage of pulmonary veins into the right atri-um (versus the left atrium)
  – Ostium primum defect: occurs in the inferior portion of the septum primum and is usually associated with atri-oventricular valve abnormalities (cleft mitral valve) and conduction defects
■ Accounts for about 10% of congenital heart defects

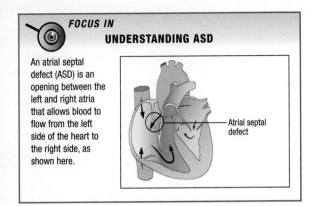

FOCUS IN
UNDERSTANDING ASD

An atrial septal defect (ASD) is an opening between the left and right atria that allows blood to flow from the left side of the heart to the right side, as shown here.

Atrial septal defect

- Twice as common in females as in males, with a possible familial tendency; usually associated with genetic syndrome, such as Holt-Oram syndrome or trisomy 21

PATHOPHYSIOLOGY

- Blood shunts from the left atrium to the right atrium because left atrial pressure is normally slightly higher than the right atrial pressure. (See *Understanding ASD*.)
- The difference in pressure forces large amounts of blood through the defect.
- Shunt results in right heart volume overload, affecting the right atrium, right ventricle, and pulmonary arteries.
- Eventually, the right atrium enlarges, and the right ventricle dilates to accommodate the increased blood volume.
- If pulmonary artery hypertension develops, increased pulmonary vascular resistance and right ventricular hypertrophy result.
- Pulmonary artery hypertension may cause reversal of the shunt direction in some adults, which results in deoxygenated blood entering the systemic circulation, ultimately causing cyanosis.

CAUSES

- No known cause
- Ostium primum defects commonly occurring in patients with Down syndrome

> **ALERT** *An infant may be cyanotic because he has a cardiac or pulmonary disorder. Cyanosis that worsens with crying most likely has a cardiac cause because crying increases pulmonary resistance to blood flow, resulting in an increased right-to-left shunt. Cyanosis that improves with crying most likely has a pulmonary cause because deep breathing improves tidal volume.*

ASSESSMENT FINDINGS

- Fatigue after exertion
- S_1 is normal or split
- Fixed, widely split S_2
- Systolic click or late systolic murmur at the apex
- Clubbing and cyanosis, if a right-to-left shunt develops
- Early to midsystolic murmur at the second or third left intercostal space
- May be asymptomatic in infancy and early childhood
- Frequent respiratory infections
- Dyspnea, shortness of breath, and palpitations
- Low-pitched diastolic murmur at the left lower sternal border, more pronounced on inspiration
- Peripheral edema
- Cyanosis
- Distended jugular veins

TEST RESULTS

- Chest X-ray shows cardiomegaly (related to right atrial and ventricular enlargement), a prominent pulmonary artery, and increased pulmonary vascular markings.
- Electrocardiography may appear normal, but commonly shows right axis deviation, a prolonged PR interval, varying degrees of right bundle branch block, right ventricu-

lar hypertrophy, atrial fibrillation and, in ostium primum defect, left axis deviation.

- Echocardiography measures right ventricular enlargement, possibly locating the defect and determining its size, as well as the amount and direction of blood flow. It can also show volume overload in the right side of the heart. (It may reveal right ventricular and pulmonary artery dilation.)
- Two-dimensional echocardiography with color Doppler flow and contrast echocardiography confirms the diagnosis of atrial septal defect (ASD). (Cardiac catheterization may be used if inconsistencies exist in the clinical data or if significant pulmonary hypertension is suspected.)

TREATMENT

- Activity, as tolerated
- Low-fat, low-cholesterol diet
- Diuretics
- Antibiotics
- Analgesics
- Minimally invasive heart surgery possibly required for the patient with an uncomplicated ASD with evidence of significant left-to-right shunting
- Large defect possibly needing immediate surgical closure with sutures or a patch graft
- Small defects may close spontaneously without intervention
- Cardiac catheterization closure, inserting an umbrella-like patch or septal occluder through a cardiac catheter, possibly performed

KEY PATIENT OUTCOMES

The patient will:
- maintain an optimal cardiac output
- maintain hemodynamic stability
- experience no cardiac arrhythmias.

NURSING INTERVENTIONS

- Encourage the child to engage in any activity he can tolerate.
- Give the patient prescribed drugs.
- Monitor the patient's vital signs, central venous and intra-arterial pressures, intake and output, cardiac rhythm, and oxygenation.

PATIENT TEACHING

Be sure to cover:
- pretest and posttest procedures with the child and his parents (If possible, use drawings or other visual aids to explain them to the child.)
- postoperative procedures, tubes, dressings, and monitoring equipment.

Attention deficit hyperactivity disorder

DESCRIPTION

- Behavioral problem characterized by difficulty with inattention, impulsivity, hyperactivity, and boredom
- The most common neurobehavioral disorder of childhood
- Difficult to diagnose before age 4 or 5; some patients not diagnosed until adulthood
- Varied symptoms
- Occurs in 3% to 5% of school-age children
- Affects males three to four times more commonly than females
- Also called *ADHD* and *ADD*

PATHOPHYSIOLOGY

- Alleles of dopamine genes may alter dopamine transmission in the neural networks.

■ During fetal development, bouts of hypoxia and hypo-tension may selectively damage neurons located in some of the critical regions of the anatomical networks.

CAUSES

■ Exact cause unknown
■ Believed to have genetic and neurobiological causes
■ Risk factors may include a family history of ADHD, history of learning disability, or a mood or conduct disorder
■ Some studies indicating that it may result from altered neurotransmitter levels in the brain

ASSESSMENT FINDINGS

■ Impulsive behavior
■ Inattentiveness
■ Disorganization in school
■ Tendency to jump quickly from one partly completed project, thought, or task to another
■ Difficulty meeting deadlines and keeping track of school or work tools and materials
■ Symptoms of inattention
  – Makes careless mistakes
  – Struggles to sustain attention
  – Fails to finish activities
  – Difficulty with organization
  – Avoids tasks that require sustained mental effort
  – Distracted or forgetful
■ Symptoms of hyperactivity
  – Fidgets
  – Can't sit still for sustained period
  – Difficulty playing quietly
  – Talks excessively
■ Symptoms of impulsivity
  – Interrupts
  – Can't wait patiently

■ The *Diagnostic and Statistical Manual of Mental Disorders,*
  Fourth Edition, Text Revision criteria; these criteria con-
  firming diagnosis:
  – Six symptoms or more from the inattention or hyper-
    activity-impulsivity categories
  – Symptoms present for at least 6 months
  – Some symptoms evident before age 7
  – Some impairment from symptoms present in two or
    more settings
  – Clear evidence of clinically significant impairment in
    social, academic, or occupational functioning
  – Symptoms aren't accounted for by another mental dis-
    order

TEST RESULTS

■ Complete psychological, medical, and neurologic evalua-
  tions rule out other problems; specific tests include continuous performance test, behavior rating scales, and
  learning disability.

TREATMENT

■ Education regarding the nature and effect of the disorder
■ Behavior modification
■ External structure
■ Supportive psychotherapy
■ Trial elimination of sugar, dyes, and additives from diet
  may result in change
■ Monitor activity (for safety purposes)
■ Stimulants for core symptoms (first-line treatment)
■ Tricyclic antidepressants considered after the failure of
  two or three stimulants (second-line treatment)
■ Mood stabilizers for the treatment of co-existing condi-
  tions such as bipolar disorder
■ Referral for family therapy

KEY PATIENT OUTCOMES

The patient (or his family) will:
- demonstrate effective social interaction skills in one-on-one and group settings
- demonstrate a decrease in disruptive behavior
- report improvement in family and social interactions
- demonstrate increasing independence and improved self-esteem
- demonstrate effective coping behavior.

NURSING INTERVENTIONS

- Set realistic expectations and limits.
- Maintain a calm and consistent manner.
- Keep all instructions short and simple — make one-step requests.
- Provide praise, rewards, and positive feedback whenever possible.
- Provide diversional activities suited to a short attention span.
- Monitor the patient's activity level, nutritional status, adverse drug reactions, response to treatment, and activity (for safety purposes).

PATIENT TEACHING

Be sure to cover (with parents):
- behavior therapy
- reinforcement of good behavior
- realistic expectations
- medication regimen and possible adverse reactions
- nutrition.

Autistic disorder

DESCRIPTION

- Severe, pervasive developmental disorder that affects social interactions and communication

- Degree of impairment varying
- Usually apparent before age 3
- Poor prognosis
- Affects approximately 1 in 1,000 children
- Four to five times more likely in males than in females, usually the firstborn male
- Sometimes called *Kanner's autism*

PATHOPHYSIOLOGY

- Central nervous system (CNS) defects may arise from prenatal complications.

CAUSES

- Exact cause unknown
- Defects in CNS from prenatal complications such as rubella
- Hypotheses include genetic or chromosomal abnormalities, obstetric complications, and exposure to toxic agents
- Theorized association with vaccinations — remains controversial

ASSESSMENT FINDINGS

- Becoming rigid or flaccid when held
- Crying when touched
- Showing little or no interest in human contact
- Delayed smiling response
- Severe language impairment
- Lack of socialization and imaginative play
- Echolalia
- Pronoun reversal
- Bizarre or self-destructive behavior
- Extreme compulsion for sameness
- Abnormal reaction to sensory stimuli
- Cognitive impairment
- Eating, drinking, and sleeping problems

- Mood disorders
- Possible seizures

DSM-IV-TR *criteria*
At least 6 of these 12 characteristics must be present, including at least two items from the first section, one from the second, and one from the third.
- Qualitative impairment in social interaction:
  – Impaired nonverbal behavior
  – Absence of peer relationships
  – Failure to seek or share enjoyment, interests, or achievements
  – Lack of social or emotional reciprocity
- Qualitative impairment in communication:
  – Delay or lack of language development
  – Inability to initiate or sustain conversation
  – Idiosyncratic or repetitive language
  – Lack of appropriate imaginative play
- Restricted repetitive and stereotyped patterns of behavior, interests, and activities:
  – Abnormal preoccupation with a restricted pattern of interest
  – Inflexible routines or rituals
  – Repetitive motor mannerisms
  – Preoccupation with parts of objects
- The diagnostic criteria also include delays or abnormal functioning in at least one of these areas before age 3:
  – Social interaction
  – Language skills
  – Symbolic or imaginative play
  – Not better accounted for by Rett's syndrome or childhood disintegrative condition

TREATMENT

- Structured treatment plan
- Behavioral, educational, and psychological techniques
- Pleasurable sensory and motor stimulation
- Nutritional therapy (food intolerance, allergies, or vitamin deficiencies may contribute to behavioral issues)

- Monitor activities (for safety purposes)
- Speech therapy, sensory integration therapy, exercise, and physical therapy
- No cure

KEY PATIENT OUTCOMES

The patient (or his family) will:
- identify and contact available resources, as needed
- openly share feelings about the present situation
- as much as possible, demonstrate age-appropriate skills and behaviors
- practice safety measures and take safety precautions in the home
- interact with family or friends.

NURSING INTERVENTIONS

- Institute safety measures when appropriate.
- Provide positive reinforcement.
- Encourage development of self-esteem.
- Encourage self-care.
- Prepare the child for change by telling him about it.
- Help family members to develop strong one-on-one relationships with the patient.
- Monitor the patient's response to treatment, adverse drug reactions, behavior patterns, nutritional status, social interaction, communication skills, and activity.

PATIENT TEACHING

Be sure to cover (with parents):
- physical care for the child's needs
- importance of proper nutrition and exercise
- importance of identifying signs of excessive stress and coping skills
- referral for resource and support services.

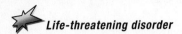 *Life-threatening disorder*

Bronchopulmonary dysplasia

DESCRIPTION

- Chronic lung disease that begins in infancy
- Also called *BPD*

PATHOPHYSIOLOGY

- Acute insult to the neonate's lungs — respiratory distress syndrome, pneumonia, or meconium aspiration — requires positive-pressure ventilation and a high concentration of oxygen over time.
- These therapies result in tissue and cellular injury and damage to the bronchiolar epithelium of the immature lung.
- Ciliary activity is inhibited; therefore, the child has trouble clearing mucus from the lungs.
- Recovery usually occurs in 6 to 12 months; however, the child may remain ventilator-dependent for years.

CAUSES

- Possible genetic factors
- Prematurity
- Ventilatory support with high positive airway pressure and oxygen in the first 2 weeks of life

ASSESSMENT FINDINGS

- Atelectasis
- Crackles, rhonchi, or wheezing
- Delayed development
- Dyspnea
- Hypoxia without ventilator assistance
- Fatigue
- Delayed muscle growth

- Pallor
- Circumoral cyanosis
- Prolonged capillary filling time
- Respiratory distress
- Right-sided heart failure
- Sternal retractions
- Weight loss or difficulty feeding

TEST RESULTS

- Arterial blood gas analysis reveals hypoxemia.
- Chest X-ray reveals such pulmonary changes as bronchiolar metaplasia or interstitial fibrosis.

TREATMENT

- Chest physiotherapy
- Continued ventilatory support and oxygen
- Enteral or total parenteral nutrition
- Supportive measures to enhance respiratory function
- Bronchodilators — albuterol to counter increased airway resistance
- Corticosteroids — dexamethasone (Decadron) therapy to reduce inflammation
- Diuretics — furosemide (Lasix)

KEY PATIENT OUTCOMES

The patient will:
- maintain respiratory rate within 5 breaths/minute of baseline
- have normal breath sounds
- maintain fluid balance, with intake equal to output
- maintain hemodynamic stability.

NURSING INTERVENTIONS

- Assess respiratory and cardiovascular status; children with BPD are susceptible to lower respiratory tract infections, hypertension, and respiratory failure.

- Monitor vital signs, pulse oximetry, and intake and output to assess and maintain adequate hydration.
- Anticipate continued ventilatory support and oxygen.
- Continue supportive measures.
- Administer bronchodilators.
- Give dexamethasone therapy.
- Be aware that because of a tendency to accumulate interstitial fluid in the lung, diuretics are given.
- Perform chest physiotherapy.
- Provide adequate time for rest.
- Provide nutritional support, including increased caloric density.
- Begin an intensive program to promote normal development.
- Encourage the parents to visit and become involved in care; the child may require lengthy hospitalization.

PATIENT TEACHING

Be sure to cover (with the parents):
- the disorder and its diagnosis and treatment
- the importance of bonding with the child and being involved with his care
- the importance of rest to avoid increased demand for oxygen
- medications and potential adverse reactions
- signs and symptoms of complications
- referral to a support group as needed.

Burns

DESCRIPTION

- Heat or chemical injury to tissue
- May be permanently disfiguring and incapacitating
- May be partial thickness or full thickness

PATHOPHYSIOLOGY

- First-degree burns (superficial, partial thickness) are localized injuries to epidermis and not life-threatening.
- Second-degree burns (deep, partial thickness) produce destruction of epidermis and some dermis with thin-walled and fluid-filled blisters. When the nerve endings are exposed to air, the blisters break causing pain and loss of barrier function of the skin.
- Third- and fourth-degree burns (full thickness) affect every body system and organ, extending into the subcutaneous tissue layer. They cause damage to muscle, bone, and interstitial tissues; interstitial fluids result in edema. Immediate immunologic response and threat of wound sepsis occurs, but is painless.

CAUSES

- Chewing electric cords
- Child abuse
- Contact with faulty electrical wiring and high voltage power lines
- Contact, ingestion, inhalation, or injection of acids, alkalies, or vesicants
- Friction or abrasion
- Improper handling of firecrackers
- Improper use or handling of matches
- Improperly stored gasoline
- Motor vehicle accidents
- Residential fires
- Scalding accidents
- Space heater or electrical malfunctions
- Sun exposure

COMMON CHARACTERISTICS OF BURNS

First-degree burns
- Localized pain
- Erythema
- Blanching
- Chills
- Headache
- Nausea and vomiting

Second-degree burns
- Thin-walled, fluid-filled blisters
- Mild to moderate pain
- White, waxy appearance of damaged area

Third- and fourth-degree burns
- Pale, white, brown, or black leathery tissue

- Visible thrombosed vessels
- No blister formation
- Painless

Electrical burns
- Silver colored, raised area at contact site
- Smoke inhalation and pulmonary damage
- Singed nasal hair

Mucosal burns
- Sores in mouth or nose
- Voice changes
- Coughing, wheezing
- Darkened sputum

ASSESSMENT FINDINGS

- Depth and size of the burn (see *Common characteristics of burns*)
- Severity of the burn estimated
- Major — more than 20% of a child's body surface area (BSA)
- Moderate — 10% to 20% of a child's BSA
- Minor — less than 10% of a child's BSA
- Respiratory distress and cyanosis
- Edema
- Alteration in pulse rate, strength, and regularity
- Stridor, wheezing, crackles, and rhonchi
- S_3 or S_4
- Hypotension

TEST RESULTS

- Arterial blood gas analysis shows evidence of smoke inhalation and may also show decreased alveolar function or hypoxia.
- Complete blood count shows decreased hemoglobin level and hematocrit (if blood loss occurs).
- Electrolytes are abnormal due to fluid losses and shifts.
- Blood urea nitrogen is increased (with fluid losses).
- In children, glucose is decreased because of limited glycogen storage.
- Urinalysis shows myoglobinuria and hemoglobinuria.
- Carboxyhemoglobin is increased.
- Electrocardiogram may show myocardial ischemia, injury, or arrhythmias, especially in electrical burns.
- Fiber-optic bronchoscopy may reveal edema of the airways.

TREATMENT

COLLABORATION *Surgeons may be needed to perform escharotomy and fasciotomy to remove burn tissue. Wound care specialists may be needed to prevent wound infections and complications (such as contractures) and promote wound healing. Respiratory therapy is needed to maximize respiratory function in cases of inhalation injury.*

As the patient improves, physical therapy is necessary to maintain or improve range of motion and prevent contractures. Nutritional therapists can prescribe an optimal diet to promote wound healing.

- Eliminating the burn source
- Securing airway
- Preventing hypoxia
- Giving I.V. fluids through a large-bore I.V. line
- Child under 66 lb (29.9 kg): maintain urine output of 1 ml/kg/hour
- Nasogastric tube and urinary catheter insertion
- Wound care

- Nothing by mouth until severity of burn is established, then high-protein, high-calorie diet
- Increased hydration with high-calorie, high-protein drinks, not free water
- Total parenteral nutrition, if unable to take food by mouth
- Activity limitation based on extent and location of burn
- Physical therapy
- Booster of tetanus toxoid
- Analgesics
- Antibiotics
- Antianxiety agents
- Loose tissue and blister debridement
- Escharotomy
- Skin grafting

KEY PATIENT OUTCOMES

The patient will:
- report increased comfort and decreased pain
- attain the highest degree of mobility
- maintain fluid balance within the acceptable range
- maintain a patent airway
- demonstrate effective coping techniques.

NURSING INTERVENTIONS

- Apply immediate, aggressive burn treatment.
- Use strict sterile technique.
- Remove clothing that's still smoldering. (Don't remove clothing that's stuck to a burn.)
- Remove constricting items.
- Perform appropriate wound care.
- Provide adequate hydration.
- Weigh the patient daily.
- Encourage verbalization and provide support.
- Refer the patient to rehabilitation if appropriate.
- Refer the patient to psychological counseling if needed.
- Refer the patient to resource and support services.

■ Monitor the patient's vital signs, respiratory status, signs
of infection, intake and output, and hydration and nutritional status.

PATIENT TEACHING

Be sure to cover:
■ the injury, diagnosis, and treatment
■ appropriate wound care
■ all medications, including administration, dosage, and
possible adverse effects
■ developing a dietary plan
■ signs and symptoms of complications.

Celiac disease

DESCRIPTION

■ Characterized by poor food absorption and intolerance of
gluten — a protein found in grains, such as wheat, rye,
oats, and barley
■ Usually becomes apparent between ages 6 and 18
months

PATHOPHYSIOLOGY

■ The amount and activity of enzymes in the intestinal
mucosal cells is decreased.
■ Villi of the proximal small intestine atrophy, decreasing
intestinal absorption.

CAUSES

■ Gluten intolerance
■ Immunoglobulin A deficiency

ASSESSMENT FINDINGS

■ Steatorrhea (fatty stools)

- Chronic diarrhea
- Anorexia
- Generalized malnutrition and failure to thrive
- Coagulation difficulty from the malabsorption of fat-soluble vitamins
- Abdominal pain and distention
- Irritability

TEST RESULTS

- Chemistry tests reveal hypocalcemia and hypoalbuminemia.
- Hemoglobin level is decreased.
- Coagulation tests reveal hypothrombinemia.
- Immunologic assay screen is positive for celiac disease.
- Stool specimen reveals high fat content.

TREATMENT

- Gluten-free diet but including corn and rice products, soy and potato flour, breast milk or soy-based formula, and fresh fruits
- Folate supplements
- Iron supplements
- Vitamins A and D in water-soluble forms

KEY PATIENT OUTCOMES

The patient will:
- maintain adequate caloric intake
- develop a normal bowel pattern
- maintain fluid volume within normal limits.

NURSING INTERVENTIONS

- Eliminate gluten from the diet.
- Give the child corn and rice products, soy and potato flour, breast milk or soy-based formula, and fresh fruits.

- Replace vitamins and calories; give small, frequent meals.
- Monitor for steatorrhea — its disappearance is a good indicator that the child's ability to absorb nutrients is improving.

PATIENT TEACHING

Be sure to cover:
- the disease and signs and symptoms of complications
- the importance of following a gluten-free diet
- that the child's weight should return to within a normal range within 6 months to 1 year after starting the diet
- how to read food labels and to avoid products with hidden gluten content such as food containing "vegetable protein."

Cerebral palsy

DESCRIPTION

- Most common crippling neuromuscular disease in children
- Comprises several neuromuscular disorders
- Results from prenatal, perinatal, or postnatal central nervous system (CNS) damage
- Three types (sometimes occurring in mixed forms):
  - spastic (affects about 70% of children with cerebral palsy)
  - athetoid (affects about 20%)
  - ataxic (affects about 10%)
- Motor impairment minimal or severely disabling
- Associated defects:
  - seizures
  - speech disorders
  - mental retardation
  - vision or hearing impairment
- Prognosis varied
- Highest in premature neonates and in those who are small for gestational age

- Slightly more common in boys than in girls
- More common in whites

PATHOPHYSIOLOGY

- A lesion or abnormality occurs in the early stages of brain development.
- Structural and functional defects occur, impairing motor or cognitive function.
- Defects may not be distinguishable until months after birth.

CAUSES

- Conditions that result in cerebral anoxia, hemorrhage, or other CNS damage

Prenatal causes
- Abnormal placental attachment
- ABO blood type incompatibility
- Anoxia
- Irradiation
- Isoimmunization
- Malnutrition
- Maternal diabetes
- Maternal infection (especially rubella in the first trimester)
- Rh factor incompatibility
- Gestational hypertension

Parturition causes
- Asphyxia from the cord wrapping around the neck
- Depressed maternal vital signs from general or spinal anesthesia
- Multiple births (neonates born last in a multiple birth have an especially high rate of cerebral palsy)
- Prematurity
- Prolonged or unusually rapid labor
- Trauma during delivery

Postnatal causes
- Any condition resulting in cerebral thrombus or embolus
- Head trauma
- Infections, such as meningitis and encephalitis
- Poisoning

ASSESSMENT FINDINGS

- Maternal or patient history revealing possible cause
- Child with retarded growth and development
- Difficulty chewing and swallowing

Spastic cerebral palsy
- Underdevelopment of affected limbs
- Characteristic scissors gait
- Walking on toes
- Crossing one foot in front of the other
- Hyperactive deep tendon reflexes
- Increased stretch reflexes
- Rapid alternating muscle contraction and relaxation
- Muscle weakness
- Impaired fine and gross motor skills
- Contractures in response to manipulation of muscles

Athetoid cerebral palsy
- Involuntary movements
- Grimacing
- Wormlike writhing
- Dystonia
- Sharp jerks impairing voluntary movement
- Involuntary facial movements (speech difficult)
- Drooling

Ataxic cerebral palsy
- Lack of leg movement during infancy
- Wide gait when child beginning to walk
- Disturbed balance
- Incoordination (especially of the arms)
- Hypoactive reflexes
- Nystagmus

- Muscle weakness
- Tremors

TEST RESULTS

- Computed tomography scan and magnetic resonance imaging of the brain may show structural abnormalities such as cerebral atrophy.
- EEG may show the source of seizure activity.

TREATMENT

- Braces or splints
- Special appliances, such as adapted eating utensils and low toilet seat with arms
- Range-of-motion (ROM) exercises
- Prescribed exercises to maintain muscle tone
- Anticonvulsants
- Muscle relaxants such as botulinum toxin (Botox) injections
- Antianxiety agents
- Orthopedic surgery
- Neurosurgery
- Eyeglasses, vision correction surgery, or hearing aids, as needed

KEY PATIENT OUTCOMES

The patient will:
- consume calorie requirements daily
- express positive feelings about self
- maintain joint mobility and ROM
- develop adequate coping mechanisms
- develop effective communication skills.

NURSING INTERVENTIONS

- Speak slowly and distinctly.
- Give all care in an unhurried manner.
- Allow participation in care decisions.

- Provide a diet with adequate calories. Stroking the throat may aid swallowing.
- Provide frequent mouth and dental care.
- Provide skin care.
- Perform prescribed exercises.
- Care for associated hearing and vision disturbances, as necessary.
- Postoperatively, give analgesics as ordered.
- Provide a safe physical environment.
- Monitor the patient's pain relief, seizure activity, speech, visual and auditory acuity, respiratory status, swallowing function, reflexes, nutritional status, skin integrity, motor development, and muscle strength.

PATIENT TEACHING

Be sure to cover:
- the prescribed medication regimen
- adverse drug reactions
- daily skin inspection and massage
- the need to place food far back in patient's mouth to facilitate swallowing
- the need to chew food thoroughly
- drinking through a straw
- sucking lollipops to develop muscle control
- proper nutrition
- opportunities for learning, such as summer camps or Special Olympics
- correct use of assistive devices.

Cleft lip and cleft palate

DESCRIPTION

- Front and sides of the face and palatine shelves imperfectly fused during pregnancy
- Twice as common in males as in females
- More common in children with a family history of cleft defects

- Cleft lip with or without cleft palate: occurs in about 1 in 1,000 births among Whites; higher incidence in Asians (1.7 in 1,000) and Native Americans (more than 3.6 in 1,000), but lower in Blacks (1 in 2,500)
- May occur separately or in combination
- Occurs unilaterally, bilaterally or, rarely, in the midline
- May affect just the lip or extend into the upper jaw or nasal cavity (see *Types of cleft deformities*, pages 58 and 59)
- Increases susceptibility to middle ear infections and potential hearing loss

PATHOPHYSIOLOGY

- Chromosomal abnormality, exposure to teratogens, genetic abnormality, or environmental factors cause the lip or palate to fuse imperfectly during the second month of pregnancy.
- Complete cleft includes the soft palate, bones of the maxilla, and alveolus on one or both sides of the premaxilla.
- Double cleft runs from the soft palate to either side of the nose, separating the maxilla and premaxilla into freely moving segments; the tongue and other muscles may displace the segments, thus enlarging the cleft.

ALERT *Isolated cleft palate occurs more commonly with congenital defects other than isolated cleft lip. The constellation of U-shaped cleft palate, mandibular hypoplasia, and glossoptosis known as Robin sequence, can occur as an isolated defect or one feature of many different syndromes. These infants should have comprehensive genetic evaluation. Because of their mandibular hypoplasia and glossoptosis, the airway in infants with Robin sequence must be carefully evaluated and managed.*

CAUSES

- Chromosomal or Mendelian syndrome (cleft defects caused by more than 300 syndromes)

FOCUS IN

TYPES OF CLEFT DEFORMITIES

These illustrations show variations of cleft lip and cleft palate.

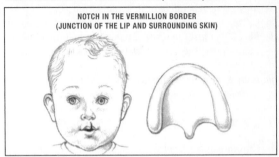

NOTCH IN THE VERMILLION BORDER
(JUNCTION OF THE LIP AND SURROUNDING SKIN)

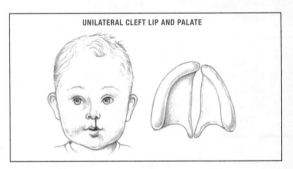

UNILATERAL CLEFT LIP AND PALATE

- Combined genetic and environmental factors
- Exposure to teratogens during fetal development

ASSESSMENT FINDINGS

- Family history of cleft defects
- Maternal exposure to teratogens during pregnancy
- Cleft running from the soft palate forward to either side
  of the nose

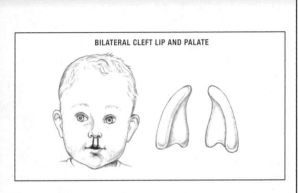

BILATERAL CLEFT LIP AND PALATE

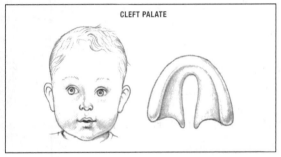

CLEFT PALATE

TEST RESULTS

■ Prenatal targeted ultrasound reveals abnormality.
■ Clinical presentation is obvious at birth.

TREATMENT

▶ **COLLABORATION** *The patient may need to see a speech therapist to correct speech patterns. Refer the parents to a social worker who can guide them to community resources, if needed, and to a genetic counselor to determine the recurrence risk.*

- Orthodontic prosthesis improves sucking
- Use of a contoured speech bulb attached to the posterior of a denture occludes the nasopharynx when a wide horseshoe defect makes surgery impossible (helps the child develop intelligible speech)
- Use of a large, soft nipple with large holes, such as a lamb's nipple improves feeding patterns and promotes adequate nutrition

ALERT *Daily use of folic acid before conception decreases the risk for isolated (not associated with another genetic or congenital malformation) cleft lip or palate by up to 25%. Women of childbearing age should be encouraged to take a daily multivitamin containing folic acid until menopause or until they're no longer fertile.*

- Surgical correction of cleft lip in the first few days of life and again at age 12 to 18 months, after the infant is gaining weight and being infection-free

KEY PATIENT OUTCOMES

The patient (or his family) will:
- exhibit normal growth and development patterns within the confines of the disorder
- not aspirate feedings
- express an understanding of the condition and treatment
- seek appropriate resources to assist with coping.

NURSING INTERVENTIONS

- Encourage the mother of an infant with cleft lip to breast-feed if the cleft doesn't prevent effective sucking.
- Suction the patient as necessary.
- Help the parents deal with their feelings about the child's deformity.

ALERT *Never place a child with Robin sequence on his back because his tongue could fall back and obstruct his airway. Place the infant on his side for sleeping. Most other infants with a cleft palate can sleep on their backs without difficulty.*

■ Monitor the patient's swallowing ability, weight gain, and intake and output.

PATIENT TEACHING

Be sure to cover:
■ treatment plan
■ how to best feed the infant
■ burping the infant frequently
■ gently cleaning the palatal cleft with a cotton-tipped applicator dipped in half-strength hydrogen peroxide or water after each feeding.

Clubfoot

DESCRIPTION

■ Congenital disorder in which the foot and ankle are twisted and can't be manipulated into the correct position
■ Unilateral clubfoot more common than bilateral
■ Also known as *talipes*

PATHOPHYSIOLOGY

■ Abnormal development of the foot during fetal growth leads to abnormal muscles and joints and contracture of soft tissue.
■ Apparent clubfoot
  – Results when a fetus maintains a position that gives his feet a clubfoot appearance at birth; it's usually corrected manually.
  – Another form of apparent clubfoot includes inversion of the feet, resulting from the denervation type of progressive muscular atrophy and progressive muscular dystrophy.

CAUSES

- Arrested development during the 9th and 10th weeks of embryonic life, when the feet are formed
- Deformed talus and shortened Achilles tendon
- Possible genetic predisposition

ASSESSMENT FINDINGS

- Deformity usually obvious at birth (see *Types of clubfoot*)
- Inability to correct deformity manually (distinguishes true clubfoot from apparent clubfoot)

TEST RESULTS

- X-rays show superimposition of the talus and calcaneus and a ladderlike appearance of the metatarsals.

TREATMENT

- Correction of the deformity
  - Series of casts to gradually stretch and realign the angle of the foot and, after cast removal, application of Denis Browne splint at night until age 1
  - Surgical correction
- Possible improvement with good function but can't correct it
- Affected calf muscle remaining slightly underdeveloped
  - Correction usually occurring in sequential order (correcting all three deformities at once results in a misshapen, rocker-bottomed foot)
- Forefoot adduction
- Varus (inversion)
- Equinus (plantar flexion)
- Maintenance of the correction until the foot gains normal muscle balance
- Close observation of the foot for several years to prevent the deformity from recurring

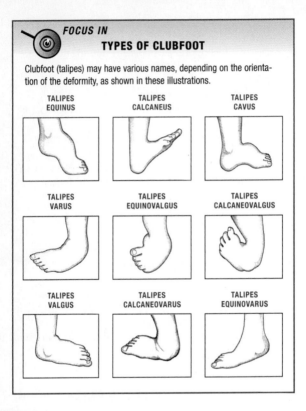

FOCUS IN

TYPES OF CLUBFOOT

Clubfoot (talipes) may have various names, depending on the orientation of the deformity, as shown in these illustrations.

TALIPES EQUINUS

TALIPES CALCANEUS

TALIPES CAVUS

TALIPES VARUS

TALIPES EQUINOVALGUS

TALIPES CALCANEOVALGUS

TALIPES VALGUS

TALIPES CALCANEOVARUS

TALIPES EQUINOVARUS

KEY PATIENT OUTCOMES

The patient (or his family) will:
- demonstrate appropriate use of corrective devices
- comply with prescribed exercise regimen and demonstrate proper technique
- remain free from complications.

NURSING INTERVENTIONS

- For the patient with a cast:
  - Assess neurovascular status.

- Use a blow dryer on the cool setting to provide relief of itching.
- Discuss the importance of placing nothing inside the cast.
- Make sure that shoes fit correctly.
- Prepare the patient for surgery, if necessary.
- Keep corrective devices on the patient as much as possible.
- Encourage the patient to walk as exercise after surgical repair.
- Perform passive range-of-motion exercises; don't use excessive force when trying to manipulate the foot.

PATIENT TEACHING

Be sure to cover:
- the need for immediate therapy and orthopedic supervision throughout the growth process
- cast care and signs of circulatory impairment
- that correction of this defect takes time and patience
- exercises that the parents and child can perform at home to help maintain the correction
- how to apply corrective shoes and splints when the child takes naps and goes to sleep at night.

Coarctation of the aorta

DESCRIPTION

- Narrowing of the aorta, usually just below the left subclavian artery, near the site where the ligamentum arteriosum (the remnant of the ductus arteriosus, a fetal blood vessel) joins the pulmonary artery to the aorta
- May occur with aortic valve stenosis (usually of a bicuspid aortic valve) and with severe cases of hypoplasia of the aortic arch, patent ductus arteriosus (PDA), and ventricular septal defect

- Ineffective pumping of the heart and increased risk of heart failure due to the obstruction of blood flow
- Accounts for about 7% of all congenital heart defects in children
- Twice as common in males as in females
- In females, commonly linked to Turner's syndrome

PATHOPHYSIOLOGY

- This disorder may develop as a result of spasm and constriction of the smooth muscle in the ductus arteriosus as it closes.
- Contractile tissue extends into the aortic wall, causing narrowing.
- This obstructive process causes hypertension in the aortic branches above the constriction (arteries that supply the arms, neck, and head) and diminished pressure in the vessel below the constriction.
- Restricted blood flow through the narrowed aorta increases the pressure load on the left ventricle and causes dilation of the proximal aorta and ventricular hypertrophy.
- As oxygenated blood leaves the left ventricle, a portion travels through the arteries that branch off the aorta proximal to the coarctation.
- If PDA is present, the rest of the blood travels through the coarctation, mixes with deoxygenated blood from the PDA, and travels to the legs.
- If the PDA is closed, the legs and lower portion of the body rely solely on the blood that gets through the coarctation.

CAUSES

- Unknown
- Turner's syndrome

ASSESSMENT FINDINGS

- Tachypnea
- Dyspnea
- Failure to thrive
- Headache
- Vertigo
- Epistaxis
- Claudication
- Pallor
- Hypertension
- Crackles
- Edema
- Tachycardia
- Cardiomegaly
- Hepatomegaly
- Hypertension
- Pink upper arms and cyanotic legs
- Absent or diminished femoral pulses
- Arm blood pressure greater than leg blood pressure
- Chest and arms more developed than legs

TEST RESULTS

- Chest X-ray may show left ventricular hypertrophy, indications of left-sided heart failure (enlarged heart, fluid in or around lungs), a wide ascending and descending aorta, and notching of the ribs' undersurfaces due to erosion by collateral circulation. (See *Recognizing coarctation of the aorta.*)
- Echocardiography may show increased left ventricular muscle thickness, coexisting aortic valve abnormalities, and the coarctation site.
- Electrocardiography may reveal left ventricular hypertrophy.
- Cardiac catheterization evaluates collateral circulation and measures pressure in the right and left ventricles and in the ascending and descending aortas (on both sides of the obstruction).
- Aortography locates the site and extent of coarctation.

RECOGNIZING COARCTATION OF THE AORTA

Collateral circulation develops to bypass the occluded aortic lumen and can be seen on X-ray as notching of the ribs. By adolescence, palpable, visible pulsations may be evident.

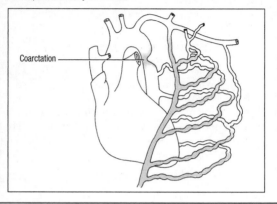

Coarctation

TREATMENT

- Low-sodium diet
- Fluid restrictions
- Limited activity
- Digoxin
- Diuretics
- Oxygen
- Sedatives
- Prostaglandin infusion to keep the ductus open
- Antibiotic prophylaxis
- Antihypertensive therapy
- Flap of the left subclavian artery may be used to reconstruct the aorta
- Balloon angioplasty or resection with end-to-end anastomosis or use of a tubular graft may also be performed

KEY PATIENT OUTCOMES

The patient will:
- carry out activities of daily living without weakness or fatigue
- maintain hemodynamic stability
- remain free from signs and symptoms of infection.

NURSING INTERVENTIONS

- Offer emotional support.
- Regulate environmental temperature.
- Give prescribed drugs.
- Monitor the patient's vital signs, intake and output, oxygenation, and blood glucose levels. Also monitor for postoperative pain and signs of infection.

PATIENT TEACHING

Be sure to cover:
- the disorder and its diagnosis and treatment
- exercise restrictions
- endocarditis prophylaxis
- the need for follow-up care, as ordered.

Croup

DESCRIPTION

- Viral infection that causes severe inflammation and obstruction of the upper airway
- Childhood disease manifested by acute laryngotracheobronchitis (most commonly), laryngitis, acute spasmodic laryngitis, and febrile rhinitis
- Incubation period about 3 to 6 days; contagious while febrile
- Recovery usually complete
- Occurs mainly in children ages 3 months to 5 years
- Affects boys more commonly than girls

- Usually occurs in late autumn and early winter
- Acute spasmodic laryngitis: usually affects children between ages 1 and 3

PATHOPHYSIOLOGY

- Viral invasion of the laryngeal mucosa leads to inflammation, hyperemia, edema, epithelial necrosis, and shedding.
- This leads to irritation and cough, reactive paralysis and continuous stridor, or collapsible supraglottic or inspiratory stridor and respiratory distress.
- A thin, fibrinous membrane covers the mucosa of the epiglottis, larynx, and trachea. (See *How croup affects the upper airways*, page 70.)

CAUSES

- Adenoviruses
- Allergies
- Bacteria (pertussis and diphtheria)
- Influenza viruses
- Measles viruses
- Parainfluenza viruses
- Respiratory syncytial virus (RSV)

ASSESSMENT FINDINGS

- Rhinorrhea
- Use of accessory muscles
- Nasal flaring
- Barklike cough
- Hoarse, muffled vocal sounds
- Inspiratory stridor
- Diminished breath sounds
- Symptoms worse at night

Laryngotracheobronchitis
- Edema of bronchi and bronchioles

FOCUS IN

HOW CROUP AFFECTS THE UPPER AIRWAYS

In croup, inflammatory swelling and spasms constrict the larynx, thereby reducing airflow. This cross-sectional drawing (from chin to chest) shows the upper airway changes caused by croup. Inflammatory changes almost completely obstruct the larynx (which includes the epiglottis) and significantly narrow the trachea.

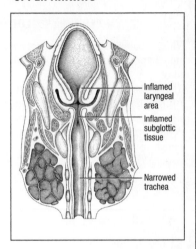

Inflamed laryngeal area

Inflamed subglottic tissue

Narrowed trachea

- Decreased breath sounds
- Expiratory rhonchi
- Scattered crackles

Laryngitis
- Suprasternal and intercostal retractions
- Inspiratory stridor
- Dyspnea, tachypnea
- Diminished breath sounds
- Severe dyspnea and exhaustion in later stages

Acute spasmodic laryngitis
- Labored breathing with retractions
- Clammy skin
- Rapid pulse rate

TEST RESULTS

- Throat cultures show bacteria and sensitivity to antibiotics.
- Neck X-ray may reveal upper airway narrowing and edema in subglottic folds and helps to differentiate croup from bacterial epiglottiditis.
- Computed tomography scan helps differentiate between croup, epiglottitis, and noninfection.
- Laryngoscopy may reveal inflammation and obstruction in epiglottal and laryngeal areas.

TREATMENT

- Home or hospitalized care
- Humidification during sleep
- Intubation if other means of preventing respiratory failure are unsuccessful
- Diet, as tolerated
- Parenteral fluids if required
- Rest periods
- Oxygen therapy as needed
- Antipyretics
- Antibiotics (if bacterial cause)
- Aerosolized racemic epinephrine for moderately severe croup
- Corticosteroids for acute laryngotracheobronchitis (controversial)

Surgery
- Tracheostomy (rare)

KEY PATIENT OUTCOMES

The patient (or his family) will:
- maintain adequate ventilation
- maintain normal temperature
- maintain a patent airway
- use effective coping strategies
- verbalize understanding of the disorder.

NURSING INTERVENTIONS

- Give prescribed drugs.
- Provide quiet diversional activities.
- Engage parents in the care of the infant or child.
- Position an infant in an infant seat or prop him up with a pillow.
- Position an older child in Fowler's position.
- Provide humidification.
- Avoid mild-based fluids if the patient has thick mucus or swallowing difficulties.
- Provide frequent mouth care.
- Isolate patients with RSV and parainfluenza infections.
- Use sponge baths and hypothermia blanket, as ordered, for temperatures above 102° F (38.9° C).
- Monitor the patient's vital signs, intake and output, and respiratory status. Also monitor for signs and symptoms of dehydration.

PATIENT TEACHING

Be sure to cover:
- the disorder and its diagnosis and treatment
- medications and possible adverse reactions
- when to notify the physician
- humidification
- hydration
- signs and symptoms of ear infection
- signs and symptoms of pneumonia.

Cryptorchidism

DESCRIPTION

- Congenital disorder in which one or both testes fail to descend into the scrotum, remaining in the abdomen or inguinal canal or at the external ring
- May be bilateral, but more commonly affects the right testis (see *Types of cryptorchidism*)

FOCUS IN

TYPES OF CRYPTORCHIDISM

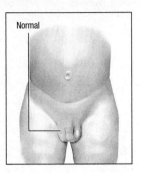

Normal

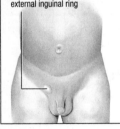

Descent interrupted beyond external inguinal ring

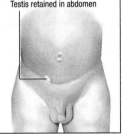

Testis retained in abdomen

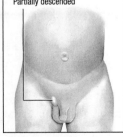

Partially descended

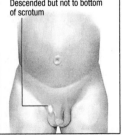

Descended but not to bottom of scrotum

- Occurs in 30% of premature male neonates, but in only 3% of those born at term
- In about 80% of affected infants, testes descending spontaneously during the first year; in the rest, testes possibly descending later

PATHOPHYSIOLOGY

- In the male fetus, testosterone normally stimulates the formation of the gubernaculum, a fibromuscular band that connects the testes to the scrotal floor.
- This band probably helps pull the testes into the scrotum by shortening as the fetus grows.
- Disorder may result from inadequate testosterone levels or a defect in the testes or the gubernaculum.
- Spermatogenesis is impaired (leading to reduced fertility) because the undescended testes are exposed to a higher temperature.
- True undescended testes remain along the path of normal descent, while ectopic testes deviate from that path.

CAUSES

- Genetic predisposition
- Hormonal factors
- Structural factors
- Testosterone deficiency

ASSESSMENT FINDINGS

- Nonpalpable testes
- Underdeveloped scrotum

TEST RESULTS

- Buccal smear (cells from oral mucosa) determines gender (a male sex chromatin pattern).
- Serum gonadotropin confirms the presence of testes by showing evidence of circulating hormone.
- Physical examination reveals disorder.

TREATMENT

- Human chorionic gonadotropin
- Orchiopexy

KEY PATIENT OUTCOMES

The patient will:
- express or demonstrate feelings of increased comfort
- remain free from complications.

NURSING INTERVENTIONS

- Encourage the parents of the child with undescended testes to express their concern about his condition.
- Tell the parents that a rubber band may be taped to the patient's thigh for about 1 week after surgery to keep the testis in place. Explain that his scrotum may swell but shouldn't be painful.
- After surgery, monitor the patient's vital signs, intake and output, and the operative site.

PATIENT TEACHING

Be sure to cover:
- the disorder, treatment, and effect on reproduction
- surgery or medications prescribed.

Life-threatening disorder

Cystic fibrosis

DESCRIPTION

- Chronic, progressive, inherited, incurable disease that affects exocrine (mucus-secreting) glands
- Transmitted as an autosomal recessive trait
- Genetic mutation involving chloride transport across epithelial membranes (more than 100 specific mutations of the gene identified)

- Most common fatal genetic disease of White children
- Twenty-five percent chance of transmission with each pregnancy when both parents are carriers of the recessive gene
- Highest in people of northern European ancestry
- Less common in Blacks, Native Americans, and people of Asian ancestry
- Equally common in both sexes
- Characterized by major aberrations in sweat gland, respiratory, and GI functions
- Accounts for almost all cases of pancreatic enzyme deficiency in children
- Clinical effects appearing soon after birth or taking years to develop
- Death from pneumonia, emphysema, or atelectasis

PATHOPHYSIOLOGY

- Viscosity of bronchial, pancreatic, and other mucous gland secretions increases, obstructing glandular ducts.
- Accumulation of thick, tenacious secretions in the bronchioles and alveoli causes respiratory changes, eventually leading to severe atelectasis and emphysema.
- This disorder also causes characteristic GI effects in the intestines, pancreas, and liver.
- Obstruction of the pancreatic ducts results in a deficiency of trypsin, amylase, and lipase; it prevents the conversion and absorption of fat and protein in the intestinal tract and interferes with the digestion of food and absorption of fat-soluble vitamins.
- In the pancreas, fibrotic tissue, multiple cysts, thick mucus, and fat replaces the acini, producing signs of pancreatic insufficiency.

CAUSES

- Autosomal recessive mutation of gene on chromosome 7

■ Causes of symptoms: increased viscosity of bronchial, pancreatic, and other mucous gland secretions and consequent destruction of glandular ducts

ASSESSMENT FINDINGS

■ Recurring bronchitis and pneumonia
■ Nasal polyps and sinusitis
■ Wheezing
■ Coughing
■ Shortness of breath
■ Abdominal distention, vomiting, constipation
■ Frequent, bulky, foul-smelling, and pale stool with a high fat content
■ Poor weight gain
■ Poor growth
■ Ravenous appetite
■ Hematemesis

> **ALERT** *Neonates may exhibit meconium ileus and develop symptoms of intestinal obstruction: abdominal distention, vomiting, constipation, dehydration, and electrolyte imbalance.*

■ Wheezy respirations
■ Dry, nonproductive, paroxysmal cough
■ Dyspnea
■ Tachypnea
■ Bibasilar crackles and hyperresonance
■ Barrel chest
■ Cyanosis, and clubbing of the fingers and toes
■ Distended abdomen
■ Thin extremities
■ Sallow skin with poor turgor
■ Delayed sexual development
■ Neonatal jaundice
■ Hepatomegaly
■ Rectal prolapse
■ Failure to thrive
■ Parents report salty-tasting skin

TEST RESULTS

- Sweat test reveals sodium and chloride values.
- Stool specimen analysis shows absence of trypsin.
- Deoxyribonucleic acid testing shows presence of the delta F 508 deletion.
- Liver enzyme tests may reveal hepatic insufficiency.
- Sputum culture may show such organisms as *Pseudomonas* and *Staphylococcus*.
- Serum albumin level is decreased.
- Serum electrolytes may show hypochloremia and hyponatremia.
- Arterial blood gas analysis shows hypoxemia.
- Chest X-ray may reveal early signs of lung obstruction.
- High-resolution chest computed tomography scan shows bronchial wall thickening, cystic lesions, and bronchiectasis.
- Pulmonary function tests show decreased vital capacity, elevated residual volume, and decreased forced expiratory volume in 1 second.

TREATMENT

COLLABORATION *Pulmonary specialists and respiratory therapists assist with clearing airway secretions and maintaining a patent airway. An endocrinologist may assist with managing diabetes as well as other pancreatic disorders. Nutritional specialists may be consulted to help with dietary measures (such as providing high-calorie meals that include the appropriate level of salt needed) and fluid therapy. Physical and occupational therapists may be needed to help with activity management and energy conservation.*

- Based on organ systems involved
- Chest physiotherapy, nebulization, and breathing exercises several times per day
- Postural drainage
- Gene therapy (experimental)
- Annual influenza vaccination

- Salt supplements
- High-fat, high-protein, high-calorie diet
- Activity as tolerated
- Dornase alfa, a pulmonary enzyme given by aerosol nebulizer
- Antibiotics
- Oxygen therapy as needed
- Oral pancreatic enzymes
- Bronchodilators
- Prednisone
- Vitamin A, D, E, and K supplements
- Lung transplantation

KEY PATIENT OUTCOMES

The patient (or his family) will:
- maintain a patent airway and adequate ventilation
- consume adequate calories daily
- use a support system to assist with coping
- express an understanding of the illness.

NURSING INTERVENTIONS

- Give prescribed drugs.
- Administer pancreatic enzymes with meals and snacks.
- Perform chest physiotherapy and postural drainage.
- Administer oxygen therapy as needed.
- Provide a well-balanced, high-calorie, high-protein diet; include adequate fats.
- Provide vitamin A, D, E, and K supplements, if indicated.
- Ensure adequate oral fluid intake.
- Provide exercise and activity periods.
- Encourage breathing exercises.
- Provide the young child with play periods.
- Enlist the help of the physical therapy department and play therapists, if available.
- Provide emotional support.
- Include family members in all phases of the child's care.

■ Monitor the patient's vital signs, intake and output, daily
   weight, hydration, pulse oximetry, and respiratory status.

PATIENT TEACHING

Be sure to cover with patient (or family):
■ the disorder and its diagnosis and treatment
■ medications and potential adverse reactions
■ when to notify the physician
■ aerosol therapy
■ chest physiotherapy
■ signs and symptoms of infection
■ complications.

Developmental dysplasia of the hip

DESCRIPTION

■ Abnormal formation of the hip joint present at birth
■ Most common disorder affecting the hip joints in chil-
   dren younger than age 3 years
■ Can be unilateral or bilateral
■ About 85% of affected infants are females
■ Occurs in three forms of varying severity (see *Degrees of
   hip dysplasia*)
■ Also called *DDH*

PATHOPHYSIOLOGY

■ Normal fetal development of the hip joint requires that
   the femoral head be seated tightly within the acetabulum.
■ Any situation that disrupts this intimate relationship increases the risk of hip dysplasia, and may occur in utero,
   perinatally, or during infancy and childhood.
■ Displacement of the femoral head from within the acetabulum may damage joint structures, including articu-
   lating surfaces, blood vessels, tendons, ligaments, and
   nerves.

FOCUS IN

DEGREES OF HIP DYSPLASIA

Normally, the head of the femur fits snugly into the acetabulum, allowing the hip to move properly. In congenital hip dysplasia, flattening of the acetabulum prevents the head of the femur from rotating adequately. The child's hip may be unstable, subluxated (partially dislocated), or completely dislocated, with the femoral head lying totally outside the acetabulum. The degree of dysplasia and the child's age are considered in determining the treatment choice.

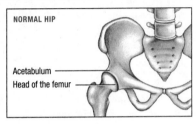

NORMAL HIP

Acetabulum
Head of the femur

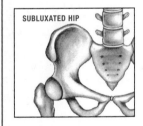

SUBLUXATED HIP

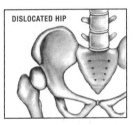

DISLOCATED HIP

- Disruption of blood flow to the joint may lead to ischemic necrosis of the femoral head.

CAUSES

- Exact cause unknown
- Risk factors: breech delivery, elevated maternal relaxin (hormone secreted by the corpus luteum during pregnancy that causes relaxation of pubic symphysis and cervical dilation), and large neonates and twins

- Additional risk factors: female gender, first-born child, and a family history of DDH

ASSESSMENT FINDINGS

- History of traumatic birth, large birth size, or twin pregnancy
- Extra skin fold on the thigh of the affected side
- Limited hip abduction on the dislocated side
- Level of knees uneven
- Swaying from side to side ("duck waddle") because of uncorrected bilateral dysplasia
- Limp due to uncorrected unilateral dysplasia

TEST RESULTS

- X-rays show the location of the femur head and a shallow acetabulum (after age 4 to 6 months).
- Sonography and magnetic resonance imaging assess for reduction.
- Physical examination reveals DDH. (See *Ortolani's and Trendelenburg's signs of DDH.*)

TREATMENT

- Varying with the patient's age
- Treatment after age 5 rarely restoring satisfactory hip function
- Referral (for child and parents) to a child life specialist to ensure continued developmental progress
- Younger than age 3 months:
  - Gentle manipulation to reduce the dislocation, followed by splint-brace or harness
  - Splint-brace or harness worn continuously for 2 to 3 months, then a night splint for another month
- Bilateral skin traction (in infants) or skeletal traction (in children who have started walking) for children over age 3 months

ORTOLANI'S AND TRENDELENBURG'S SIGNS OF DDH

A positive Ortolani's or Trendelenburg's sign confirms developmental dysplasia of the hip (DDH).

Ortolani's sign
- Place the infant on her back, with hip flexed and in abduction. Adduct the hip while pressing the femur downward. This will dislocate the hip.
- Next, abduct the hip while moving the femur upward. A click or a jerk (produced by the femoral head moving over the acetabular rim) indicates subluxation in an infant younger than 1 month. The sign indicates subluxation or complete dislocation in an older infant.

Trendelenburg's sign
- When the child rests her weight on the side of the dislocation and lifts her other knee, the pelvis drops on the normal side because abductor muscles in the affected hip are weak.
- However, when the child stands with her weight on the normal side and lifts the other knee, the pelvis remains horizontal.

- Bryant's traction or divarication traction (both extremities placed in traction, even if only one is affected, to help maintain immobilization) for 2 to 3 weeks for children younger than age 3 and weighing less than 35 lb (15.9 kg)
- Immobilization in a spica cast for approximately 3 months for children ages 6 to 12 months
- Gentle closed reduction under general anesthesia to further abduct the hips, followed by a spica cast for 3 months (if traction fails)
- In children older than age 18 months, open reduction and pelvic or femoral osteotomy to correct bony deformity followed by immobilization in a spica cast for 6 to 8 weeks
- In children ages 2 to 5 years, skeletal traction and subcutaneous adductor tenotomy (surgical cutting of the tendon)

KEY PATIENT OUTCOMES

The patient will:
- maintain joint mobility and range of motion
- maintain muscle strength
- achieve the highest level of mobility possible within the confines of the disease.

NURSING INTERVENTIONS

- Provide reassurance to the parents.
- Turn the child every 2 hours.
- Provide appropriate cast care.
- Monitor the parental care of cast or equipment; skin integrity, color, and sensation; motion of the infant's legs and feet; and patient comfort.

PATIENT TEACHING

Be sure to cover:
- how to correctly splint or brace the hips, as ordered
- importance of strict compliance with harnesses or external traction devices, where appropriate
- good hygiene
- signs and symptoms of cast compression (cyanosis, cool extremities, or pain)
- the need for frequent checkups.

Diabetes mellitus

DESCRIPTION

- Chronic disease of absolute or relative insulin deficiency or resistance
- Type 1 diabetes mellitus: most common childhood endocrine disorder
- Type 2 diabetes mellitus: rising incidence due to childhood obesity and sedentary lifestyles

PATHOPHYSIOLOGY

- Diabetes mellitus is characterized by disturbances in carbohydrate, protein, and fat metabolism.
- Insulin:
  - Allows glucose transport into the cells for use as energy or storage as glycogen.
  - Stimulates protein synthesis and free fatty acid storage in adipose tissues.
  - Deficiency compromises the body tissues' access to essential nutrients for fuel and storage.
- Two primary forms:
  - Type 1, characterized by absolute insulin insufficiency.
  - Type 2, characterized by insulin resistance with varying degrees of insulin secretory defects.

CAUSES

- Autoimmune factors (type 1)
- Genetic factors
- Viral infection
- Risk factors (type II): family history, obesity, sedentary lifestyle, hypertension, and dyslipidemia

ASSESSMENT FINDINGS

- Polyuria
- Polydipsia
- Polyphagia
- Nocturia
- Weight loss and hunger
- Weakness and fatigue
- Dehydration
  - Dry mucous membranes
  - Poor skin turgor
- Vision changes
  - Retinopathy or cataract formation
  - Possibly leading to blindness
- Frequent skin and urinary tract infections

- Skin changes
  - Dry, itchy skin (especially on the hands and feet)
  - Cool temperature
- Numbness or pain in the hands or feet
- Postprandial feeling of nausea or fullness
- Nocturnal diarrhea
- Decreased peripheral pulses
- Diminished deep tendon reflexes
- Orthostatic hypotension
- Characteristic "fruity" breath odor in ketoacidosis
- Possible hypovolemia and shock in ketoacidosis and hyperosmolar hyperglycemic state
- Type 1 specific
  - Rapidly developing symptoms
  - Muscle wasting and loss of subcutaneous fat
  - Honeymoon period
    - One-time remission of the symptoms, occurring shortly after insulin treatment started
    - Last effort by pancreas to produce insulin
    - Child can be insulin-free for up to 1 year but possibly needing oral hypoglycemics
    - Symptoms of hyperglycemia reappearing, and the child will be insulin-dependent for life
- Type 2 specific
  - Vague, long-standing symptoms developing gradually
  - Severe viral infection
  - Other endocrine diseases
  - Recent stress or trauma
  - Use of medications increasing blood glucose levels
  - Obesity, particularly in the abdominal area

TEST RESULTS

- Fasting plasma glucose level is greater than or equal to 126 mg/dl on at least two occasions.
- Random blood glucose level is greater than or equal to 200 mg/dl.
- Two-hour postprandial blood glucose level is greater than or equal to 200 mg/dl.
- Glycosylated hemoglobin (HbA_{1C}) is increased.

- Urinalysis may show acetone or glucose.
- Ophthalmologic examination may show diabetic retinopathy.

> ▶ **COLLABORATION** *The child with diabetes mellitus will need to be monitored by an endocrinologist as well as a dietitian for nutritional support. Family support counselors should be available to aid the patient and family with emotional issues associated with a long-term illness.*

TREATMENT

- Glycemic control to prevent complications
- Insulins
  - Regular (Humulin-R)
  - NPH (Humulin-N)
  - Lente (Humulin-L)
  - Ultralente (Humulin-U Ultralente)
  - Lispro (Humalog)
- Most common insulin regimen for children consisting of a combination of rapid-acting (regular) and intermediate-acting (NPH or Lente) insulins mixed in one syringe and administered twice daily, before breakfast and before dinner
- Oral antidiabetic drugs (type 2); insulin possibly required
- Pancreas transplantation
- Modest caloric restricted diet for weight loss or maintenance
- Follow American Diabetes Association recommendations to reach target glucose, HbA_{1C}, lipid, and blood pressure levels
- Regular aerobic exercise

KEY PATIENT OUTCOMES

The patient will:
- maintain optimal body weight
- remain free from infection

- avoid complications
- verbalize understanding of the disorder and treatment
- demonstrate adaptive coping behaviors.

NURSING INTERVENTIONS

- Administer medications as ordered.
- Monitor for signs and symptoms of hypoglycemia (insulin shock), such as:
  - behavioral changes (belligerence, confusion, slurred speech)
  - diaphoresis
  - palpitations
  - tachycardia
  - tremors.
- For hypoglycemia give rapidly absorbed carbohydrates such as orange juice or, if the child is unconscious, glucagon or I.V. dextrose, as ordered.
- Monitor for signs and symptoms of hyperglycemia, such as:
  - abdominal cramping
  - dry, flushed skin
  - fatigue
  - fruity breath odor
  - headache
  - mental status changes
  - nausea
  - thin appearance and possible malnourishment
  - vomiting
  - weakness.
- Administer I.V. fluids and insulin replacement for hyperglycemic crisis, as ordered.
- If it can't be determined whether a stuporous diabetic is suffering from hypoglycemia or hyperglycemia, treat for hypoglycemia.
- Provide meticulous skin care, especially to the feet and legs.
- Treat all injuries, cuts, and blisters immediately.
- Avoid constricting hose, slippers, or bed linens.

- Encourage adequate fluid intake.
- Consult a nutritionist.
- Encourage verbalization of feelings.
- Offer emotional support.
- Help to develop effective coping strategies.

PATIENT TEACHING

Be sure to cover:
- the disorder, diagnostic studies, and treatment
- insulin
- drawing up clear insulin first to prevent contamination (when giving a combination of clear and cloudy insulins)
- how to prevent air bubbles, to not shake the vial, and to gently rotate intermediate forms because they are suspensions
- administration of insulin as ordered (commonly twice daily; however, more injections per day may be ordered), 30 minutes before breakfast and 30 minutes before dinner; know that both injections will include a combination of fast-acting and intermediate-acting insulin
- varying insulin dosages (The dosage for one day is based on blood glucose levels of the previous day, with two-thirds of the daily dose usually given in the morning injection and one-third in the evening injection.)
- watching for hypoglycemic reactions during the peak action times for fast-acting and intermediate-acting insulins
- rotating injection sites to prevent lipodystrophy
- making sure the child eats when the insulin peaks by giving a midafternoon or bedtime snack for example
- keeping in mind that insulin requirements may be altered with illness, stress, growth, food intake, and exercise (Blood glucose measurements are the best way to determine insulin adjustments.)
- instructions (to parents) in all aspects of insulin therapy
- when to notify the physician
- appropriate exercise plan
- self-monitoring of glucose

- signs and symptoms of hyperglycemia, hypoglycemia, infection, and diabetic neuropathy
- foot care
- safety precautions.

Down syndrome

DESCRIPTION

- Chromosomal aberration that results in mental retardation, abnormal facial features, and other distinctive physical abnormalities
- Commonly associated with heart defects and other congenital disorders
- Average IQ between 30 and 50 (some higher)
- Occurs in 1 per 800 to 1,000 live births
- Maternal age above 35 considered a risk factor for having a child with Down syndrome
- Also known as *mongolism* and *trisomy 21 syndrome*

PATHOPHYSIOLOGY

- There are three main types of chromosome abnormalities in Down syndrome:
  - The vast majority of children with Down syndrome have three copies of chromosome 21 instead of the normal two because of faulty meiosis (nondisjunction) of the ovum or, sometimes, the sperm. Each cell in this individual has 47 chromosomes instead of 46. This is known as *trisomy 21*.
  - Three to four percent have translocation Down syndrome where the extra chromosome 21 is attached to another chromosome.
  - In Mosiac Down syndrome, which is noted in about 1% of Down syndrome infants, some cells have 47 chromosomes and some have 46.

CAUSES

- Deterioration of the oocyte resulting from age or cumulative effects of radiation and viruses
- Trisomy 21

ASSESSMENT FINDINGS

- Lethargy and poor feeding (in a neonate)
- Slanting, almond-shaped eyes
- Small, open mouth, protruding tongue
- Single transverse palmar crease
- Brushfield's spots on the iris
- Small skull
- Flat bridge across the nose
- Flattened face
- Small external ears
- Short neck with excess skin
- Dry, sensitive skin with decreased elasticity
- Umbilical hernia
- Short stature
- Short extremities with broad, flat, and squarish hands and feet
- Dysplastic middle phalanx of the fifth finger
- Wide space between the first and second toes
- Abnormal fingerprints and footprints
- Impaired reflex development
- Absent Moro's reflex and hyperextensible joints
- Impaired posture, coordination, and balance
- Imperforate anus and other intestinal abnormalities

TEST RESULTS

- Karyotype analysis or chromosome mapping show the chromosomal abnormality and confirm the diagnosis of Down syndrome.
- Maternal serum alpha-fetoprotein reveals reduced levels of alpha-fetoprotein prenatally.

- Prenatal ultrasonography can suggest, but not definitively diagnose, Down syndrome if a duodenal obstruction or an atrioventricular canal defect is present.
- Chorionic villus sampling (at 9 to 14 weeks' gestation) and amniocentesis (at 16 to 18 weeks' gestation) allow for prenatal diagnosis.

> **COLLABORATION** *The parents and other siblings should be referred for genetic and psychological counseling as appropriate. Social services or community support groups may be beneficial to the parents to help them utilize available resources. As the child develops, he may benefit from special education programs such as vocational training for adolescents or special athletic programs.*

- Developmental screening tests show severity and progress of retardation.

TREATMENT

- Referral for infant stimulation classes
- Maximal environmental simulation for infants
- Safety precautions for children and adults in a controlled environment
- Antibiotic therapy for recurrent infections
- Thyroid hormone replacement for hypothyroidism
- Open-heart surgery to correct cardiac defects, such as ventricular septal defects or atrial septal defects

KEY PATIENT OUTCOMES

The patient (or his family) will:

- demonstrate age-appropriate skills and behaviors to the extent possible
- perform health maintenance activities according to level of ability
- participate in developmental stimulation programs to increase skill levels.

NURSING INTERVENTIONS

- Establish a trusting relationship with the child's parents.
- Encourage verbalization and provide support.
- Encourage the parents to hold and nurture their child.
- Monitor for signs and symptoms of infection and the presence of complications. Also monitor the child's nutritional status, growth and development, thyroid function test results, heart sounds, and response to treatment.

PATIENT TEACHING

Be sure to cover:
- the need for adequate exercise and maximal environmental stimulation
- realistic goals for the parents and child
- information about a balanced diet
- the importance of remembering the emotional needs of other children in the family.

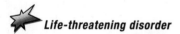 *Life-threatening disorder*

Epiglottiditis

DESCRIPTION

- Acute inflammation of the epiglottis and surrounding area
- Life-threatening emergency that rapidly causes edema and induration
- If left untreated, complete airway obstruction
- In children ages 2 to 8, mortality 8% to 12%
- Occurs from infancy to adulthood
- Occurs in any season

PATHOPHYSIOLOGY

- Infection of the epiglottis and surrounding area leads to intense inflammation of the supraglottic region.
- Swelling of the epiglottis, aryepiglottic folds, arytenoid cartilage, and ventricular bands lead to acute airway obstruction.

CAUSES

- Bacterial infection, usually *Haemophilus influenzae* type B
- *Streptococcus pneumoniae, Staphylococcus aureus*, or group A *streptococci*

ASSESSMENT FINDINGS

- Recent upper respiratory tract infection
- Sore throat
- Dysphagia
- Sudden onset of high fever
- Red and inflamed throat
- Fever
- Drooling
- Dyspnea
- Pale or cyanotic skin
- Restlessness and irritability
- Nasal flaring
- Patient may sit in tripod position
- Thick and muffled voice sounds

TEST RESULTS

- Arterial blood gas (ABG) analysis may show hypoxia.
- Lateral neck X-rays show an enlarged epiglottis and distended hypopharynx.
- Blood culture reveals *H. influenzae* or other bacteria.

AIRWAY CRISIS

Epiglottiditis can progress to complete airway obstruction within minutes. To prepare for this medical emergency, keep these tips in mind:

- Watch for the inability to speak; weak, ineffective cough; high-pitched sounds or no sounds while inhaling; increased difficulty breathing; and possible cyanosis. These are warning signs of total airway obstruction and the need for an emergency tracheotomy.
- Keep the following equipment available at the patient's bedside in case of sudden, complete airway obstruction: a tracheotomy tray, endotracheal tubes, a handheld resuscitation bag, oxygen equipment, and a laryngoscope with blades of various sizes.
- Remember that using a tongue blade or throat culture swab can initiate sudden, complete airway obstruction.
- Before examining the patient's throat, request trained personnel, such as an anesthesiologist, to stand by if emergency airway insertion is needed.

TREATMENT

- Direct laryngoscopy showing swollen, beefy-red epiglottis
- Pulse oximetry showing decreased oxygen saturation
- Emergency hospitalization
- Humidification of airway
- Parenteral fluids
- Activity as tolerated
- Parenteral antibiotics
- Corticosteroids
- Oxygen therapy
- Possible tracheotomy

KEY PATIENT OUTCOMES

The patient will:
- maintain adequate ventilation
- maintain adequate fluid volume
- maintain a patent airway (see *Airway crisis*)
- use alternate means of communication.

NURSING INTERVENTIONS

- Give prescribed drugs.
- Place the patient in a sitting position.
- Place the patient in a cool-mist tent.
- Encourage the parents to remain with their child.
- Offer reassurance and support.
- Ensure adequate fluid intake.
- Minimize external stimuli.
- Monitor the patient's vital signs, intake and output, respiratory status, ABG results, pulse oximetry, and signs and symptoms of secondary infection and dehydration.

PATIENT TEACHING

Be sure to cover:
- the disorder and its diagnosis and treatment
- prescribed drugs and potential adverse reactions
- when to call the physician
- humidification
- signs and symptoms of respiratory distress
- signs and symptoms of dehydration
- referral for *Haemophilus influenzae* b conjugate vaccine, preferably at age 2 months, if indicated.

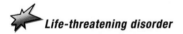 *Life-threatening disorder*

Ewing's sarcoma

DESCRIPTION

- Highly malignant, nonosseous tumor that arises from cells within the bone marrow
- Usually affects lower extremities, but can occur in the arms, pelvis, or chest
- Occurs between ages 4 and 25, usually in males ages 10 to 20
- Highly metastatic to lungs and bones with a poor prognosis
- Rare in Black and Asian children

PATHOPHYSIOLOGY

- Malignant cells originate in the bone marrow and invade the shafts of the long and flat bones.
- This disorder occurs most commonly in the diaphysis (midshaft) of long bones.
- Metastasis usually occurs in the lungs and bones.

CAUSES

- Unknown

ASSESSMENT FINDINGS

- Pain and swelling at the site becoming increasingly severe and persistent
- Pain possibly becoming so severe that the child can't sleep at night

TEST RESULTS

- Biopsy (by incision or by aspiration) confirms the diagnosis.
- Bone X-rays have a "moth-eaten" or "onionskin" appearance.
- Body computed tomography scans show tumor size.

TREATMENT

- Radiation
- Chemotherapy to slow growth using dactinomycin (Actinomycin D), doxorubicin (Adriamycin), cyclophosphamide, ifosfamide (Ifex), vincristine, and etoposide (VP-16)
- Amputation only if there's no evidence of metastases or the tumor appears unresectable
- Surgical removal of the primary tumor

KEY PATIENT OUTCOMES

The patient (or his family) will:
■ maintain optimal activity level
■ verbalize feelings and concerns
■ express feelings of increased comfort and decreased pain
■ use effective coping strategies.

NURSING INTERVENTIONS

■ Assist with radiation and chemotherapy.
■ Note that amputation isn't routine because the tumor spreads easily through the bone marrow.
■ Express the need for long-term follow up

PATIENT TEACHING

Be sure to cover (with the patient or his parents):
■ the disorder, its diagnosis, and treatment
■ possible adverse effects of chemotherapy and radiation
■ importance of consistent follow-up care
■ referral to a local support group.

Gastroesophageal reflux

DESCRIPTION

■ Return of gastric or duodenal contents into the esophagus from an incompetent or poorly developed esophageal sphincter
■ Also called *GERD*

PATHOPHYSIOLOGY

■ Lower esophageal sphincter (LES) function prevents gastric contents from backing up into the esophagus.
■ LES normally creates pressure, closing the lower end of the esophagus, but relaxing after each swallow to allow food into the stomach.

■ Reflux occurs with deficient LES pressure or when pressure within the stomach exceeds LES pressure.

CAUSES

■ Predisposing factors: administration of agents decreasing LES pressure, hiatal hernia with incompetent sphincter, long-term nasogastric intubation, prematurity

ASSESSMENT FINDINGS

■ Vomiting, possibly related to feedings, positioning, and activity level immediately after feedings (in infants)
■ Occurring most immediately after eating
■ Typically affecting infants but also seen in young children with spastic cerebral palsy due to decreased muscle tone
■ Esophagitis, indicated by blood in the emesis or stool
■ Weight loss
■ Aspiration of feedings
■ Recurrent pneumonia
■ Apnea (many infants may require apnea monitoring)

TEST RESULTS

■ A 24-hour pH probe study measures acid exposure of the esophagus.
■ Endoscopy and biopsy confirm pathologic changes in the mucosa.

TREATMENT

■ Positional therapy (especially useful in infants and children)
■ Small, frequent feedings of thickened liquids and frequent burping helping to lessen chances of regurgitation
■ Metoclopramide (Reglan) increasing LES tone and stimulating upper GI motility

- Ranitidine (Zantac) inhibiting gastric acid secretion, lessening inflammation of the esophagus
- Surgery to repair incompetent LES to prevent pulmonary aspiration
- Nissen fundoplication (surgical procedure involving wrapping the stomach fundus around the lower esophagus to increase the pressure necessary for food to enter the esophagus from the stomach)
- Placement of a jejunostomy tube (alternative for patients requiring long-term, continuous tube feedings)

KEY PATIENT OUTCOMES

The patient (or his family) will:
- state and demonstrate understanding of the disorder and its treatment
- express feelings of increased comfort
- show no signs of aspiration
- have minimal or no complications.

NURSING INTERVENTIONS

- To maximize the benefits of medications, administer them 30 minutes before meals.
- Provide formula thickened with cereal.
- Enlarge the bottle's nipple opening to allow for easier delivery of formula.
- Feed the infant in an upright position, burping frequently.
- Hold the infant in an upright position for 15 to 30 minutes after feeding.
- Give the infant small, frequent feedings.
- Prepare for surgery (Nissen fundoplication), if necessary.

PATIENT TEACHING

Be sure to cover (with the parents):
- the causes of reflux, how to avoid it, and what symptoms to watch for and report.

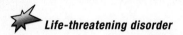
Life-threatening disorder

Hemophilia

DESCRIPTION

- Hereditary bleeding disorder
- Characterized by greatly prolonged coagulation time
- Results from deficiency of specific clotting factors
- Hemophilia A (classic hemophilia: affects more than 80% of hemophiliacs, resulting from factor VIII deficiency
- Hemophilia B (Christmas disease): affects 15% of hemophiliacs, resulting from factor IX deficiency
- Most common X-linked genetic disease
- Occurs in about 1.25 of 10,000 live male births
- Incurable

PATHOPHYSIOLOGY

- A low level or absence of the blood protein necessary for clotting causes disruption of normal intrinsic coagulation cascade.
- This produces abnormal bleeding, which may be mild, moderate, or severe, depending on the degree of protein factor deficiency.
- After a platelet plug forms at a bleeding site, the lack of clotting factors impairs formation of a stable fibrin clot.
- Hemorrhage isn't always immediate; delayed bleeding is common.

CAUSES

- Acquired immunologic process
- Hemophilia A and B inherited as X-linked recessive traits
- Spontaneous mutation

ASSESSMENT FINDINGS

- Familial history of bleeding disorders
- Prolonged bleeding with circumcision
- Concomitant illness
- Pain and swelling in a weight-bearing joint, such as the hip, knee, or ankle
- With mild hemophilia or after minor trauma, lack of spontaneous bleeding, but prolonged bleeding with major trauma or surgery
- Moderate hemophilia producing only occasional spontaneous bleeding episodes
- Severe hemophilia causing spontaneous bleeding
- Prolonged bleeding after surgery or trauma or joint pain in spontaneous bleeding into muscles or joints
- Signs of internal bleeding, such as abdominal, chest, or flank pain; episodes of hematuria or hematemesis; and tarry stools
- Activity or movement limitations and need for assistive devices, such as splints, canes, or crutches
- Hematomas on extremities, torso, or both
- Joint swelling in episodes of bleeding into joints
- Limited and painful joint range of motion (ROM) in episodes of bleeding into joints

TEST RESULTS

Hemophilia A
- Factor VIII assay is 0% to 25% of normal.
- Partial thromboplastin time (PTT) is prolonged.
- Platelet count and function, bleeding time, and prothrombin time are normal.

Hemophilia B
- Factor IX assay is deficient.
- Baseline coagulation results are similar to those of hemophilia A, with normal factor VIII.

Hemophilia A or B
- Degree of factor deficiency defines severity:

– Mild hemophilia — factor levels are 5% to 25% of normal.
– Moderate hemophilia — factor levels are 1% to 5% of normal.
– Severe hemophilia — factor levels are less than 1% of normal.

TREATMENT

■ Correct treatment to quickly stop bleeding by increasing plasma levels of deficient clotting factors
■ Diet consisting of foods high in vitamin K (such as dark green leafy vegetables and soybeans)
■ Activity guided by degree of factor deficiency
■ Aminocaproic acid

Hemophilia A
■ Cryoprecipitated antihemophilic factor (AHF), lyophilized AHF, or both
■ Desmopressin (DDAVP)

Hemophilia B
■ Factor IX concentrate

KEY PATIENT OUTCOMES

The patient (or his family) will:
■ maintain hemodynamic stability
■ have peripheral pulses that remain palpable and strong
■ express feelings of increased comfort and decreased pain
■ maintain ROM and joint mobility
■ demonstrate adequate coping skills
■ verbalize understanding of disease process and treatment regimen.

NURSING INTERVENTIONS

■ Follow standard precautions.
■ Provide emotional support, and reassurance when indicated.

During bleeding episodes
- Apply pressure to bleeding sites.
- Give the deficient clotting factor or plasma, as ordered, until bleeding stops.
- Apply cold compresses or ice bags, and elevate the injured part.
- To prevent recurrence of bleeding, restrict activity for 48 hours after bleeding is under control.
- Control pain with prescribed analgesics.
- Avoid I.M. injections.
- Avoid aspirin, aspirin-containing drugs, and over-the-counter anti-inflammatory agents.

During bleeding into a joint
- Immediately elevate the joint.
- To restore joint mobility, begin ROM exercises at least 48 hours after the bleeding is controlled.
- Restrict weight bearing until bleeding stops and swelling subsides.
- Give prescribed analgesics for pain.
- Apply ice packs and elastic bandages to alleviate pain.
- Monitor the patient's PTT, adverse reactions to blood products, signs and symptoms of decreased tissue perfusion, vital signs, and bleeding from the skin, mucous membranes, and wounds.

PATIENT TEACHING

Be sure to cover:
- the benefits of regular isometric exercises
- how parents can protect their child from injury while avoiding unnecessary restrictions that impair normal development
- the need to avoid contact sports
- if an injury occurs, directions for parents to apply cold compresses or ice bags and to elevate the injured part or apply light pressure to bleeding
- the need to notify the physician immediately after even a minor injury

- need for parents to watch for signs of internal bleeding
- importance of avoiding aspirin, combination medications that contain aspirin, and over-the-counter anti-inflammatory agents (use acetaminophen instead)
- the importance of good dental care and the need to check with the physician before dental extractions or surgery
- need to wear medical identification jewelry at all times
- how to administer blood factor components at home, if appropriate
- need to keep blood factor concentrate and infusion equipment available at all times
- adverse reactions that can result from replacement factor procedures
- signs, symptoms, and treatment of anaphylaxis
- need for the patient or parents to watch for early signs of hepatitis
- need to follow standard precautions
- referral for new patients to a hemophilia treatment center for evaluation
- referral for the patient's family to the National Hemophilia Foundation.

Hirschsprung's disease

DESCRIPTION

- Absence of parasympathetic ganglionic cells in a segment of the colon (usually at the distal end of the large intestine)
- Lack of nerve innervation leading to lack of, or alteration in, peristalsis in the affected part (see *A look at Hirschsprung's disease*, page 106)

PATHOPHYSIOLOGY

- Stool enters the affected part and remains there until additional stool pushes it through.
- The affected part of the colon dilates, possibly resulting in a mechanical obstruction.

FOCUS IN

A LOOK AT HIRSCHSPRUNG'S DISEASE

Hirschsprung's disease is a congenital disorder of the large intestine characterized by the absence or marked reduction of parasympathetic ganglion cells in the colorectal wall.

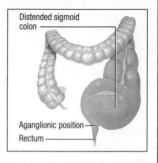

Distended sigmoid colon

Aganglionic position

Rectum

CAUSES

- Commonly coexisting with other congenital anomalies, particularly Down syndrome (trisomy 21) and anomalies of the urinary tract
- Familial, congenital defect

ASSESSMENT FINDINGS

- Failure to pass meconium and stool
- Liquid or ribbonlike stools
- Distended abdomen and easily palpable stool masses
- Bile-stained or fecal vomiting
- Irritability and lethargy
- Failure to thrive and weight loss
- Signs of dehydration (pallor, dry mucous membranes, sunken eyes)

TEST RESULTS

- Rectal biopsy provides definitive diagnosis by showing the absence of ganglion cells.

- Suction aspiration determines the absence of ganglion cells.
- Rectal manometry detects failure of the internal anal sphincter to relax and contract.
- Abdominal X-rays show colon distention.

TREATMENT

- Daily colonic lavage to empty the bowel until surgery
- Digital examination (performed by a physician to expand the anus enough to release the impacted stool and provide temporary relief if megacolon located near the rectum)
- Preoperative bowel prep with an antibiotic (neomycin [Neo-fradin] or nystatin [Mycostatin])
- Surgical treatment involving pulling the normal ganglionic segment through to the anus
- Surgery usually delayed until at least age 10 months
- Temporary colostomy or ileostomy possibly necessary to decompress the colon in total obstruction

KEY PATIENT OUTCOMES

The patient will:
- maintain adequate caloric intake
- avoid complications
- have bowel function return to normal patterns
- maintain fluid balance.

NURSING INTERVENTIONS

Preoperative
- Maintain fluid and electrolyte balance to prevent dehydration and shock.
- Monitor vital signs to prevent sepsis and enterocolitis.
- Administer isotonic enemas (normal saline solution or mineral oil) to evacuate the bowel; don't administer tap water because of the risk of water intoxication.

After colostomy or ileostomy

■ Monitor fluid intake and output (ileostomy is especially likely to cause excessive electrolyte loss).

■ Keep the area around the stoma clean and dry; use colostomy or ileostomy appliances to collect drainage.

■ Monitor for return of bowel sounds to begin diet.

After corrective surgery

■ Keep the wound clean and dry to prevent infection.

■ Don't use a rectal thermometer or suppositories.

■ Begin oral feedings when active bowel sounds begin and nasogastric drainage decreases.

PATIENT TEACHING

Be sure to cover (with the parents):

■ the disease

■ appropriate preoperative teaching (reinforcing the physician's explanation about the procedure and its possible complications)

■ the signs of fluid loss and dehydration (decreased urine output, sunken eyes, and sudden, marked abdominal distention)

■ before discharge, if possible, consultation with an enterostomal therapist for valuable tips on colostomy or ileostomy care

■ the importance of watching for foods that increase the number of stools and to avoid offering these foods, reassuring that their child will, in time, probably gain sphincter control and eat a normal diet

■ that complete continence can take years to develop and that constipation may recur.

Hodgkin's lymphoma

DESCRIPTION

■ Malignant neoplasm of the lymphoid tissue

■ Commonly seen in adolescents and young adults

■ Excellent prognosis

PATHOPHYSIOLOGY

- This disorder may originate in a localized group of lymph nodes.
- It proliferates by way of lymphocytes to other sites, including bone marrow, the liver, the lungs, the mediastinum, and the spleen.

CAUSES

- Unknown; suspected viral etiology, particularly with the Epstein-Barr virus
- Environmental and immunologic factors

ASSESSMENT FINDINGS

- Painless, firm, persistently enlarged lymph nodes
  - Appearing insidiously
  - Most commonly occurring in the lower cervical region
- Night sweats
- Pruritus
- Recurrent fever
- Weight loss

TEST RESULTS

- Lymph node and bone marrow biopsies confirm diagnosis by revealing Reed-Sternberg cells (enlarged, abnormal histiocytes).
- Chest X-ray, abdominal computed tomography scan, ultrasound, or lymphangiogram detect lymph node or organ involvement.
- I.V. dye is injected into the feet (with X-rays tracking it) and travels up the body where it's absorbed by the lymphatic system (cancerous nodes differ in appearance from normal lymph nodes).
- Blood tests show mild to severe normocytic anemia and elevated serum alkaline phosphatase, which indicates liver or bone involvement.

STAGING HODGKIN'S LYMPHOMA

Treatment of Hodgkin's lymphoma depends on the stage it has reached — that is, the number, location, and degree of involved lymph nodes.

Stage I
Hodgkin's lymphoma appears in a single lymph node region or a single extralymphatic organ.

Stage II
The disease appears in two or more nodes on the same side of the diaphragm and in an extralymphatic organ.

Stage III
Hodgkin's lymphoma spreads to lymph node regions on both sides of the diaphragm and perhaps to an extralymphatic organ, the spleen, or both.

Stage IV
The disease disseminates, involving one or more extralymphatic organs or tissues, with or without associated lymph node involvement.

TREATMENT

- Depending on the number, location, and degree of involved lymph nodes (see *Staging Hodgkin's lymphoma*)
- Radiation therapy or chemotherapy alone for stages I and II and in combination for stage III
- Chemotherapy for stage IV, sometimes inducing a complete remission
  - MOPP protocol — mechlorethamine (Mustargen), vincristine (Oncovin), procarbazine (Matulane), and prednisone
  - ABVD protocol — doxorubicin (Adriamycin), bleomycin (Blenoxane), vinblastine, and dacarbazine (DTIC-Dome)
  - High-dose chemotherapy with autologous bone marrow transplant or autologous peripheral blood stem cell

transfusions for a patient unresponsive to radiation therapy or chemotherapy

KEY PATIENT OUTCOMES

The patient will:
- have no further weight loss
- express feelings of increased energy
- demonstrate adequate skin integrity
- demonstrate effective coping mechanisms
- express feelings of increased comfort and decreased pain.

NURSING INTERVENTIONS

- Assess for adverse effects of radiation and chemotherapy, including anorexia, nausea, vomiting, diarrhea, fever, and bleeding.
- Control pain and bleeding of stomatitis by using a soft toothbrush, applying petroleum jelly to the lips, and avoiding astringent mouthwashes.
- Offer the patient and his family appropriate emotional support, including information on the local chapter of the American Cancer Society.

PATIENT TEACHING

Be sure to cover:
- the disorder and its diagnosis and treatment
- signs and symptoms of infection
- the importance of maintaining good nutrition
- the pacing of activities to counteract therapy-induced fatigue
- the importance of good oral hygiene
- the avoidance of crowds and people with known infection
- the importance of checking the lymph nodes
- all prescribed drugs, including administration, dosage, and possible adverse effects.

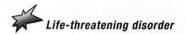 *Life-threatening disorder*

Hydrocephalus

DESCRIPTION

■ Variety of conditions characterized by an excess of fluid within the cranial vault, subarachnoid space, or both
■ Occurs because of interference with cerebrospinal fluid (CSF) flow caused by increased fluid production, obstruction within the ventricular system, or defective reabsorption of CSF
■ Types:
  – Noncommunicating hydrocephalus — obstruction within the ventricular system
  – Communicating hydrocephalus — impaired absorption of CSF

PATHOPHYSIOLOGY

■ Obstruction of CSF flow associated with hydrocephalus produces dilation of the ventricles proximal to the obstruction.
■ Obstructed CSF under pressure causes atrophy of the cerebral cortex and degeneration of the white matter tracts; selective preservation of gray matter also occurs.
■ When excess CSF fills a defect caused by atrophy, a degenerative disorder, or a surgical excision, the fluid isn't under pressure and atrophy and degenerative changes aren't induced.

CAUSES

Communicating hydrocephalus
■ Adhesions from inflammation, such as with meningitis or subarachnoid hemorrhage
■ Cerebral atrophy
■ Compression of the subarachnoid space by a mass such as a tumor

- Congenital abnormalities of the subarachnoid space
- Head injury
- High venous pressure within the sagittal sinus

Noncommunicating hydrocephalus
- Aqueduct stenosis
- Arnold-Chiari malformation
- Congenital abnormalities in the ventricular system
- Mass lesions such as a tumor compressing one of the structures of the ventricular system

ASSESSMENT FINDINGS

Infants
- Enlarged head clearly disproportionate to the infant's growth
- Head possibly appearing normal in size with bulging fontanels
- Distended scalp veins
- Thin, fragile, and shiny scalp skin
- Underdeveloped neck muscles
- Displacement of the eyes downward (sunset sign)
- Abnormal leg muscle tone

Older children
- Decreased level of consciousness (LOC)
- Ataxia
- Impaired intellect
- Incontinence
- Signs of increased intracranial pressure (ICP) (such as headache, nausea, vomiting, lethargy, and irritability)

TEST RESULTS

- Skull X-rays show thinning of the skull with separated sutures and widened fontanels in infants.
- Angiography, computed tomography scan, and magnetic resonance imaging show differentiation between hydrocephalus and intracranial lesions and Arnold-Chiari malformation.

TREATMENT

- Shunting of CSF directly from the ventricular system to some point beyond the obstruction
- Small, frequent feedings
- Slow feeding of infant
- Decreased movement during and immediately after meals
- Possible preoperative and postoperative antibiotics
- Surgical correction (the only treatment for hydrocephalus) including:
  - removal of obstruction to CSF flow
  - implantation of a ventriculoperitoneal shunt to divert CSF flow from the brain's lateral ventricle into the peritoneal cavity
  - with concurrent abdominal problem, ventriculoatrial shunt to divert CSF flow from the brain's lateral ventricle into the right atrium of the heart

KEY PATIENT OUTCOMES

The patient will:
- maintain adequate ventilation
- develop no signs and symptoms of infection
- maintain and improve current LOC
- develop no signs and symptoms of increased ICP.

NURSING INTERVENTIONS

- Elevate the head of the bed to 30 degrees or put an infant in an infant seat.
- Give prescribed oxygen, as needed.
- Provide small, frequent feedings.
- Decrease the patient's movement during and immediately after meals.
- Provide skin care.

After shunt surgery

- Place the infant or child on the side opposite the operative site.
- Give prescribed I.V. fluids and analgesics.

- Refer the patient and his parents to special education programs, as appropriate.
- Monitor the patient's fontanels for tension or fullness, head circumference, signs and symptoms of increased ICP, growth and development, neurologic status, and intake and output.
- After surgery, monitor the patient's dressing for drainage and redness, swelling, and other signs and symptoms of local infection. Also monitor the patient for response to analgesics and for signs and symptoms of meningitis.

 ALERT *Monitor the patient for vomiting, which may be an early sign of shunt malfunction.*

PATIENT TEACHING

Be sure to cover:
- the disorder and its diagnosis and treatment
- shunt surgery (hair loss and the visibility of a mechanical device)
- postoperative shunt care
- signs and symptoms of increased ICP or shunt malfunction, infection, and paralytic ileus
- the need for periodic shunt surgery to lengthen the shunt as the child grows older.

Hyperbilirubinemia

DESCRIPTION

- Excessive serum bilirubin levels and jaundice
- Result of hemolytic processes in the neonate
- Can be physiologic (with jaundice the only symptom) or pathologic (resulting from an underlying disease)
- Also called *neonatal jaundice*

PATHOPHYSIOLOGY

- As erythrocytes break down at the end of their neonatal life cycle, hemoglobin separates into globin (protein) and heme (iron) fragments.

■ Heme fragments form unconjugated (indirect) bilirubin, which binds with albumin for transport to liver cells to conjugate with glucuronide, forming direct bilirubin.

■ Fat-soluble unconjugated bilirubin not excreted in the urine or bile may possibly escape to extravascular tissue, especially fatty tissue and the brain.

■ May develop when:
  – certain factors disrupt conjugation and usurp albumin-binding sites, including drugs (such as aspirin, tranquilizers, and sulfonamides) and conditions (such as hypothermia, anoxia, hypoglycemia, and hypoalbuminemia)
  – decreased hepatic function results in reduced bilirubin conjugation
  – increased erythrocyte production or breakdown results from hemolytic disorders or Rh or ABO incompatibility
  – biliary obstruction or hepatitis results in blockage of normal bile flow
  – maternal enzymes present in breast milk inhibit the infant's glucuronosyltransferase conjugating activity (rare).

CAUSES

See *Onset-related causes of hyperbilirubinemia.*

ASSESSMENT FINDINGS

■ Yellowish skin, usually appearing in head-to-toe manner
■ Yellowing of the eyes

TEST RESULTS

■ Serum bilirubin levels are elevated.

TREATMENT

■ Phototherapy
■ Exchange transfusions
■ Albumin

ONSET-RELATED CAUSES OF HYPERBILIRUBINEMIA

The infant's age at onset of hyperbilirubinemia may provide clues to the source of this jaundice-causing disorder.

Day 1
- Blood type incompatibility (Rh, ABO, other minor blood groups)
- Intrauterine infection (rubella, cytomegalic inclusion body disease, toxoplasmosis, syphilis and, occasionally, such bacteria as *Escherichia coli*, *Staphylococcus*, *Pseudomonas*, *Klebsiella*, *Proteus*, and *Streptococcus*)

Day 2 or 3
- Infection (usually from gram-negative bacteria)
- Polycythemia
- Enclosed hemorrhage (skin bruises, subdural hematoma)
- Respiratory distress syndrome (hyaline membrane disease)
- Heinz body anemia from drugs and toxins (vitamin K_3, sodium nitrate)
- Transient neonatal hyperbilirubinemia
- Abnormal red blood cell morphology
- Red cell enzyme deficiencies (glucose-6-phosphate dehydrogenase, hexokinase)
- Physiologic jaundice
- Blood group incompatibilities

Day 4 and 5
- Breast-feeding, respiratory distress syndrome, maternal diabetes
- Crigler-Najjar syndrome (congenital nonhemolytic icterus)
- Gilbert syndrome

Day 7 and later
- Herpes simplex
- Pyloric stenosis
- Hypothyroidism
- Neonatal giant cell hepatitis
- Infection (usually acquired in neonatal period)
- Bile duct atresia
- Galactosemia
- Choledochal cysts

- Phenobarbital (rarely used)
- $Rh_o(D)$ immune globulin (human) (RhoGAM) (given to Rh-negative mother)

KEY PATIENT OUTCOMES

The patient will:
- exhibit normal body temperature
- maintain normal fluid balance
- maintain skin integrity
- have a reduced bilirubin level.

NURSING INTERVENTIONS

- Reassure the parents that most infants experience some degree of jaundice.
- Keep emergency equipment available when transfusing blood.
- Administer $Rh_o(D)$ immune globulin (human), to an Rh-negative mother after amniocentesis, or — to prevent hemolytic disease in subsequent infants — to an Rh-negative mother during the third trimester, after the birth of an Rh-positive infant, or after spontaneous or elective abortion.
- Monitor the patient's bilirubin levels, body temperature, intake and output.
- Also monitor for jaundice, bleeding, and possible complications.

PATIENT TEACHING

Be sure to cover:
- the disorder and its diagnosis and treatment
- that the infant's stool contains some bile and may be greenish.

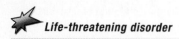

Life-threatening disorder

Hypoplastic left heart syndrome

DESCRIPTION

- Underdevelopment of the left side of the heart
- Types of defects:
  - Aortic valve atresia or stenosis
  - Mitral valve atresia or stenosis
  - Diminutive or absent left ventricle
  - Severe hypoplasia of the ascending aorta and aortic arch (see *Looking at hypoplastic left heart syndrome*)

PATHOPHYSIOLOGY

- Blood from the left atrium travels through a patent foramen ovale to the right ventricle and pulmonary artery,

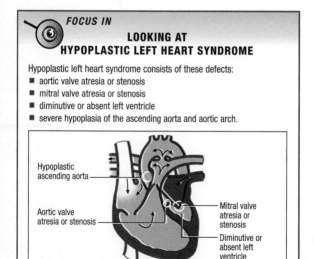

FOCUS IN

LOOKING AT HYPOPLASTIC LEFT HEART SYNDROME

Hypoplastic left heart syndrome consists of these defects:
- aortic valve atresia or stenosis
- mitral valve atresia or stenosis
- diminutive or absent left ventricle
- severe hypoplasia of the ascending aorta and aortic arch.

Hypoplastic ascending aorta

Aortic valve atresia or stenosis

Mitral valve atresia or stenosis

Diminutive or absent left ventricle

where it enters the systemic circulation via the ductus arteriosus.

■ Patency of the ductus arteriosus allows blood to flow to the systemic circulation (necessary to sustain life).

CAUSES

■ Unknown

ASSESSMENT FINDINGS

■ Normal appearance at birth; symptoms developing in 24 to 48 hours
■ Cyanosis and pallor
■ Tachypnea
■ Dyspnea
■ Lethargy
■ Difficulty feeding
■ Poor peripheral perfusion with diminished pulses
■ Hypothermia
■ Tachycardia
■ Loud second heart sound (S_2)

TEST RESULTS

■ Echocardiography shows the defect.

TREATMENT

■ Prostaglandin E to maintain patency of the ductus arteriosus
■ Ventilator support, if necessary
■ Digoxin and diuretics to control heart failure
■ Surgical repair
■ Heart transplantation
■ Norwood procedure (three-stage procedure involving restructuring the heart)
■ Without surgery, death occurring in early infancy

KEY PATIENT OUTCOMES

The patient will:
- maintain hemodynamic stability
- foster improved cardiac blood flow
- have no signs of heart failure.

NURSING INTERVENTIONS

- Monitor the patient's vital signs, pulse oximetry, and intake and output.
- Assess cardiovascular and respiratory status.
- Monitor fluid status, enforcing fluid restrictions as appropriate.
- Take the patient's apical pulse for 1 minute before giving digoxin, and withhold the drug to prevent toxicity if the patient's heart rate is below 100 beats/minute.
- Weigh the child daily.
- Weigh soiled diapers.
- Organize physical care and anticipate the need to reduce the child's oxygen demands.

PATIENT TEACHING

Be sure to cover (with the parents):
- the heart defect and answer any questions to prepare the child for surgery.

Hypospadias and epispadias

DESCRIPTION

- Hypospadias — congenital anomaly of the penis in which the urethral meatus opens on the ventral surface (underside) of the penis; occurs in 1 in 300 live male births
- Epispadias — rare condition in which the urinary meatus opens on the dorsal surface (top side) of the penis; occurs in 1 in 200,000 live male births

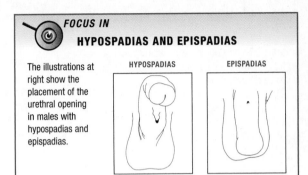

FOCUS IN

HYPOSPADIAS AND EPISPADIAS

The illustrations at right show the placement of the urethral opening in males with hypospadias and epispadias.

HYPOSPADIAS

EPISPADIAS

- Both conditions: shortened distance to the bladder, offering bacteria easier access

PATHOPHYSIOLOGY

- Hypospadias — The urethral opening is located on the ventral surface of the penis. In severe cases, the urethral opening is located on the perineal or scrotal region.
- Epispadias — The urethral opening is located on the dorsal surface of the penis. (See *Hypospadias and epispadias.*)

CAUSES

- Exact cause unknown
- Possible genetic factors

ASSESSMENT FINDINGS

- Hypospadias
  - Altered angle of urination
  - Normal urination impossible with penis elevated due to chordee (band of fibrous tissue causing penis curvature)
  - Urethral opening located on underside of penis
- Epispadias
  - Urethral opening located on topside of penis

– Exstrophy of the bladder
– Exposed bladder appearing bright red and obvious at birth
– Urine seeping onto the abdominal wall from abnormal ureteral openings

TEST RESULTS

■ Physical observation confirms the diagnosis.

TREATMENT

■ Hypospadias

ALERT Avoid circumcision because the foreskin may be needed later for surgical repair.

– No treatment necessary in mild disorder
– Meatotomy (surgical procedure performed to extend the urethra into a normal position)
– Surgery to release the chordee
– Typically performed when the child is between ages 12 and 18 months
– If extensive repair necessary, surgery delayed until age 4

■ Epispadias

– Surgery typically requiring multiple procedures
– Associated bladder exstrophy closed preferably within the first few days of life
– Second phase of surgery involving the lengthening and straightening of the penis and the creation of a more distal urethral opening

KEY PATIENT OUTCOMES

The patient will:

■ remain free from infection
■ maintain fluid balance
■ maintain urinary continence.

NURSING INTERVENTIONS

- Keep the area clean.
- Be aware that surgery involving implants or reconstruction may be needed.
- Encourage the parents to express their feelings and concerns, and provide emotional support.

PATIENT TEACHING

Be sure to cover (with the parents):
- the disorder and its treatment options
- proper cleaning techniques for infection prevention
- realistic postsurgical expectations
- importance of skin care and methods of handling urinary incontinence
- importance of providing child with emotional support
- referral to support group, as appropriate.

Impetigo

DESCRIPTION

- Contagious, superficial bacterial skin infection
- Nonbullous and bullous forms
- May complicate chickenpox, eczema, and other skin disorders marked by open lesions
- Most commonly appears on face, arms, and legs

PATHOPHYSIOLOGY

Nonbullous impetigo
- Eruption occurs when bacteria inoculate traumatized skin cells.
- Lesions begin as small vesicles, which rapidly erode.
- Honey-colored crusts are surrounded by erythema.

Bullous impetigo
- Eruption occurs in nontraumatized skin via bacterial toxin or exotoxin.

FOCUS IN

RECOGNIZING IMPETIGO

When the vesicles break, crust forms from the exudate. This infection is especially contagious among young children.

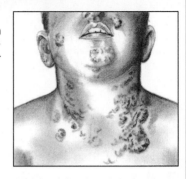

- Lesions begin as thin-walled bullae and vesicles.
- Lesions contain clear to turbid yellow fluid; some crusting exists. (See *Recognizing impetigo*.)

CAUSES

- Bacterial infection (commonly *Staphylococcus aureus* or Group A streptococci)
- Spread by autoinoculation through scratching

ASSESSMENT FINDINGS

Nonbullous impetigo
- Small, red macule or vesicle becoming pustular within a few hours
- Characteristic thick, honey colored crust forming from the exudate
- Satellite lesions caused by autoinoculation

Bullous impetigo
- Thin-walled vesicle
- Thin, clear crust forming from exudate

■ Lesion appearing as a central clearing circumscribed by an outer rim

TEST RESULTS

■ Gram stain of vesicular fluid shows infecting organism.
■ Culture and sensitivity testing of exudate or denuded crust shows infecting organism.

TREATMENT

■ Antibiotics (oral and topical)
■ Removal of exudate and crusts by washing lesions two to three times per day with antibacterial soap and water and a clean washcloth
■ Warm soaks or compresses of normal saline solution or a diluted soap solution for stubborn crusts
■ Prevention by benzoyl peroxide soap
■ Antihistamines

KEY PATIENT OUTCOMES

The patient will:
■ exhibit improved or healed wounds or lesions
■ report feelings of increased comfort
■ demonstrate proper skin care regimen
■ verbalize feelings about changed body image.

NURSING INTERVENTIONS

■ Use meticulous hand-washing technique.
■ Follow standard precautions.
■ Remove crusts by gently washing with bactericidal soap and water.
■ Soften stubborn crusts with cool compresses.
■ Give prescribed drugs.
■ Encourage verbalization of feelings about body image.
■ Comply with local public health standards and guidelines.

- Monitor the patient's response to treatment and for possible adverse drug reactions, or complications.

PATIENT TEACHING

Be sure to cover:
- the disorder and its diagnosis and treatment
- meticulous hand-washing technique
- trimming fingernails short
- regular bathing with bactericidal soap
- avoiding sharing clothes and linens
- identification of characteristic lesions
- completion of prescribed medications
- potential adverse reactions
- lesion care.

Juvenile rheumatoid arthritis

DESCRIPTION

- Refers to several conditions characterized by chronic synovitis and joint swelling, pain, and tenderness
- Pauciarticular JRA: asymmetrical involvement of less than five joints; usually affects large joints, such as the knees, ankles, and elbows, and causes eye complications, such as iridocyclitis
- Polyarticular JRA: symmetrical involvement of five or more joints, especially the hands and weight-bearing joints, such as the hips, knees, and feet; involves the temporomandibular joint, possibly causing earache; also involves the sternoclavicular joint, possibly causing chest pain
- Systemic disease with polyarthritis: involves the lining of the heart and lungs, blood cells, and abdominal organs; exacerbations possibly lasting for months; fever, rash, and lymphadenopathy possibly occurring
- Also called *JRA*

PATHOPHYSIOLOGY

- If JRA isn't arrested, the inflammatory process occurs in four stages:
  - Synovitis develops from congestion and edema of the synovial membrane and joint capsule.
  - Pannus covers and invades cartilage, eventually destroying the joint capsule and bone.
  - Fibrous tissue and ankylosis occludes the joint space.
  - Fibrous tissue calcifies, resulting in bony ankylosis and total immobility.

CAUSES

- Unknown
- Suggested link to genetic factors or an abnormal immune response
- Viral or bacterial (streptococcal) infection, trauma, and emotional stress

ASSESSMENT FINDINGS

- Inflammation around the joints
- Stiffness, pain, and guarding of the affected joints

TEST RESULTS

- Serum hemoglobin levels are decreased and neutrophil (neutrophilia) and platelet (thrombocytosis) levels are increased; other findings include increased erythrocyte sedimentation rate and elevated levels of C-reactive protein, serum haptoglobin, immunoglobulin, and C3 complement.
- Antinuclear antibody test is positive in patients with polyarticular JRA and in those with pauciarticular JRA with chronic iridocyclitis.
- Rheumatoid factor (RF) appears in about 15% of patients with JRA; patients with polyarticular JRA may test positive for RF.
- HLA-B27 forecasts later development of ankylosing spondylitis.

- X-ray demonstrates early structural changes associated with JRA, including soft-tissue swelling, effusion, and periostitis in affected joints.

TREATMENT

- Heat therapy including warm compresses, baths
- Splint application
- Low-dose corticosteroids
- Low-dose methotrexate (used as a second-line medication)
- Nonsteroidal anti-inflammatory drugs (NSAIDs): naproxen (Aleve, Naprosyn), ibuprofen (Advil, Motrin)
- Physical therapy

KEY PATIENT OUTCOMES

The patient will:
- express feelings of increased comfort and decreased pain
- maintain skin integrity
- attain the highest degree of mobility within the constrains of the disease
- verbalize feelings about limitations.

NURSING INTERVENTIONS

- Focus your care on reducing pain and promoting mobility.
- During inflammatory exacerbations, administer NSAIDs or prescribed medications on a regular schedule.
- Allow the patient to rest frequently throughout the day.
- Encourage feelings of accomplishment by arranging the patient's environment for participation in activities of daily living.

PATIENT TEACHING

Be sure to cover:
- instructions for receiving regular slit-lamp examinations to enable early diagnosis and treatment of iridocyclitis.

Lead poisoning

DESCRIPTION

- Lead: heavy metal that's poorly absorbed in the body and slowly excreted; replaces calcium in the bones and increases the permeability of central nervous system membranes
- In children, obtained by teething on or eating lead-based paint or inhaling lead dust
- Most common in toddlers
- Confirmed when the child has two successive blood lead levels greater than 10 mcg/dl

PATHOPHYSIOLOGY

- Lead has an affinity for bone and acts by replacing calcium.
- When high concentrations of lead are deposited in growing bone, the greatest concentration occurs in the metaphysis and (in children) affects the distal femur, both ends of the tibia, and distal radius.

CAUSES

- Ingestion of lead through oral route or by inhalation
  - Sources: lead-based paint, soil, drinking water, and certain folk remedies such as alarcon, alkohl, azarcon, bali goli, coral, ghasard, greta, liga, paylooah, and rueda, and traditional cosmetics such as kohl

ASSESSMENT FINDINGS

- Bone pain
- Increased intracranial pressure
- Cortical atrophy
- Behavioral changes
- Altered cognition and motor skills (lethargy and clumsiness) and seizures
- Lead lines seen along gums and recorded on X-rays

- GI distress, abdominal pain, constipation, vomiting, and weight loss
- Peripheral neuritis from calcium release into the blood

TEST RESULTS

- The Centers for Disease Control and Prevention has defined an elevated blood lead level as greater than 10 mcg/dl for children younger than age 6 years. A blood lead level greater than 20 mcg/dl in a child requires medical and environmental intervention. Children who have blood concentrations just under the emergency cutoff of 70 mcg/dl or higher should be treated and tested again within 24 hours.
- X-ray reveals lead lines near the epiphyseal lines (areas of increased density) of long bones.
- Blood tests show anemia from inhibition of hemoglobin formation.
- Erythrocyte protoporphin tests show elevated blood lead levels.
- Urinalysis reveals increased levels of coproporphyrin.

TREATMENT

- Removal of child from the source of lead poisoning
- Chelation therapy using EDTA
- Oral administration of succimer (Chemet)

KEY PATIENT OUTCOMES

The patient will:
- maintain adequate fluid volume
- maintain adequate hydration
- maintain hemodynamic status.

NURSING INTERVENTIONS

- Monitor fluid and electrolyte levels carefully because fluid shifts may occur during chelation therapy.

- Institute seizure precautions especially if the child's blood lead levels are high.
- Provide adequate fluids and hydration.
- Monitor intake and output.
- Monitor blood lead levels and liver function studies.

PATIENT TEACHING

Be sure to cover (with the parents):
- the disorder
- that succimer capsules may be opened and sprinkled on the child's food
- that the succimer bottle, upon opening, has an unpleasant odor, which is normal
- encouragement of the child to drink plenty of water while taking succimer
- identification of areas of lead poisoning sites within their home and environment and how to prevent it.

Legg-Calvé-Perthes disease

DESCRIPTION

- Ischemic necrosis that leads to eventual flattening of the head of the femur due to vascular interruption
- Typically unilateral, occurring bilaterally in 20% of patients
- Usually runs its course in 3 to 4 years
- Occurs most commonly in boys ages 4 to 10
- Tends to occur in families
- May lead to premature osteoarthritis later in life from misalignment of the acetabulum and flattening of the femoral head
- Also called *coxa plana*

PATHOPHYSIOLOGY

- Occurs in four stages:
  - The first stage, synovitis, is characterized by synovial inflammation and increased joint fluid. It typically lasts 1 to 3 weeks.
  - In the second (avascular) stage, vascular interruption causes necrosis of the ossification center of the femoral head (usually in several months to 1 year).
  - In the third stage, revascularization, new blood supply causes bone resorption and deposition of immature bone cells; new bone replaces necrotic bone and the femoral head gradually reforms.
  - The final, or residual stage, involves healing and regeneration; immature bone cells are replaced with normal bone cells, thereby fixing the joint's shape (there may be residual deformity, based on the degree of necrosis that occurred in the second stage).

CAUSES

- Exact cause unknown
- Current theories:
  - Increased blood viscosity resulting in stasis and decreased blood flow
  - Trauma to retinacular vessels
  - Vascular irregularities (congenital or developmental)
  - Vascular occlusion secondary to increased intracapsular pressure from acute transient synovitis
  - Venous obstruction with secondary intraepiphyseal thrombosis

ASSESSMENT FINDINGS

- Muscle atrophy of proximal thigh
- Slight shortening of the affected leg
- Restricted hip abduction and internal rotation
- Adductor muscle spasm in the affected hip

TEST RESULTS

- Hip X-rays taken every 3 to 4 months confirm the diagnosis, with findings varying according to the stage of the disease.
- Anterior-posterior X-rays and magnetic resonance imaging enhances early diagnosis of necrosis and visualization of articular surface.
- Physical examination and clinical history reveals the disorder.

TREATMENT

- Protection of the femoral head from further stress and damage by containing it within the acetabulum
- Reduced weight bearing by means of bed rest in bilateral split counterpoised traction, then application of hip abduction splint or cast, or weight bearing while a splint, cast, or brace holds the leg in abduction (braces may remain in place for 6 to 18 months)
- Physical therapy with passive and active range-of-motion exercises after cast removal
- Well-balanced diet
- Analgesics
- Pelvic or femoral osteotomy
- Postoperatively, patient requiring a spica cast for about 2 months

KEY PATIENT OUTCOMES

The patient will:
- express feelings of increased comfort and decreased pain
- perform activities of daily living within the confines of the disease
- express understanding of the disorder and treatment regimen.

NURSING INTERVENTIONS

- Provide cast care.

- Give prescribed analgesics.
- Provide emotional support.
- Monitor the patient's intake and output, neurovascular status of affected extremity, and skin integrity.

PATIENT TEACHING

Be sure to cover:
- the disorder and its diagnosis and treatment
- proper cast care and monitoring of skin integrity.

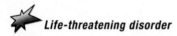 *Life-threatening disorder*

Leukemia

DESCRIPTION

- Abnormal, uncontrolled proliferation of white blood cells (WBCs)
- Acute lymphocytic leukemia (ALL) most common type of leukemia and cancer in children
  - Peak age 2 to 5
  - 90% to 95% of children achieving a first remission
  - Almost 80% living 5 years
  - Child between ages 3 and 7 and an initial WBC count of less than 10,000/µl at the time of diagnosis having the best prognosis
- Acute myeloblastic (myelogenous) leukemia (AML) more common than ALL in adolescents
  - 50% to 70% of adolescents achieving a first remission
  - 40% living 5 years

PATHOPHYSIOLOGY

- WBCs produce so rapidly that immature cells (blast cells) release into the circulation.
- Blast cells are nonfunctional, can't fight infection, and multiply continuously without respect to the body's

needs; they appear in the peripheral blood (where they normally don't appear).

- Blast cells are as high as 95% in the bone marrow (normally less than 5%), as measured by marrow aspiration in the posterior iliac crest (the sternum can't be used in children).
- Increased proliferation of WBCs robs healthy cells of nutrition.
- Bone marrow first undergoes hypertrophy, possibly resulting in pathologic fractures.
- Bone marrow then undergoes atrophy, which results in a decrease in all blood cells, leading to anemia, bleeding disorders, and immunosuppression.

CAUSES

- Exact cause unknown
- Increasing evidence suggesting a combination of contributing factors
- Predisposing factors:
  - Congenital disorders, such as Down syndrome, Bloom syndrome, and ataxia-telangiectasia
  - Exposure to the chemical benzene and cytotoxins such as alkylating agents
  - Familial tendency
  - Ionizing radiation
  - Monozygotic twin with leukemia
  - Viruses

ASSESSMENT FINDINGS

- High fever
- Thrombocytopenia
- Abdominal, bone, or joint pain
- Pallor, chills, and recurrent infections
- Petechiae and ecchymosis
- Abnormal bleeding, such as nosebleeds, poor wound healing, and oral lesions

■ Confusion, lethargy, and headache if the blood-brain barrier has been crossed

TEST RESULTS

■ Bone marrow aspirate shows a proliferation of immature WBCs.
■ Bone marrow biopsy of the posterior superior iliac spine helps to confirm diagnosis.
■ Blood counts show thrombocytopenia, neutropenia, and anemia.
■ Differential leukocyte count determines cell type.
■ Lumbar puncture detects meningeal involvement.

TREATMENT

■ Systemic chemotherapy aiming to eradicate leukemic cells and inducing remission
   – ALL — combination therapy including vincristine, prednisone, high-dose cytarabine (Cytosar-U), L-asparaginase (Elspar), and daunorubicin (Cerubidine)
   – AML — combination of I.V. daunorubicin and cytarabine; combination of cyclophosphamide (Neosar), vincristine, prednisone, or methotrexate; high-dose cytarabine alone or with other drugs; etoposide (Toposar); and azacitidine (Vidaza) and mitoxantrone (Novantrone)
■ Intrathecal chemotherapy to prevent central nervous system (CNS) infiltration by leukemic cells
■ Antibiotic, antifungal, and antiviral drugs and granulocyte injections to control infection
■ Transfusions of platelets to prevent bleeding and of red blood cells to prevent anemia
■ Possible bone marrow transplant

KEY PATIENT OUTCOMES

The patient will:
■ have no further weight loss
■ exhibit intact mucous membranes

- experience no chills, fever, or other signs and symptoms of illness
- express feelings of increased comfort
- utilize available support systems.

NURSING INTERVENTIONS

- Prevent infection by placing the patient in a private room, giving special attention to mouth care, and screening staff and visitors for contagious diseases.
- Inspect the skin frequently; avoid taking a rectal temperature or administering rectal medications.
- Use interventions for anemia and thrombocytopenia.
- Give increased fluids to flush chemotherapy through the kidneys.
- Provide a high-protein, high-calorie, and bland diet.
- Provide pain relief.
- Monitor CNS for involvement (confusion, lethargy, and headache).
- Gear nursing measures toward easing the adverse effects of radiation and chemotherapy.
- Help the child and the family verbalize their fears and guilt; allow the family to participate in the patient's care, as appropriate.
- Help the child adjust to changes in body image.

PATIENT TEACHING

Be sure to cover:
- the disorder and its diagnosis and treatment
- medication, including administration, dosage, and possible adverse effects
- use of a soft toothbrush and avoidance of hot, spicy foods and commercial mouthwashes
- signs and symptoms of infection and abnormal bleeding
- planned rest periods during the day
- need for long-term follow-up.

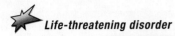 *Life-threatening disorder*

Meningitis

DESCRIPTION

- Inflammation of brain and spinal cord meninges
- Usually follows onset of respiratory symptoms
- Sudden onset, causing serious illness within 24 hours
- Good prognosis with viral meningitis; complications rare
- If bacterial, causes acute infection in the subarachnoid space
- Good prognosis if rare complications recognized early and infecting organism responsive to antibiotic therapy
- In 10% to 15% of cases, bacterial meningitis fatal; sequelae common when occurring in the first 2 months of life
- Condition common in infants and toddlers; incidence now greatly decreased with the routine administration of *Haemophilus influenzae* type B (Hib) vaccine

PATHOPHYSIOLOGY

- Viral or bacterial agents are transmitted by the spreading of droplets; organisms enter the blood from the nasopharynx or middle ear.
- Inflammation may involve all three meningeal membranes — the dura mater, the arachnoid, and the pia mater.

CAUSES

- Aseptic meningitis — viral (see *Aseptic meningitis*, page 140)
- Vascular dissemination from focus of infection elsewhere in the body; infections possibly including or resulting from:
  - Bacteremia
  - Brain abscesses

ASEPTIC MENINGITIS

Aseptic meningitis is a benign syndrome characterized by headache, fever, vomiting, and meningeal symptoms. It results from some form of viral infection, including enteroviruses (most common), arboviruses, herpes simplex virus, mumps virus, or lymphocytic choriomeningitis virus.

Signs and symptoms

Aseptic meningitis begins suddenly with a fever up to 104° F (40° C), alterations in consciousness (drowsiness, confusion, stupor), and neck or spine stiffness, which is slight at first. (The patient experiences such stiffness when bending forward.) Other signs and symptoms include headaches, nausea, vomiting, abdominal pain, poorly defined chest pain, and sore throat.

Diagnostic tests

Patient history of recent illness and knowledge of seasonal epidemics are essential in differentiating among the many forms of aseptic meningitis. Negative bacteriologic cultures and cerebrospinal (CSF) analysis showing pleocytosis and increased protein levels suggest the diagnosis. Isolation of the virus from CSF confirms it.

Treatment

Treatment is supportive, including bed rest, maintenance of fluid and electrolyte balance, analgesics for pain, and exercises to combat residual weakness. Isolation isn't necessary. Careful handling of excretions and good hand-washing technique prevent spreading the disease.

- Empyema
- Encephalitis
- Endocarditis
- *H. influenzae* (in children and young adults)
- Lumbar puncture
- Myelitis
- *Neisseria meningitides*
- Osteomyelitis
- Otitis media
- Penetrating head wound
- Pneumonia
- Sinusitis
- Skull fracture

- *Streptococcus pneumoniae*
- Ventricular shunting procedures

ASSESSMENT FINDINGS

- Coma
- Delirium
- Fever
- Headache
- High-pitched cry
- Irritability
- Nuchal rigidity possibly progressing to opisthotonos (arching of the back)
- Gradual or abrupt onset after an upper respiratory infection
- Petechial or purpuric lesions possibly presenting in bacterial meningitis
- Positive Brudzinski's sign (the child flexes the knees and hips in response to passive neck flexion)
- Positive Kernig's sign (the child is unable to extend the leg when the hip and knee are flexed)
- Projectile vomiting causing dehydration; dehydration possibly preventing a bulging fontanel and thus masking an important sign of increased intracranial pressure (ICP)
- Seizures
- Bulging fontanels, separated sutures
- Chills
- Malaise
- Sinus arrhythmias
- Diplopia

ALERT *Meningismus and fever are commonly absent in neonates and the only clinical clues may be nonspecific, such as refusal to feed, high-pitched cry, and irritability.*

TEST RESULTS

- Lumbar puncture shows increased cerebrospinal fluid pressure, cloudy color, increased white blood cell count and protein level, and decreased glucose level (if meningitis is caused by bacteria).

TREATMENT

- Analgesics to treat pain of meningeal irritation
- Corticosteroids — dexamethasone (Decadron)
- Parenteral antibiotics — ceftazidime (Fortaz), ceftriaxone (Rocephin); possibly intraventricular administration of antibiotics
- Burr holes to evacuate subdural effusion, if present
- Oxygen therapy (possible intubation and mechanical ventilation to induce hyperventilation to decrease ICP)

KEY PATIENT OUTCOMES

The patient will:
- maintain adequate ventilation
- have normal temperature
- express feelings of increased comfort and pain relief
- maintain normal fluid volume
- have intact skin.

NURSING INTERVENTIONS

- Follow standard precautions.
- Maintain respiratory isolation for first 24 hours (with meningococcal meningitis).
- Give prescribed oxygen.
- Position the patient in proper body alignment.
- Encourage active range-of-motion (ROM) exercises when appropriate.
- Provide passive ROM exercises when appropriate.
- Maintain adequate nutrition.
- Give prescribed laxatives or stool softeners.
- Provide meticulous skin and mouth care.
- Give prescribed drugs.
- Monitor the patient's neurologic status, vital signs, level of consciousness, respiratory status, arterial blood gas results, fluid balance, and response to medications.

■ Monitor for signs and symptoms of cranial nerve involvement, presence of seizures, and increased ICP.

PATIENT TEACHING

Be sure to cover:
■ the disorder and its diagnosis and treatment
■ contagion risks for close contacts
■ medication regimen
■ adverse drug effects
■ signs and symptoms of meningitis
■ polysaccharide meningococcal vaccine, pneumococcal vaccine, and Hib vaccine.

Mumps

DESCRIPTION

■ Acute inflammation of one or both parotid glands or the sublingual or submaxillary glands
■ Also called *infectious* or *parotitis*

PATHOPHYSIOLOGY

■ Paramyxovirus is found in the saliva of an infected person.
■ It's transmitted by droplets or by direct contact with the saliva of an infected person.

CAUSES

■ Necrosis of acinar and epithelial duct cells in the salivary glands and germinal epithelium of the seminiferous tubules
■ Perivascular and interstitial mononuclear cell infiltrating with edema, due to infection of the central nervous system (CNS) or glandular tissues (or both)
■ Virus replication in the epithelium of the upper respiratory tract, leading to viremia

FOCUS IN
PAROTID INFLAMMATION IN MUMPS

The mumps virus
(paramyxovirus) attacks
the parotid glands—
the main salivary
glands. Inflammation
causes characteristic
swelling and discomfort
associated with eating,
swallowing, and talk-
ing.

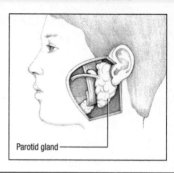

Parotid gland

ASSESSMENT FINDINGS

- Swelling and tenderness of the parotid glands
- Simultaneous or subsequent swelling of one or more other salivary glands (see *Parotid inflammation in mumps*)

TEST RESULTS

- Glandular swelling confirms the diagnosis.
- Serologic testing shows mumps antibodies.

TREATMENT

- Rest
- Cold compresses for swollen glands
- Use of athletic supporter if testicles are tender
- Liquid to mechanical soft diet until able to swallow
- Increased fluid intake
- Bed rest until fever resolves
- Rest periods when fatigued
- Analgesics
- Antipyretics

KEY PATIENT OUTCOMES

The patient will:
- remain afebrile
- express feelings of increased comfort and decreased pain
- maintain adequate fluid volume
- achieve adequate nutritional intake.

NURSING INTERVENTIONS

- Apply warm or cool compresses to the neck area to relieve pain.
- Give prescribed drugs.
- Provide scrotal support, if needed.
- Report all cases of mumps to local public health authorities.
- Disinfect articles soiled with nose and throat secretions.
- Monitor the patient's response to treatment, auditory acuity, and for signs of CNS involvement or complications.

PATIENT TEACHING

Be sure to cover:
- the disorder and its diagnosis and treatment
- need to stay away from day care or school during the infectious period (typically not returning until 9 days after parotid swelling began)
- importance of immunization with live attenuated mumps vaccine at age 15 months or older, if applicable
- if epididymoorchitis occurs, reassurance that it won't cause impotence and sterility (occurs only with bilateral orchitis)
- need for bed rest during febrile period
- need to avoid spicy, irritating foods, and those that require much chewing; advise a soft, bland diet
- need for family members to follow respiratory isolation precautions until symptoms subside.

Muscular dystrophy

DESCRIPTION

- Hereditary disorder characterized by progressive symmetrical wasting of skeletal muscles
- No neural or sensory defects
- Four main types: Duchenne's (pseudohypertrophic), Becker's (benign pseudohypertrophic), Landouzy-Dejerine (facioscapulohumeral), and Erb's (limb-girdle) dystrophies
- Duchenne's beginning in early childhood; death within 10 to 15 years

PATHOPHYSIOLOGY

- Muscle fibers necrotize and regenerate in various states.
- As regeneration slows down, degeneration dominates.
- Fat and connective tissue replace muscle fibers, with ensuing weakness.

CAUSES

- Duchenne's and Becker's X-linked recessive
- Erb's usually autosomal recessive
- Landouzy-Dejerine autosomal dominant
- Various genetic mechanisms (band Xp 21)

ASSESSMENT FINDINGS

Duchenne's and Becker's

- Wide stance and waddling gait
- Gowers' sign when rising from a sitting or supine position
- Muscle hypertrophy and atrophy
- Calves enlarging because of fat infiltration into the muscle
- Posture changes
- Lordosis and a protuberant abdomen
- Scapular "winging" or flaring when raising arms

- Contractures
- Tachypnea and shortness of breath

Landouzy-Dejerine
- Pendulous lower lip
- Possible disappearance of nasolabial fold
- Diffuse facial flattening leading to a masklike expression
- Inability to suckle (infants)
- Scapulae with a winglike appearance; inability to raise arms above head

Erb's
- Effects of muscle weakness apparent
- Muscle wasting
- Winging of the scapulae
- Lordosis with abdominal protrusion
- Waddling gait
- Poor balance
- Inability to raise the arms

TEST RESULTS

- Urine creatinine, serum creatine kinase, lactate dehydrogenase, alanine aminotransferase, and aspartate aminotransferase levels are elevated.
- Muscle biopsy confirms diagnosis.
- Immunologic and biologic results facilitate prenatal and postnatal diagnosis.
- Electromyography shows abnormal muscle movements.
- Amniocentesis detects gender of fetus for high-risk family.
- Genetic testing may be used to detect the gene defect that leads to muscular dystrophy in some families.

TREATMENT

- No known treatment to stop progression
- Orthopedic appliances
- Low-calorie, high-protein, high-fiber diet
- Tube feedings, as needed

- Exercise, as tolerated
- Physical therapy
- Stool softeners
- Possible steroids
- Surgery to correct contractures
- Spinal fusion

KEY PATIENT OUTCOMES

The patient will:
- perform activities of daily living without muscle fatigue or intolerance
- maintain muscle strength, joint mobility, and range of motion
- show no evidence of complications
- maintain respiratory rate within 5 breaths/minute of baseline.

NURSING INTERVENTIONS

- Encourage coughing and deep-breathing exercises.
- Take steps to prevent muscle atrophy.
- Use splints, braces, grab bars, and overhead slings.
- Use a footboard or high topped shoes and a foot cradle.
- Provide a low-calorie, high-protein, and high-fiber diet.
- Monitor the patient's intake and output, respiratory status, joint mobility, and muscle weakness.

PATIENT TEACHING

Be sure to cover (with the parents):
- the disorder and its diagnosis and treatment
- maintenance of peer relationships
- how to maintain mobility and independence
- possible complications and prevention
- signs and symptoms of respiratory tract infections
- need for a low-calorie, high-protein, and high-fiber diet
- need to avoid long periods of bed rest and inactivity
- referral for physical therapy, vocational rehabilitation, social services, and financial assistance

■ referral to the Muscular Dystrophy Association
■ referral for genetic counseling.

Nephrotic syndrome

DESCRIPTION

■ Kidney disorder characterized by marked proteinuria, hypoalbuminemia, hyperlipidemia, increased coagulation, and edema
■ Results from a glomerular defect that affects permeability, indicating renal damage
■ Prognosis highly variable, depending on underlying cause
■ Some forms possibly progressing to end-stage renal failure
■ In children, 1 in 50,000 new cases per year
■ In children, peak incidence between ages 2 and 3
■ Slightly more common in males than in females

PATHOPHYSIOLOGY

■ Glomerular protein permeability increases.
■ Urinary excretion of protein, especially albumin, increases.
■ Hypoalbuminemia develops and causes decreased colloidal oncotic pressure.
■ Leakage of fluid into interstitial spaces leads to acute, generalized edema.
■ Vascular volume loss leads to increased blood viscosity and coagulation disorders.
■ Renin-angiotensin system is triggered, causing tubular reabsorption of sodium and water and contributing to edema.

CAUSES

■ Certain neoplastic diseases such as multiple myeloma
■ Circulatory diseases

- Collagen-vascular disorders
- Focal glomerulosclerosis (developing spontaneously at any age, occurring after kidney transplantation, or resulting from heroin injection; developing in about 10% of childhood cases and up to 20% of adult cases)
- Lipid nephrosis (main cause in children younger than age 8)
- Membranoproliferative glomerulonephritis (possibly following infection, particularly streptococcal infection; occurring primarily in children and young adults)
- Membranous glomerulonephritis (most common lesion in adult idiopathic nephrotic syndrome)
- Metabolic diseases
- Primary (idiopathic) glomerulonephritis (about 75% of cases)

ASSESSMENT FINDINGS

- Periorbital edema
- Mild to severe dependent edema
- Orthostatic hypotension
- Ascites
- Swollen external genitalia
- Signs of pleural effusion
- Pallor
- Frothy or foamy urine

TEST RESULTS

- Urinalysis reveals an increased number of hyaline, granular, waxy, fatty casts, and oval fat bodies; consistent, heavy proteinuria (levels over 3.5 mg/dl for 24 hours) strongly suggests nephrotic syndrome.
- Serum cholesterol, serum phospholipids, and serum triglycerides are increased; serum albumin levels are decreased.
- Renal biopsy allows for histologic identification of the lesion.

TREATMENT

- Correction of the underlying cause if possible
- Diet consisting of 0.6 g of protein per kilogram of body weight
- Restricted sodium intake
- Frequent rest periods
- Diuretics
- Antibiotics (for infection)
- Glucocorticoids
- Possible alkylating agents
- Possible cytotoxic agents

KEY PATIENT OUTCOMES

The patient will:
- avoid or have minimal complications
- maintain fluid balance
- identify risk factors that worsen tissue perfusion, and modify lifestyle appropriately
- maintain hemodynamic stability.

NURSING INTERVENTIONS

- Offer the patient reassurance and support, especially during the acute phase, when severe edema changes body image.
- Monitor the patient's urine for protein, intake and output, daily weight, plasma albumin and transferrin levels, and for signs of edema.

PATIENT TEACHING

Be sure to cover:
- the disorder and its diagnosis and treatments
- signs of infection that should be reported
- adherence to diet
- medication administration, dosage, and possible adverse effects.

Neural tube defects

DESCRIPTION

- Birth defects that involve the spine or skull
- Result from neural tube's failure to close approximately 28 days after conception
- Spina bifida (50% of cases), anencephaly (40%), and encephalocele (10%)
- Also called *NTD*

PATHOPHYSIOLOGY

- Spina bifida occulta (least severe NTD) is characterized by incomplete closure of one or more vertebrae without protrusion of the spinal cord or meninges; more severe forms have incomplete closure of one or more vertebrae, causing protrusion of the spinal contents in an external sac or cystic lesion (spina bifida cystica). (See *Types of spinal cord defects.*)
- Anencephaly is a closure defect that occurs at the cranial end of the neuroaxis and results in missing a part or the entire top of the skull, severely damaging the brain; portions of the brain stem and spinal cord may also be missing (fatal).
- Encephalocele is a saclike portion of the meninges and brain that protrudes through a defective opening in the skull; it usually occurs in the occipital area, but may also occur in the parietal, nasopharyngeal, or frontal area.

CAUSES

- Combination of genetic and environmental factors; possibly a lack of folic acid in the mother's diet
- Exposure to a teratogen
- Part of a multiple malformation syndrome such as trisomy 18 or 13 syndrome

FOCUS IN
TYPES OF SPINAL CORD DEFECTS

There are three major types of spinal cord defects. Spina bifida occulta is characterized by a depression or raised area and a tuft of hair over the defect. In myelomeningocele, an external sac contains meninges, cerebrospinal fluid, and a portion of the spinal cord or nerve roots. In meningocele, an external sac contains only meninges and cerebrospinal fluid.

SPINA BIFIDA OCCULTA

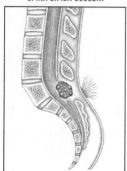

MYELOMENINGOCELE

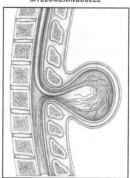

MENINGOCELE

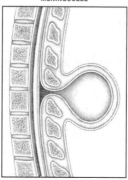

ASSESSMENT FINDINGS

Spina bifida

- Possibly a depression or dimple, tuft of hair, soft fatty deposit, port wine nevi, or a combination of these abnormalities on the skin over the spinal area
- Saclike protrusion over the spinal cord
- Flaccid or spastic paralysis

Anencephaly

- Part or entire top of skull missing

Encephalocele

- Saclike protrusion through a defective opening in the skull
- Paralysis

TEST RESULTS

- Elevated maternal alpha-fetoprotein (AFP), amniotic fluid AFP, and amniotic fluid acetylcholinesterase levels require further testing.
- Fetal karyotype detects chromosomal abnormalities (present in 5% to 7% of NTDs).
- Maternal serum AFP screening in combination with other serum markers, such as human chorionic gonadotropin (hCG), free beta-hCG, or unconjugated estriol (for patients with a lower risk of NTDs and those who will be younger than age 34½ at the time of delivery) estimates a fetus's risk of NTD as well as possible increased risk for perinatal complications, such as premature rupture of membranes, abruptio placentae, or fetal death.
- Ultrasound is indicated when increased risk of open NTD exists, based on family history or abnormal serum screening results; it isn't conclusive for open NTDs or ventral wall defects.
- Spinal X-rays reveal spina bifida occulta.
- Myelography differentiates spina bifida occulta from other spinal abnormalities, especially spinal cord tumors.

- Skull X-rays, cephalic measurements, and computed tomography (CT) scan demonstrate associated hydrocephalus.
- X-rays show a basilar bony skull defect (CT scan and ultrasonography further define the defect [with encephalocele]).
- Transillumination of the protruding sac distinguishes between myelomeningocele (typically doesn't transilluminate) and meningocele (typically transilluminates).

TREATMENT

- Symptomatic according to neurologic effects of defect
- Assessment of growth and development throughout lifetime
- Diet, as tolerated
- Physical therapy
- Antibiotics, as indicated
- Surgical closure of the protruding sac
- Shunt to relieve associated hydrocephalus
- Surgery during infancy to place protruding tissues back in the skull, excise the sac, and correct associated craniofacial abnormalities (encephalocele)

▶ **COLLABORATION** *A patient with an NTD may require the collaboration of a surgeon to perform a surgical repair. Depending on the extent of the defect, the patient may have multiple handicaps requiring collaboration with occupational and physical therapists, dietitians for nutritional support, and community and social services for family support.*

KEY PATIENT OUTCOMES

The patient will:
- maintain intact skin integrity
- maintain joint mobility and range of motion
- attain appropriate growth and development for age.

NURSING INTERVENTIONS

- Provide psychological support.

Before surgery
- Clean the defect gently with sterile normal saline solution or other solutions, as ordered.
- Handle the infant carefully, and don't apply pressure to the defect.
- Provide adequate time for parent-child bonding, if possible.

After surgery
- Change the dressing regularly, as ordered, and check and report signs of drainage, wound rupture, and infection.
- Place the infant in a prone position.
- If leg casts have been applied, watch for signs that the child is outgrowing the cast. Ensure adequate circulation by regularly checking distal pulses.
- Before surgery, monitor the patient's neurologic status, feeding ability, and nutritional status.
- After surgery, monitor the patient's intake and output, vital signs, and for signs of infection or increased intracranial pressure.

PATIENT TEACHING

Be sure to cover:
- the disorder and its diagnosis and treatment
- how to prevent contractures, pressure ulcers, and urinary tract infections.

 Life-threatening disorder

Neuroblastoma

DESCRIPTION

- Most common extracranial solid tumor diagnosed in infancy

- Usually arises from the adrenal gland but may also arise at multiple sites, usually within the abdomen
- Usually metastasizes before it's diagnosed
- Highly malignant
- Poor prognosis (less than 50% chance of survival) for the child older than age 1; prognosis approaches 75% chance of survival for children diagnosed younger than age 1
- If tumor occurs in the abdomen, resembles Wilms' tumor

PATHOPHYSIOLOGY

- Tumors originate from embryonic cells in the neural crest, giving rise to the adrenal medulla and the sympathetic nervous system.
- Tumors occur most commonly in the abdomen near the adrenal gland or spinal ganglia.
- The most common sites of metastasis are the bone marrow, liver, and subcutaneous tissue.
- Stages
  - In stage I, the tumor is confined to the organ or structure of origin and is completely removable by surgery.
  - In stage II, continuity extends beyond the primary site but not across the midline; the tumor isn't completely removable by surgery.
  - In stage III, the tumor extends beyond the midline, with bilateral regional lymph node involvement.
  - In stage IV, the tumor metastasizes.

CAUSES

- Unknown

ASSESSMENT FINDINGS

- Be aware that symptoms varying and typically resulting from compression of the tumor on adjacent structures
- Firm abdominal mass crossing the midline
- Urinary frequency or retention
- Bone pain
- Weakness and lethargy

- Anorexia and weight loss

TEST RESULTS

- Ultrasound and computed tomography scan confirm diagnosis.
- 24-hour urine collection measures catecholamines, preceded by a vanillylmandelic acid diet for 3 days (eliminate bananas, nuts, chocolate, vanilla).

TREATMENT

- Complete surgical removal for stage I
- Complete or partial surgical removal for stage II
- Radiation for stage III possibly not improving survival rate but possibly alleviating pain from metastasis
- Chemotherapy for treatment of extensive disease, including vincristine, doxorubicin (Rubex), cyclophosphamide (Neosar), and cisplatin (Platinol)

KEY PATIENT OUTCOMES

The patient (or his family) will:
- communicate understanding of the condition and treatment regimen
- remain free from signs and symptoms of infection
- remain free from postsurgical complications (stage I or II)
- maintain adequate nutrition
- express or indicate feelings of increased comfort and decreased pain
- use support systems and to help cope effectively.

NURSING INTERVENTIONS

- Provide adequate time for parent-child bonding, if possible.
- Before surgery, monitor the patient's neurologic status, feeding ability, and nutritional status.

- After surgery, monitor the patient's intake and output, vital signs, and for signs of infection or increased intracranial pressure.

PATIENT TEACHING

Be sure to cover (with the parents):
- treatment options to the patient and family, including possible adverse effects from radiation and chemotherapy
- preparation for operative procedures
- emotional support for the family (due to the high degree of mortality associated with the disease).

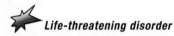 *Life-threatening disorder*

Non-Hodgkin's lymphoma

DESCRIPTION

- Includes lymphosarcoma, reticulum cell sarcoma, and Burkitt's lymphoma
- Prognosis for aggressively treated localized disease: nearly 90% survival; for advanced disease, survival greater than 60%
- Also known as *malignant lymphoma*

PATHOPHYSIOLOGY

- Although similar to Hodgkin's disease, Reed-Sternberg cells aren't present, and lymph node destruction is different.
- Lymphoid tissue is defined by the pattern of infiltration as diffuse or nodular; nodular lymphomas yield a better prognosis than the diffuse form, but prognosis (for both forms) is less hopeful than in Hodgkin's disease.

CAUSES

- Unknown, although some theories suggesting a viral source for some cases

ASSESSMENT FINDINGS

- Varied symptoms depending on the organ involved
- Enlarged lymph nodes, most commonly in the lower cervical region, including tonsils and adenoids
- Dyspnea and coughing
- Night sweats, fatigue, malaise, weight loss, and fever

TEST RESULTS

- Biopsy of lymph nodes confirms diagnosis.
- Bone and chest X-rays, lymphangiography, liver and spleen scan, abdominal computed tomography scan, and excretory urography detect organ involvement.
- Blood tests show anemia, increased uric acid, and an elevated calcium level (if bone lesions are present).

TREATMENT

- Radiation therapy mainly in the early localized stage of the disease
- Chemotherapy most effective with multiple combinations of drugs
  - CHOP — cyclophosphamide (Neosar), doxorubicin (Rubex, also known as *hydroxydaunorubicin*), vincristine (Oncovin), and prednisone
  - M-BACOP — methotrexate, bleomycin (Blenoxane), doxorubicin (Adriamycin), cyclophosphamide, vincristine, and prednisone

▶ **COLLABORATION** *The patient will require a consultation with a dietitian for nutritional support during chemotherapy as well as support from social services and community resources for the patient and his family.*

KEY PATIENT OUTCOMES

The patient will:
- have no further weight loss
- demonstrate effective coping mechanisms
- express feelings of increased comfort and decreased pain.

NURSING INTERVENTIONS

- Give prescribed drugs.
- Provide time for rest periods.
- Encourage verbalization and provide support.
- Assess for adverse effects of radiation and chemotherapy, including anorexia, nausea, vomiting, diarrhea, fever, and bleeding.

PATIENT TEACHING

Be sure to cover:
- the disorder and its diagnosis and treatment
- how to keep irradiated skin dry
- preoperative and postoperative procedures
- dietary plan
- mouth care using a soft bristled toothbrush and avoidance of commercial mouthwashes
- relaxation and comfort measures
- medication, including administration, dosage, and possible adverse effects
- symptoms that require immediate attention.

Osteogenesis imperfecta

DESCRIPTION

- Genetic disease in which bones are thin, poorly developed, and fracture easily
- Expression dependent on whether defect is carried as a trait or clinically obvious

- Autosomal dominant disorder occurring in about 1 in 30,000 live births
- Affects males and females equally
- Also called *little bone disease*

PATHOPHYSIOLOGY

- Pathogenesis begins when mutations in the genes change the structure of collagen.
- Possible mutations in other genes may cause variations in the assembly and maintenance of bone and other connective tissues.
- Collectively or alone, these mutated genes lead to pathologic fractures and impaired healing.

CAUSES

- Autosomal recessive carriage of gene defects producing osteogenesis imperfecta in homozygotes (osteoporosis in some)
- Genetic disease, typically autosomal dominant (characterized by a defect in the synthesis of connective tissue)

 ALERT *Age of onset of symptoms ranges from in utero to infancy.*

ASSESSMENT FINDINGS

- Blue sclerae, showing mutation expressed in more than one connective tissue
- Short trunk
- Hearing loss
- Fractures
- Kyphoscoliosis

TEST RESULTS

- Serum alkaline phosphatase levels are elevated (during periods of rapid bone formation and cellular injury).
- Skin culture shows reduced quantity of fibroblasts.

- Echocardiography may show mitral insufficiency or floppy mitral valves.
- Prenatal ultrasound (during second trimester) reveals bowing of long bones, fractures, limb shortening, and decreasing skull echogenicity.
- Skull, long bone, and pelvis X-rays reveal thin bones, fractures with deformities, beaded ribs, and osteopenia.

TREATMENT

- Prevention of fractures
- Nutritious, well-balanced diet
- Safety during periods of activity
- Physical therapy
- Antibiotics (when infection occurs)
- Stabilization and deformity prevention (through internal fixation of fractures)
- Spinal fusion (for scoliosis)

▶ **COLLABORATION** *A multidisciplinary team approach is needed with referrals to a dietitian for nutritional support, physical therapy, and social services to help the family utilize community resources.*

KEY PATIENT OUTCOMES

The patient (or his family) will:
- follow safety measures to prevent fractures
- understand the disorder and its treatment
- demonstrate effective coping mechanisms.

NURSING INTERVENTIONS

- Ensure a safe environment.
- Encourage activities based on ability.
- Provide psychological support.
- Monitor the patient's environment and bone condition.

PATIENT TEACHING

Be sure to cover:
- safe handling of an infant
- how to recognize fractures and correctly splint them
- how to protect the child during diapering, dressing, and other activities of daily living
- encouraging interests that don't require strenuous physical activity
- the importance of good nutrition to heal bones and promote growth
- use of shock-absorbing footwear
- importance of not letting infants younger than age 1 sit upright.

Osteogenic sarcoma

DESCRIPTION

- Most common bone cancer in children
- Peak age late adolescence; rare in young children
- Usually involves the diaphyseal long bones; about 50% of cases occur in femur but may also occur in tibia, humerus, fibula, ileum, vertebra, or mandible
- Highly malignant; metastasizes quickly to the lungs
- Survival rate about 60%; increases to 85% if nonmetastasized

PATHOPHYSIOLOGY

- Tumor arises from bone-forming osteoblast and bone-digesting osteoclast.

CAUSES

- Unknown
- Current theories: heredity, trauma, and excessive radiotherapy

ASSESSMENT FINDINGS

- Impaired mobility
- Pain and swelling at the site
- Pain more intense at night and not usually associated with mobility
- Absence of infection or trauma at the site preceding the pain
- Pathologic fractures, possibly resulting from bone marrow involvement

TEST RESULTS

- Biopsy (by incision or by aspiration) confirms the diagnosis.
- Body computed tomography scan determines extent of the lesion.
- Sunburst appearance is noted on X-ray due to new bone formations growing at right angles to one another.
- Alkaline phosphatase is elevated.
- Lung tomography reveals lung metastasis.

TREATMENT

- Amputation at the joint proximal to the tumor; some health care facilities removing only the bone and salvage the limb
- Chemotherapy agents either alone or in combination with one another
- Doxorubicin (Rubex), bleomycin (Blenoxane), cyclophosphamide (Neosar), and high-dose methotrexate infused intra-arterially into the long bones of the legs
- Thoracotomy followed by chemotherapy if lung metastasis present

KEY PATIENT OUTCOMES

The patient (or his family) will:
- communicate understanding of the condition and treatment regimen

- remain free from complications and signs and symptoms of infection
- achieve the highest level of mobility possible
- express or indicate feelings of increased comfort and decreased pain
- express positive feelings about self
- use support systems and to help cope effectively.

NURSING INTERVENTIONS

- Provide support if patient has phantom limb pain.
- Provide stump care and help the child prepare for a prosthesis.
- Assist with chemotherapy.

PATIENT TEACHING

Be sure to cover:
- the fact that the child didn't cause the tumor
- stump care
- psychological support and reinforcement of the child's strengths.

Otitis media

DESCRIPTION

- Inflammation of the middle ear associated with fluid accumulation
- Peaks between ages 6 and 24 months
- Subsides after age 3
- Occurs most commonly during winter months
- Can be suppurative or secretory (acute or chronic)

PATHOPHYSIOLOGY

- Suppurative otitis media occurs when nasopharyngeal flora reflux through the eustachian tube and colonize in the middle ear.

- Risk factors of suppurative otitis media include:
  - respiratory tract infection
  - allergic reaction
  - nasotracheal intubation
  - positional changes.
- Predisposing factors of suppurative otitis media include:
  - wider, shorter, more horizontal eustachian tubes and increased lymphoid tissue in children
  - anatomic anomalies.
- Chronic suppurative otitis media results with inadequate treatment of acute otitis episodes, infections by resistant strains of bacteria, or, rarely, tuberculosis.
- Secretory otitis media results from obstruction of the eustachian tube:
  - Buildup of negative pressure in the middle ear permits sterile serous fluid from blood vessels to pass through the membrane of the middle ear.
  - Effusion may be secondary to eustachian tube dysfunction from viral infection or allergy.
  - Effusion may follow barotraumas (pressure injury caused by inability to equalize pressures between the environment and the middle ear).
- Occurs during rapid aircraft descent in a person with an upper respiratory tract infection.
- Chronic secretory otitis media follows persistent eustachian tube dysfunction, possibly resulting from mechanical obstruction (adenoidal tissue overgrowth, tumors), edema (allergic rhinitis, chronic sinus infection), or inadequate treatment of acute suppurative otitis media.

CAUSES

- Bacteria
  - Gram-negative bacteria
  - *Haemophilus influenzae*
  - *Moraxella catarrhalis*
  - *Staphylococci*
  - *Streptococcus pneumoniae*

- Disruption of eustachian tube patency

ASSESSMENT FINDINGS

- Suppurative otitis media
  - Severe, deep, throbbing pain (from pressure behind the tympanic membrane)
  - Signs of upper respiratory tract infection (sneezing and coughing)
  - Mild to very high fever
  - Hearing loss (usually mild and conductive)
  - Tinnitus
  - Dizziness
  - Nausea
  - Vomiting
  - Bulging of the tympanic membrane with erythema
  - Purulent drainage in the ear canal if tympanic membrane ruptures
  - Some patients asymptomatic
  - Ruptured tympanic membrane accompanied by sudden stopping of pain
- Acute secretory otitis media
  - Possibly not causing any symptoms in the first few months of life; irritability may be the only indication of earache
  - Severe conductive hearing loss; varying from 15 to 35 dB, depending on the thickness and amount of fluid in the middle ear cavity
  - Sensation of fullness in the ear and popping, crackling, or clicking sounds on swallowing or with jaw movement
  - Echo when speaking and vague feeling of top-heaviness due to the accumulation of fluid
  - Ruptured tympanic membrane accompanied with sudden stopping of pain
- Chronic otitis media
  - Thickening and scarring of the tympanic membrane
  - Decreased or absent tympanic membrane mobility
  - Cholesteatoma (a cystlike mass in the middle ear)
  - Painless purulent discharge

- Hearing loss
- Ruptured tympanic membrane accompanied with sudden stopping of pain

TEST RESULTS

■ Acute suppurative otitis media
- Otoscopy shows obscured or distorted bony landmarks of the tympanic membrane.
- Pneumatoscopy reveals decreased tympanic membrane mobility.
- Culture of ear drainage identifies the causative organism.
■ Acute secretory otitis media
- Otoscopy shows how bony landmarks appear more prominent because of tympanic membrane retraction.
- Clear or amber fluid appears behind the tympanic membrane.
- If hemorrhage has occurred, the membrane is blue-black.
■ Chronic otitis media
- Otoscopy shows thickening, scarring (sometimes), and decreasing mobility of the tympanic membrane.
- Pneumatoscopy reveals decreased or absent tympanic membrane movement.

TREATMENT

■ Acute suppurative otitis media
- Antibiotic therapy — ampicillin or amoxicillin (Amoxil)
- Myringotomy to treat severe, painful bulging of the tympanic membrane
- Single dose of ceftriaxone (Rocephin) effective against major pathogens (expensive and reserved for extremely sick infants)
- In recurring infection, antibiotics must be used with discretion, which prevents the development of resistant strains of bacteria

- Acute secretory otitis media
  - Inflation of the eustachian tube using Valsalva's maneuver several times per day
  - Nasopharyngeal decongestant therapy
  - Possible myringotomy and aspiration of middle ear fluid followed by insertion of a polyethylene tube into the tympanic membrane for immediate and prolonged equalization of pressure
- Chronic otitis media
  - Broad-spectrum antibiotics, such as amoxicillin/clavulanate potassium (Augmentin) or cefuroxime (Ceftin)
  - Elimination of eustachian tube obstruction
  - Treatment of otitis externa
  - Myringoplasty and tympanoplasty, which reconstructs middle ear structures when thickening and scarring is present
  - Possibly, mastoidectomy
  - Excision of cholesteatoma

KEY PATIENT OUTCOMES

The patient will:
- express feelings of increased comfort
- exhibit no signs or symptoms of infection
- verbalize understanding of the disorder and treatment regimen
- regain hearing or develop compensatory mechanisms
- experience no injury or harm.

NURSING INTERVENTIONS

After tympanoplasty
- Reinforce dressings.
- Observe for excessive bleeding from the ear canal.
- Administer analgesics, as needed.

With hearing loss
- Offer reassurance, when appropriate, that hearing loss caused by serious otitis media is temporary.

- Provide clear, concise explanations.
- Face the patient when speaking and enunciate clearly and slowly.
- Allow time for the patient to grasp what was said.
- Provide a pencil and paper.
- Alert the staff to the patient's communication problem.

After myringotomy

- Wash your hands before and after ear care.
- Maintain drainage flow.
- Place sterile cotton loosely in the patient's external ear, which absorbs drainage and prevents infection. Change the cotton when damp. Avoid placing cotton or plugs deep in ear canal.
- Give prescribed analgesics.
- Give antiemetics after tympanoplasty and reinforce dressings.
- Monitor the patient's pain level, response to treatment, auditory acuity, and for excessive bleeding or discharge.

PATIENT TEACHING

Be sure to cover (with the parents):
- proper instillation of ointment, drops, and ear wash, as ordered
- drug administration, dosage, and possible adverse effects
- importance of taking antibiotics
- adequate fluid intake
- correct instillation of nasopharyngeal decongestants
- use of fitted earplugs for swimming and bathing after myringotomy and tympanostomy tube insertion
- notification of the physician if the tube falls out and for ear pain, fever, or pus-filled discharge
- preventing recurrence.

ALERT *Instruct parents not to feed their infant when he's lying in a supine position and not to put him in his crib or bed with a bottle — doing so could cause reflux of nasopharyngeal flora.*

Patent ductus arteriosus

DESCRIPTION

- Heart condition in which the lumen of the ductus (fetal blood vessel connecting the pulmonary artery to the descending aorta) remains open after birth (see *Anatomy of patent ductus arteriosus*)
- Good prognosis if shunt is small or surgical repair is effective; otherwise, may advance to intractable heart failure, which may be fatal
- Twice as common in females as in males
- Also called *PDA*

PATHOPHYSIOLOGY

- The lumen of the ductus remains open after birth and creates a left-to-right shunt of blood from the aorta to the pulmonary artery, resulting in recirculation of arterial blood through the lungs.
- PDA is prevalent in premature neonates; it probably results from abnormalities in oxygenation or the relaxant action of prostaglandin E, which prevents ductal spasm and contracture necessary for closure.

CAUSES

- Associated with other congenital defects, such as coarctation of the aorta, pulmonary and aortic stenoses, and ventricular septal defect
- Prematurity
- Rubella syndrome

ASSESSMENT FINDINGS

- History of premature birth, rubella, or difficulty breathing
- In infants: respiratory distress, signs and symptoms of heart failure, slow motor development, failure to thrive,

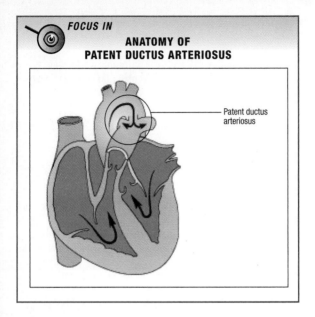

FOCUS IN

ANATOMY OF
PATENT DUCTUS ARTERIOSUS

Patent ductus arteriosus

and heightened susceptibility to respiratory tract infections
- Gibson murmur during systole and diastole
- Thrill at the left sternal border
- Prominent left ventricular impulse
- Bounding peripheral arterial pulses (Corrigan's pulse)
- Widened pulse pressure

TEST RESULTS

- Chest X-rays may show increased pulmonary vascular markings, prominent pulmonary arteries, and an enlarged left ventricle and aorta.
- Echocardiography detects and helps estimate the size of a PDA; it also reveals an enlarged left atrium and left ventricle or right ventricular hypertrophy from pulmonary vascular disease.

- Electrocardiogram may be normal or indicate left atrial or ventricular hypertrophy and, in pulmonary vascular disease, biventricular hypertrophy.
- Cardiac catheterization shows pulmonary arterial oxygen content higher than right ventricular content because of the influx of aortic blood.

TREATMENT

- No immediate treatment (if asymptomatic)
- Fluid restriction
- Activity, as tolerated
- Diuretics
- Cardiac glycosides
- Antibiotics (preoperatively)
- Surgical ligation of the ductus

   ALERT If symptoms are mild, surgical correction is usually delayed until at least age 1. Before surgery, children with PDA require antibiotics to protect against infective endocarditis.

- Alprostadil (Prostin VR/Pediatric) may be used as palliative treatment until surgery can be performed
- Coil occlusion via cardiac catheterization to deposit a plug in the ductus to stop shunting
- Indomethacin I.V. (Indocin I.V.), a prostaglandin inhibitor that's an alternative to surgery in premature neonates, to induce ductus spasm and closure

KEY PATIENT OUTCOMES

The patient will:
- maintain adequate ventilation
- maintain hemodynamic stability
- remain free from signs and symptoms of infection
- utilize support groups to help cope effectively.

NURSING INTERVENTIONS

- Monitor vital signs, respiratory status, heart rhythm, and intake and output.
- Give prescribed drugs.
- Provide emotional support to the patient and her family.
- Stress the need for regular medical follow-up examinations.

PATIENT TEACHING

Be sure to cover:
- activity restrictions based on the child's tolerance and energy levels
- importance of informing any physician who treats the child about her history of surgery for PDA — even if the child is being treated for an unrelated medical problem.

Pyloric stenosis

DESCRIPTION

- Hyperplasia (increased mass) and hypertrophy (increased size) of the circular and longitudinal muscle layers at the pylorus, which narrows the pyloric canal (see *Understanding pyloric stenosis*, page 176)
- Most commonly seen in male infants between ages 1 and 6 months

PATHOPHYSIOLOGY

- The passageway between the stomach and the duodenum is narrowed.
- Swelling and inflammation further reduce the size of the lumen, possibly resulting in complete obstruction; thus, normal emptying of the stomach is prevented.

FOCUS IN

UNDERSTANDING PYLORIC STENOSIS

In pyloric stenosis, hyperplasia (increased mass) and hypertrophy (increased size) of the circular and longitudinal muscle layers at the pylorus (the lower opening of the stomach leading into the duodenum) prevent the stomach from emptying normally.

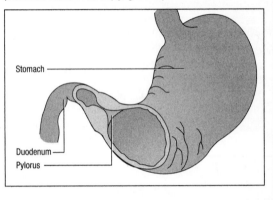

Stomach

Duodenum
Pylorus

CAUSES

- Exact cause unknown
- May be associated with anorectal abnormalities, esophageal atresia, urinary tract obstruction, and malrotation
- Not an inherited disorder

ASSESSMENT FINDINGS

- Olive-sized bulge below the right costal margin
- Projectile vomiting during or shortly after feedings preceded by reverse peristaltic waves (going left to right), but not by nausea
- Child resumes eating after vomiting
- Poor weight gain

■ Symptoms of malnutrition and dehydration despite the child's apparent adequate intake of food
■ Tetany

TEST RESULTS

■ Arterial blood gas analysis reveals metabolic alkalosis.
■ Blood chemistry tests reveal hypocalcemia, hypokalemia, and hypochloremia.
■ Hematest shows blood in the vomitus.
■ Ultrasound and endoscopy reveal a hypertrophied sphincter.

TREATMENT

■ Nothing-by-mouth status before surgery
■ I.V. therapy to correct fluid and electrolyte imbalances
■ Insertion of nasogastric tube, kept open for gastric decompression
■ Surgery: pyloromyotomy performed by laparoscopy

KEY PATIENT OUTCOMES

The patient will:
■ maintain adequate nutrition
■ achieve balanced fluid and electrolytes
■ remain free from postoperative infections or complications.

NURSING INTERVENTIONS

■ Weigh the child daily.
■ Monitor vital signs and intake and output.
■ Assess for metabolic alkalosis and dehydration from frequent vomiting.
■ Assess abdominal and cardiovascular status.
■ Provide small, frequent, thickened feedings with the head of the bed elevated; burp the child frequently.
■ Position the child, preferably on his right side.

Preoperative care
- Maintain nothing-by-mouth status.
- Provide I.V. therapy to maintain fluid and electrolyte balance.

Postoperative care
- Feed the child small amounts of oral electrolyte solution at first; then increase the amount and concentration of food until normal feeding is achieved.
- Provide a pacifier.
- Position the child on his right side, allowing gravity to help the flow of fluid through the pyloric valve.
- Keep the incision area clean.

PATIENT TEACHING

Be sure to cover (with the parents):
- the disorder and its diagnosis and treatment
- preventing complications before surgery
- early signs and symptoms of complications that should be reported postoperatively.

 Life-threatening disorder

Respiratory distress syndrome
DESCRIPTION

- Respiratory disorder related to a developmental delay in lung maturity, involving widespread alveolar collapse
- Most common cause of neonatal death
- Affects approximately 10% of all premature neonates
- Almost exclusively affects neonates born before the 27th gestational week; occurs in about 60% of those born before the 28th week if untreated antenatally
- Most commonly occurs in neonates of mothers with diabetes, neonates delivered by cesarean birth, and neonates with perinatal asphyxia
- If mild, subsides slowly after about 3 days
- Also called *RDS* or *hyaline membrane disease*

PATHOPHYSIOLOGY

- In premature neonates, immaturity of alveoli and capillary blood supply leads to alveolar collapse from lack of surfactant (a lipoprotein normally present in alveoli and respiratory bronchioles that lowers surface tension and helps maintain alveolar patency).
- Surfactant deficiency causes alveolar collapse, resulting in inadequate alveolar ventilation and shunting of blood through collapsed lung areas (atelectasis).
- Inadequate ventilation leads to hypoxia and acidosis.
- Compensatory grunting occurs and produces positive end-expiratory pressure (PEEP), helping to prevent further alveolar collapse.

CAUSES

- Surfactant deficiency stemming from preterm birth

ASSESSMENT FINDINGS

- History of preterm birth, cesarean birth, or other stress during delivery
- Maternal history of diabetes or antepartum hemorrhage
- Rapid, shallow respirations
- Intercostal, subcostal, or sternal retractions
- Nasal flaring
- Audible expiratory grunting
- Pallor
- Frothy sputum
- Low body temperature
- Diminished gas exchange and crackles
- Possible hypotension, peripheral edema, and oliguria
- Possible apnea, bradycardia, and cyanosis

TEST RESULTS

- Partial pressure of arterial oxygen (Pao_2) is decreased; partial pressure of arterial carbon dioxide may be normal, decreased, or increased; and arterial pH is decreased (from respiratory or metabolic acidosis or both).

- Lecithin-sphingomyelin ratio shows prenatal lung development and RDS risk.
- Chest X-rays may show a fine reticulogranular pattern with a "ground glass" appearance.

COLLABORATION *The patient will need referrals to other members of the healthcare team, including a neonatal ophthalmologist to assess for retinopathy and a social worker to help the family utilize community resources.*

TREATMENT

- Mechanical ventilation with PEEP or continuous positive airway pressure (CPAP) administered by a tight-fitting face mask or, when necessary, an endotracheal tube
- For a neonate who can't maintain adequate gas exchange, high-frequency oscillation ventilation
- Radiant warmer or Isolette
- Warm, humidified, oxygen-enriched gases given by oxygen hood or mechanical ventilation
- Tube feedings or total parenteral nutrition
- I.V. fluids and sodium bicarbonate
- Pancuronium bromide
- Prophylactic antibiotics
- Diuretics
- Surfactant replacement therapy
- Vitamin E
- Antenatal corticosteroids
- Possible tracheostomy

KEY PATIENT OUTCOMES

The patient (or his family) will:
- maintain adequate ventilation
- maintain a patent airway
- remain free from infection
- maintain intact skin integrity
- identify factors that increase the risk of neonatal injury.

NURSING INTERVENTIONS

- Monitor vital signs, arterial blood gas (ABG) values, intake and output, central venous pressure, pulse oximetry, daily weight, skin color, respiratory status, and skin integrity.
- Give prescribed drugs.
- Check the umbilical catheter for arterial or venous hypotension, as appropriate.
- Suction as necessary.
- Change the transcutaneous Pao_2 monitor lead placement site every 2 to 4 hours.
- Adjust PEEP or CPAP settings as indicated by ABG values.

ALERT *In a neonate on a mechanical ventilator, watch carefully for signs of barotrauma and accidental disconnection from the ventilator. Check ventilator settings frequently. Be alert for signs of complications of PEEP or CPAP therapy, such as decreased cardiac output, pneumothorax, and pneumomediastinum.*

ALERT *Watch for evidence of complications from oxygen therapy, such as lung capillary damage, decreased mucus flow, impaired ciliary functioning, and widespread atelectasis. Also be alert for signs of patent ductus arteriosus, heart failure, retinopathy, pulmonary hypertension, necrotizing enterocolitis, and neurologic abnormalities.*

- Monitor for signs and symptoms of infection, thrombosis, and decreased peripheral circulation.
- Implement measures to prevent infection.
- Provide mouth care every 2 hours.
- Encourage parents to participate in the infant's care.
- Encourage parents to ask questions and to express their fears and concerns.
- Advise parents that full recovery may take up to 12 months.
- Offer emotional support.

PATIENT TEACHING

Be sure to cover (with the parents):
- the disorder and its diagnosis and treatment
- drugs and possible adverse effects
- explanations of respiratory equipment, alarm sounds, and mechanical noise
- potential complications
- when to notify the physician.

Respiratory syncytial virus infection

DESCRIPTION

- Leading cause of lower respiratory tract infection in infants and young children
- Suspected cause of fatal respiratory diseases in infants
- Almost exclusively affects infants (ages 1 to 6 months, peaking between ages 2 and 3 months) and young children, especially those in day-care settings
- May cause serious illness in patients with underlying cardiopulmonary disease
- Common characteristics: rhinorrhea, low-grade fever, tachypnea, shortness of breath, cyanosis, apneic episodes, and mild systemic symptoms accompanied by coughing and wheezing
- Also known as *RSV*

PATHOPHYSIOLOGY

- Virus attaches to cells, eventually resulting in necrosis of the bronchiolar epithelium; in severe infection, peribronchiolar infiltrate of lymphocytes and mononuclear cells occurs.
- Intra-alveolar thickening and resultant fluid fills the alveolar spaces.
- Airway passages narrow on expiration, preventing air from leaving the lungs and causing progressive over-inflation.

CAUSES

- Probably spread to infants and young children by school-age children, adolescents, and young adults with mild reinfections
- Reinfections are common, typically producing milder symptoms than the primary infection
- Respiratory syncytial virus, a subgroup of myxoviruses resembling paramyxovirus
- Transmitted from person to person by respiratory secretions

ASSESSMENT FINDINGS

- Nasal congestion
- Nasal and pharyngeal inflammation
- Coughing
- Wheezing, rhonchi, and crackles
- Malaise
- Sore throat
- Earache
- Dyspnea
- Fever
- Otitis media
- Severe respiratory distress (nasal flaring, retraction, cyanosis, and tachypnea)

TEST RESULTS

- Cultures of nasal and pharyngeal secretions show RSV.
- Serum RSV antibody titers are elevated.
- Arterial blood gas values show hypoxemia and respiratory acidosis.
- In dehydration, blood urea nitrogen levels are elevated.

TREATMENT

- Respiratory support
- Adequate nutrition

- Avoidance of overhydration
- Rest periods when fatigued
- Ribavirin (Virazole)
- Possible tracheostomy

KEY PATIENT OUTCOMES

The patient will:
- maintain respiratory rate that supports adequate ventilation
- express or indicate feelings of increased comfort while maintaining adequate air exchange
- cough effectively
- maintain adequate fluid volume.

NURSING INTERVENTIONS

- Institute contact isolation.
- Monitor respiratory status.
- Perform percussion, drainage, and suction when necessary.
- Give prescribed oxygen.
- Use a croup tent, as needed.
- Place the patient in semi-Fowler's position.
- Monitor fluid and electrolyte status.
- Observe for signs and symptoms of dehydration, and administer I.V. fluids accordingly.
- Promote bed rest and activity as tolerated.
- Offer diversional activities tailored to the patient's condition and age.

PATIENT TEACHING

Be sure to cover (with the parents):
- the disorder and its diagnosis and treatment
- how the infection spreads
- drugs and possible adverse effects
- importance of a nonsmoking environment in the home
- follow-up care.

Rheumatic fever

DESCRIPTION

- Systemic inflammatory disease of childhood that occurs 2 to 6 weeks after an inadequately treated upper respiratory infection with group A beta-hemolytic streptococci
- Principally involves the heart, joints, central nervous system, skin, and subcutaneous tissues
- Commonly recurs

PATHOPHYSIOLOGY

- Rheumatic fever is a hypersensitivity reaction to a group A beta-hemolytic streptococcal infection, in which antibodies are manufactured to prevent streptococci from reacting and producing characteristic lesions at specific tissue sites, especially in the heart and joints.
- Antigens of group A streptococci bind to receptors in the heart, muscle, brain, and synovial joints, causing an autoimmune response.
- Rheumatic heart disease refers to cardiac manifestations of rheumatic fever (pancarditis [myocarditis, pericarditis, and endocarditis] during the early acute phase and chronic valvular disease later).

 ALERT *In children, mitral insufficiency is the major consequence of rheumatic heart disease.*

CAUSES

- Prior group A beta-hemolytic streptococcal infection

ASSESSMENT FINDINGS

- The Jones criteria for diagnosing rheumatic fever (the patient must have two major criteria or one major and two minor criteria):
- Major criteria:
  – Carditis

- – Chorea
- – Erythema marginatum (temporary, disk-shaped, non-pruritic, reddened macules that fade in the center, leaving raised margins)
- – Migratory joint pain (polyarthritis)
- – Subcutaneous nodules
- Minor criteria:
  - – Arthralgia
  - – Prolonged PR interval
  - – Fever
  - – Elevated acute phase reactants (erythrocyte sedimentation rate [ESR] and C-reactive protein)
- To complete the diagnosis, evidence of a preceding group A streptococcal infection must also exist

TEST RESULTS

- Antistreptolysin-O titer is elevated.
- Throat culture or rapid strep antigen test for group A streptococci is positive.
- ESR may be increased.
- Electrocardiogram may show a prolonged PR interval.
- Echocardiography helps to evaluate valvular damage, chamber size, and ventricular function.
- Cardiac catheterization evaluates valvular damage and left ventricular function in severe cardiac involvement.

TREATMENT

- Analgesic, such as aspirin, for arthritis pain
- Antibiotic, such as penicillin, to prevent damage from future attacks (taken until age 20 or for 5 years after the attack, whichever is longer)
- Anti-inflammatories, such as corticosteroids
- Strict bed rest for about 5 weeks during the acute phase with active carditis, followed by a progressive increase in physical activity, depending on clinical and laboratory findings and response to treatment
- Valvular surgery for damaged valves

KEY PATIENT OUTCOMES

The patient will:
- maintain adequate ventilation
- maintain hemodynamic stability
- avoid arrhythmias
- carry out activities of daily living (ADLs) without weakness or fatigue.

NURSING INTERVENTIONS

- Monitor vital signs and intake and output.
- Institute safety measures for chorea; maintain a calm environment, reduce stimulation, avoid the use of forks or glass, and assist in walking.
- Encourage bed rest as ordered; assist in arranging for home schooling and diversified activities as needed.
- Provide appropriate passive stimulation.
- Provide emotional support for long-term convalescence.
- Note a history of and monitor for penicillin allergy.
- Promote good dental hygiene; make sure the patient and his family understand the need to comply with prolonged antibiotic therapy and follow-up care and the need for additional antibiotics during dental surgery or procedures.

PATIENT TEACHING

Be sure to cover (with the parents):
- the disorder and its diagnosis and treatment
- the importance of resuming ADLs slowly and scheduling frequent rest periods as instructed by the physician
- what to do if signs of an allergic reaction to penicillin occur
- the importance of reporting signs of recurrent pharyngeal streptococcal infection
- keeping the child away from people with respiratory tract infections
- the transient nature of chorea

- compliance with prolonged antibiotic therapy and follow-up care
- the need for certain patients to take prophylactic antibiotics before dental work or invasive procedures.

Roseola infantum

DESCRIPTION

- Commonly acute, benign, viral illness characterized by fever with subsequent rash (see *Incubation and duration of common rash-producing infections*)
- Affects infants and young children (typically from age 6 months to 3 years) and affects both sexes equally
- Most commonly occurs in the spring and fall
- Has an incubation period of 5 to 15 days
- Also known as *exanthema subitum*

PATHOPHYSIOLOGY

- Human herpesvirus (HHV) type 6B replicates in leukocytes and in the salivary glands.
- HHV-6 shows persistent and intermittent or chronic shedding in the normal population, resulting in the unusually early infection of children.

CAUSES

- HHV-6 (most common)
- May be transmitted by saliva, blood and, possibly, by genital secretions

ASSESSMENT FINDINGS

- Abruptly increasing, unexplainable fever peaking between 103° and 105° F (39.4° and 40.6° C) for 3 to 5 days and then dropping suddenly
- Anorexia
- Irritability

INCUBATION AND DURATION OF COMMON RASH-PRODUCING INFECTIONS

Infection	Incubation (days)	Duration (days)
Roseola	5 to 15	3 to 6
Varicella	10 to 14	7 to 14
Rubeola	13 to 17	5
Rubella	6 to 18	3
Herpes simplex	2 to 12	7 to 21

- Listlessness
- Cough
- When temperature dropping abruptly, maculopapular, nonpruritic rash appearing and blanching with pressure
- Profuse rash on the trunk, arms, and neck; mild rash on the face and legs; fading within 24 hours
- Nagayama spots (red papules on soft palate and uvula)
- Periorbital edema

TEST RESULTS

- Diagnosis usually results from clinical observation.
- The causative organism is present in saliva.
- HHV-6 is isolated in peripheral blood.
- Complete blood count shows leukopenia and relative lymphocytosis as temperature increases.
- Immunofluorescence or enzyme immunoassays may show seroconversion during the convalescent phase.

TREATMENT

- Supportive and symptomatic
- Increased fluid intake
- Rest until fever subsides
- Antipyretics

- Anticonvulsants, if needed for central nervous system (CNS) involvement

KEY PATIENT OUTCOMES

The patient will:
- regain a normal body temperature
- maintain adequate fluid volume
- maintain adequate nutritional intake
- exhibit improved or healed lesions or wounds.

NURSING INTERVENTIONS

- Monitor vital signs, especially temperature.
- Give tepid sponge baths and prescribed antipyretics (Tylenol or ibuprofen — *no* aspirin for viral illness).
- Monitor and replace fluids and electrolytes, as needed.
- Monitor neurologic status.
- Institute seizure precautions if there's CNS involvement.
- Provide emotional support to parents.

PATIENT TEACHING

Be sure to cover (with the parents):
- the disorder and its diagnosis and treatment
- methods to reduce fever:
  - tepid sponge baths
  - dressing the child in lightweight clothing
  - keeping a comfortable room temperature
  - use of antipyretics
- importance of adequate fluid intake
- no need for isolation
- reassurance that brief febrile seizures won't cause brain damage and will stop as the fever subsides.

Rubella

DESCRIPTION

- Acute, mildly contagious viral disease that causes a distinctive maculopapular rash (resembling measles or scarlet fever) and lymphadenopathy
- Self-limiting with excellent prognosis, except for congenital rubella, which can have disastrous consequences
- Occurs through direct contact with blood, urine, stools, or nasopharyngeal secretions of an infected person; may also occur transplacentally
- Communicable from about 10 days before until 5 days after rash appears
- Occurs worldwide; most commonly among children ages 5 to 9, adolescents, and young adults who haven't been adequately immunized
- Flourishes during spring, with limited outbreaks in schools
- Also called *German measles*

PATHOPHYSIOLOGY

- Ribonucleic acid virus enters the bloodstream, usually through the respiratory route.
- The incubation period lasts 18 days, with a duration of 12 to 23 days.
- The rash is thought to result from virus dissemination to the skin.

CAUSES

- Rubella virus (a togavirus) spreading by direct contact or contaminated airborne respiratory droplets

ASSESSMENT FINDINGS

- Inadequate immunization, exposure to a person with rubella infection within the previous 2 to 3 weeks, or re-

cent travel to an endemic area without adequate immunization
- In a child, absence of prodromal symptoms
- In an adolescent, headache, malaise, anorexia, coryza, sore throat, and cough preceding rash onset
- Rash accompanied by low-grade fever (99° to 101° F [37.2° to 38.3° C]) possibly reaching 104° F (40° C)
- Exanthematous, maculopapular, mildly pruritic rash; typically beginning on the face, and spreading rapidly, covering the trunk (may be confluent and hard to distinguish from scarlet fever rash) and limbs within hours
- Rash fading in the opposite order in which it appeared by the end of day 2, and disappearing on day 3
- Small, red, petechial macules on the soft palate (Forschheimer spots) preceding or accompanying the rash
- Coryza
- Conjunctivitis
- Suboccipital, postauricular, and postcervical lymph node enlargement

TEST RESULTS

- Diagnosis usually results from clinical observation.
- Cultures of throat, blood, urine, and cerebrospinal fluid isolate the rubella virus; convalescent serum shows a fourfold increase in antibody titers.
- Enzyme-linked immunosorbent assay for immunoglobulin (Ig) M antibodies reveals rubella-specific IgM antibody.
- In congenital rubella, rubella-specific IgM antibody is present in umbilical cord blood.

TREATMENT

- Isolation precautions
- Small, frequent meals
- Increased fluid intake
- Rest until fever subsides
- Skin care

- Antipyretics, such as acetaminophen
- Analgesics

KEY PATIENT OUTCOMES

The patient will:
- remain free from signs and symptoms of infection
- exhibit improvement or healing of lesions
- express or demonstrate feelings of increased comfort and decreased pain.

NURSING INTERVENTIONS

- Monitor vital signs.
- Give prescribed drugs.
- Institute isolation precautions until 5 days after the rash disappears. Keep an infant with congenital rubella in isolation for 3 months, until three throat cultures are negative.
- Monitor for auditory impairment in infants with congenital rubella.
- Keep the patient's skin clean and dry and monitor for signs of exanthema.
- Make sure that the patient receives care only from nonpregnant hospital workers who aren't at risk for rubella. As ordered, administer immune globulin to nonimmunized people who visit the patient. (See *Giving the rubella vaccine*, page 194.)
- Report confirmed rubella cases to local public health officials.
- Provide parents of an infant with congenital rubella with support, counseling, and referrals, as needed.
- Refer the patient to an infectious disease specialist if congenital rubella is confirmed.

PATIENT TEACHING

Be sure to cover (with the parents):
- the disorder and its diagnosis and treatment

FOCUS IN

GIVING THE RUBELLA VACCINE

Know how to manage rubella immunization before giving the vaccine. First, ask about allergies, especially to neomycin. If the person has this allergy or has had a reaction to any immunization in the past, check with the physician before giving the vaccine.

If the person is a woman of childbearing age, ask if she's pregnant. If she is or thinks she may be, don't give the vaccine.

Give the vaccine at least 3 months after any administration of immune globulin or blood. These substances may have antibodies that could neutralize the vaccine.

Don't vaccinate an immunocompromised person, a person with immunodeficiency disease, or a person receiving immunosuppressant, radiation, or corticosteroid therapy. Instead, administer immune serum globulin, as ordered, to prevent or reduce infection.

- ways to reduce fever
- devastating effects of rubella on a fetus
- importance of people with rubella avoiding pregnant women
- avoidance of aspirin in a child receiving rubella vaccine or one who has rubella.

Rubeola

DESCRIPTION

- Acute, highly contagious infection that causes a characteristic rash
- In United States, usually an excellent prognosis
- May be severe or fatal in patients with impaired cell-mediated immunity
- Affects mostly preschool children
- Peak communicability from 1 to 2 days before symptom onset until 4 days after rash appears
- Mortality highest in children younger than age 2 and in adults

- In temperate zones, most commonly seen in late winter and early spring
- Also called *measles* or *morbilli*

PATHOPHYSIOLOGY

- The virus invades the respiratory epithelium and spreads (via the bloodstream) to the reticuloendothelial system, infecting all types of white blood cells.
- Viremia and viruria develop, leading to infection of the entire respiratory tract, and spread to the integumentary system.
- In measles encephalitis, focal hemorrhage, congestion, and perivascular demyelination occur.

CAUSES

- Rubeola virus
- Spread by direct contact or by contaminated airborne respiratory droplets, with portal of entry in the upper respiratory tract

ASSESSMENT FINDINGS

- Inadequate immunization and exposure to someone with measles in the past 14 days
- Photophobia
- Malaise
- Anorexia
- Coryza
- Hoarseness
- Hacking cough
- Rhinorrhea
- Lymphadenopathy
- Temperature peaking between 103° and 105° F (39.4° C and 40.6° C)
- Periorbital edema
- Conjunctivitis

- Koplik's spots (tiny, bluish-gray specks, surrounded by red halo) on oral mucosa opposite the molars, which may bleed
- Pruritic rash starting as faint macules behind the ears and on the neck and cheeks, becoming papular and erythematous, and rapidly spreading over the face, neck, eyelids, arms, chest, back, abdomen, and thighs
- Fading of rash when it reaches the feet 2 to 3 days later, occurring in the same sequence it appeared, leaving brown discoloration that disappears in 7 to 10 days

TEST RESULTS

- Measles virus appears in blood, nasopharyngeal secretions, and urine during the febrile period.
- Serum antibodies appear within 3 days of rash onset and reach peak titers 2 to 4 weeks later.

TREATMENT

- Respiratory isolation precautions
- Use of vaporizer
- Warm environment
- Small, frequent meals
- Increased fluid intake
- Rest until symptoms improve
- Skin care
- Antipyretics, such as acetaminophen (do *not* give aspirin to children with viral illnesses)

KEY PATIENT OUTCOMES

The patient (or his family) will:
- remain free from signs and symptoms of infection
- exhibit improved or healed lesions or wounds
- remain free from complications related to oral mucous membrane trauma
- communicate an understanding of the patient's special dietary needs.

NURSING INTERVENTIONS

- Monitor vital signs.
- Institute respiratory isolation measures for 4 days after rash onset.
- Follow standard infection control precautions.
- Monitor skin for signs of exanthema, eyes for conjunctivitis, and ears for otitis media.
- Monitor mental status.
- Monitor for signs and symptoms of pneumonia.
- Give prescribed drugs.
- Encourage bed rest during the acute period.
- If photophobia occurs, darken the room or provide sunglasses.
- Administer measles vaccine, as ordered and needed.
- Report measles cases to local health authorities.

PATIENT TEACHING

Be sure to cover (with the parents):
- the disorder and its diagnosis and treatment
- supportive measures, isolation, bed rest, and increased fluids
- instructions on cleaning a vaporizer (if used) and the importance of changing the water every 8 hours
- early signs and symptoms of complications that should be reported.

Scoliosis

DESCRIPTION

- Lateral curvature of the spine that may occur in the thoracic, lumbar, or thoracolumbar spinal segment, measuring greater than 10 degrees, and associated with vertebral rotation
- Classified as nonstructural (flexible spinal curve, with temporary straightening when patient leans sideways) or structural (fixed deformity)

■ Most commonly occurs in females; typically diagnosed at puberty and throughout adolescence

PATHOPHYSIOLOGY

Nonstructural scoliosis

■ Pelvic tilt is caused by unequal leg lengths, poor posture, paraspinal inflammation, acute disk disease, or head tilt associated with poor vision leading to a spinal deviation.

■ There's little change in the shape of the vertebrae.

Structural scoliosis

■ Congenital scoliosis is usually associated with wedge vertebrae, fused ribs or vertebrae, or hemivertebrae; it may also result from trauma to the zygote or embryo.

■ Paralytic or musculoskeletal scoliosis develops several months after asymmetrical paralysis of the trunk muscles due to polio, cerebral palsy, or muscular dystrophy.

■ Idiopathic scoliosis is the most common form; it may be transmitted as an autosomal dominant or multifactorial trait.

– It appears in a previously straight spine during the growing years.

– A possible cause of idiopathic scoliosis is brain stem dysfunction, possibly due to a lesion of the posterior columns or the inner ear.

– Occurs in three classifications:

  ■ Infantile — affects mostly male infants between birth and age 3 and causes left thoracic and right lumbar curves

  ■ Juvenile — affects both sexes between ages 4 and 10 and causes varying types of curvature

  ■ Adolescent — generally affects females between ages 10 and achievement of skeletal maturity and causes varying types of curvature

■ Scoliosis stops progressing when bone growth stops.

CAUSES

■ Functional, nonstructural, or postural scoliosis
  – Acute disk disease
  – Discrepancy in leg lengths
  – Paraspinal inflammation
  – Poor posture
  – Poor vision
■ Progressive or structural scoliosis
  – Deformity of the vertebral bodies
  – Rib changes

ASSESSMENT FINDINGS

■ Backache
■ Fatigue
■ Dyspnea

Nonstructural scoliosis
■ Curve of the spine disappearing when child bends at waist to touch the toes

Structural scoliosis
■ Curve in the thoracic segment of the spine, with convexity to the right, and compensatory curves (S curves) in the cervical segment above and the lumbar segment below, both with a convexity to the left (see *Cobb method for measuring angle of curvature*, page 200)
■ Spinal curve failing to straighten when the child bends forward with the knees straight and arms hanging down toward the feet
■ Hips, ribs, shoulders, and shoulder blades asymmetrical

TEST RESULTS

■ X-rays of the spine confirm scoliosis and determine the degree of curvature and flexibility of the spine; they also determine skeletal maturity, predict remaining bone growth, and differentiate nonstructural from structural scoliosis.

FOCUS IN

COBB METHOD FOR MEASURING ANGLE OF CURVATURE

The Cobb method measures the angle of curvature in patients with scoliosis. The top vertebra in the curve (T6 in the illustration) is the uppermost vertebra whose upper face tilts toward the curve's concave side. The bottom vertebra in the curve (T12) is the lowest vertebra whose lower face tilts toward the curve's concave side. The angle at which perpendicular lines drawn from the upper face of the top vertebra and the lower face of the bottom vertebra intersect is the angle of the curve.

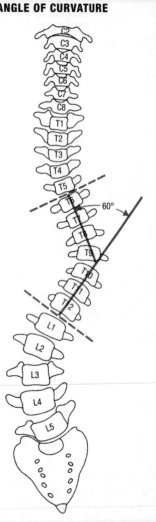

TREATMENT

Nonstructural scoliosis
■ Corrective lenses if associated problem occurs with poor vision due to the head tilting
■ Postural exercises
■ Shoe lifts

Structural scoliosis
■ Possible prolonged bracing (Milwaukee or Boston brace)
■ Electrical stimulation for mild to moderate curvatures
■ Harrington, Luque, or Cotrel-Dubousset rods for curves greater than 40 degrees (to realign the spine or when curves fail to respond to orthotic treatment)
■ Worn over a T-shirt for 23 hours per day
■ Brace adjustments every 3 months
  – Skin traction or halo femoral traction
  – Spinal fusion with bone from the iliac crest

▶ **COLLABORATION** *Scoliosis can affect numerous body systems, thereby necessitating a multidisciplinary approach to care. Orthopedic specialists, including surgeons, may be consulted to provide casting, bracing, or surgery. A physical therapist may assist with exercises to maximize mobility and prevent complications related to treatments. A respiratory therapist may provide measures to ensure adequate lung expansion if rib cage deformities are present. Social services may be needed to provide referrals for follow-up and information about community support services.*

KEY PATIENT OUTCOMES

The patient will:
■ experience feelings of increased comfort and decreased pain
■ maintain joint mobility and range of motion
■ achieve the highest level of mobility possible
■ express positive feelings about self
■ demonstrate measures to prevent injury to self.

NURSING INTERVENTIONS

■ After spinal fusion and the insertion of rods
  – Monitor vital signs and intake and output.
  – Turn the child only by logrolling.
  – Maintain correct body alignment.
  – Keep the bed in a flat position.
  – Help the child adjust to the increase in height and al-
    tered self-perception.
■ Teach the child to perform stretching exercises for the
  spine.
■ Help the child to maintain self-esteem.
■ Teach the child and parents about the brace.
  – How to apply it and how long to wear it
  – How to prevent skin breakdown
■ Keep the skin beneath the brace clean and dry.
■ Wear a tight-fitting T-shirt under the brace.

> **ALERT** *Watch for signs of cast syndrome (nausea,
> abdominal pressure, and vague abdominal pain),*
> *which may result from hyperextension of the spine.*

PATIENT TEACHING

Be sure to cover:
■ the disorder and its diagnosis and treatment
■ brace care
■ skin care
■ safe body mechanics
■ cast care, if needed
■ the signs of cast syndrome
■ the prescribed drug regimen
■ adverse drug reactions
■ relaxation techniques.

Seizure disorder

DESCRIPTION

■ Neurologic condition characterized by recurrent seizures
■ No effect on intelligence

- Usually occurs in patients of both sexes younger than age 20
- First seizure usually experienced during childhood or after age 50
- Good seizure control in about 80% of patients with strict adherence to prescribed treatment
- Also known as *epilepsy*

PATHOPHYSIOLOGY

- Seizures occur as paroxysmal events involving abnormal electrical discharges of neurons in the brain and cell membrane potential. (See *Classifying seizures*, pages 204 and 205.)
- On stimulation, the neuron fires, the discharge spreads to surrounding cells, and stimulation continues to one side or both sides of the brain, resulting in seizure activity.

CAUSES

- Idiopathic (50% cases)
- Nonidiopathic
  - Anoxia
  - Apparent familial incidence in some seizure disorders
  - Birth trauma
  - Brain tumors or other space-occupying lesions
  - Genetic abnormalities (tuberous sclerosis and phenylketonuria)
  - Ingestion of toxins, such as mercury, lead, or carbon monoxide
  - Meningitis, encephalitis, or brain abscess
  - Metabolic abnormalities (hypoglycemia, pyridoxine deficiency, hypoparathyroidism)
  - Perinatal infection
  - Perinatal injuries
  - Traumatic injury

FOCUS IN
CLASSIFYING SEIZURES

Seizures can take various forms, depending on their origin and whether they're localized to one area of the brain, as occurs in partial seizures, or occur in both hemispheres, as happens in generalized seizures. This chart describes each type of seizure and lists common signs and symptoms.

Type	Description	Signs and symptoms
Partial		
Simple partial	Symptoms confined to one hemisphere	Possibly having motor (change in posture), sensory (hallucinations), or autonomic (flushing, tachycardia) symptoms; no loss of consciousness
Complex partial	Beginning in one focal area but spreading to both hemispheres (more common in adults)	Loss of consciousness; aura of visual disturbances; postictal symptoms
Generalized		
Absence (petit mal)	Sudden onset; lasting 5 to 10 seconds; possibly having 100 daily; precipitated by stress, hyperventilation, hypoglycemia, fatigue; differentiated from daydreaming	Loss of responsiveness but continued ability to maintain posture control and not fall; twitching eyelids; lip smacking; no postictal symptoms
Myoclonic	Movement disorder (not a seizure); seen as child awakening or falling asleep; may be precipitated by touch or visual stimuli; focal or generalized; symmetrical or asymmetrical	No loss of consciousness; sudden, brief, shocklike involuntary contraction of one muscle group
Clonic	Opposing muscles contracting and relaxing alternately in rhythmic pattern; possibly occurring in one limb more than others	Mucus production

CLASSIFYING SEIZURES (continued)

Type	Description	Signs and symptoms
Generalized (continued)		
Tonic	Muscles maintained in continuous contracted state (rigid posture)	Variable loss of consciousness; pupils dilating; eyes rolling up; glottis closing; possible incontinence; possibly foaming at mouth
Tonic-clonic (grand mal, major motor)	Violent total body seizure	Aura; tonic first (20 to 40 seconds); clonic next; postictal symptoms
Atonic	Drop and fall attack; needing to wear protective helmet	Loss of posture tone
Akinetic	Sudden brief loss of muscle tone or posture	Temporary loss of consciousness
Febrile	Seizure threshold lowered by elevated temperature; only one seizure per fever; common in 4% of population under age 5; occurring when temperature is rapidly rising	Lasting less than 5 minutes; generalized, transient, and nonprogressive; doesn't generally result in brain damage; EEG normal after 2 weeks
Status epilepticus	Prolonged or frequent repetition of seizures without interruption; resulting in anoxia and cardiac and respiratory arrest	Consciousness not regained between seizures; lasting more than 30 minutes

ASSESSMENT FINDINGS

- Seizure occurrence unpredictable and unrelated to activities
- Precipitating factors or events possibly reported
- Headache
- Mood changes

- Lethargy
- Myoclonic jerking
- Description of an aura
- Pungent smell
- GI distress
- Rising or sinking feeling in the stomach
- Dreamy feeling
- Unusual taste in the mouth
- Vision disturbance
- Findings possibly normal while patient isn't having a seizure and when the cause is idiopathic
- Findings related to underlying cause of the seizure

TEST RESULTS

- Serum glucose and calcium study results rule out other diagnoses.
- Computed tomography scan and magnetic resonance imaging may indicate abnormalities in internal structures.
- Skull radiography may show certain neoplasms within the brain substance or skull fractures.
- Brain scan may show malignant lesions when X-ray findings are normal or questionable.
- Cerebral angiography may show cerebrovascular abnormalities, such as aneurysm or tumor.
- EEG shows paroxysmal abnormalities. (A negative EEG doesn't rule out seizure disorder because paroxysmal abnormalities occur intermittently.)

TREATMENT

- Airway protection during seizure
- Vagus nerve stimulation by pacemaker (see *Vagus nerve stimulation*)
- Detailed presurgical evaluation to characterize seizure type, frequency, site of onset, psychological functioning, and degree of disability to select candidates for surgery in medically intractable patients
- No dietary restrictions

FOCUS IN

VAGUS NERVE STIMULATION

The vagus nerve stimulator is a U.S. Food and Drug Administration–approved method to treat medically refractory seizure disorder. The stimulator device is about the size of a pacemaker and is surgically placed in a pocket under the skin in the upper chest. Leadwires from the stimulator are tunneled under the skin to a neck incision where the vagus nerve has been exposed. The electrode coils are then placed around the nerve. The treating physician has a computer, which can be used to alter the stimulation parameters, thereby optimizing the treatment of seizures.

The device stimulates the vagus nerve for 30 seconds every 5 minutes to prevent seizure occurrence. A magnet over the area can activate the device to give extra, on-demand stimulation if the patient feels a seizure coming on. Adverse effects of the device include voice change, throat discomfort, shortness of breath, and coughing and are usually experienced only when the device is "on."

- Safety measures
- Activity as tolerated
- Anticonvulsants
- Removal of a demonstrated focal lesion
- Correction of the underlying problem

KEY PATIENT OUTCOMES

The patient will:
- remain free from injury
- communicate understanding of the condition and treatment regimen
- use support systems and develop adequate coping
- maintain usual participation in social situations and activities.

NURSING INTERVENTIONS

- Monitor vital signs, focusing on respiratory status.
- Monitor for seizure activity and associated injuries.
- Institute seizure precautions.

- Prepare the patient for surgery if indicated.
- Give prescribed anticonvulsants and monitor patient response.
- Refer the patient to the Epilepsy Foundation of America.
- Refer the patient to his state's motor vehicle department for information about a driver's license.

PATIENT TEACHING

Be sure to cover:
- the disorder and its diagnosis and treatment
- maintenance of a normal lifestyle
- compliance with the prescribed drug schedule
- adverse drug effects
- care during a seizure
- the importance of regular meals and checking with the physician before dieting
- the importance of carrying a medical identification card or wearing medical identification jewelry.

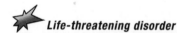 *Life-threatening disorder*

Severe combined immunodeficiency disease

DESCRIPTION

- Involves deficient or absent cell-mediated (T cell) and humoral (B cell) immunity
- Predisposes patient to infection from all classes of microorganisms during infancy
- Occurs in 1 of every 100,000 to 500,000 births, affecting more males than females, but is difficult to detect before an infant reaches age 5 months
- Also known as *SCID, graft-versus-host disease*, and *bubble-boy disease*

PATHOPHYSIOLOGY

- ▪ Three types of SCID have been identified:
- – Reticular dysgenesis (most severe) occurs when hematopoietic stem cells fail to differentiate into lymphocytes and granulocytes.
- – Swiss-type agammaglobulinemia occurs when hematopoietic stem cells fail to differentiate into lymphocytes alone.
- – Enzyme deficiency (such as adenosine deaminase deficiency) occurs when a buildup of toxic products in the lymphoid tissue causes damage and subsequent dysfunction.

CAUSES

- ▪ Failure of thymus or bursa equivalent to develop normally or possible defect in thymus and bone marrow (responsible for T- and B-cell development)
- ▪ Possible enzyme deficiency
- ▪ Transmitted as autosomal recessive trait but may be X-linked

ASSESSMENT FINDINGS

- ▪ Extreme susceptibility to infection within the first few months after birth, but probably no sign of gramnegative infection until about age 6 months because of protection by maternal immunoglobulin G
- ▪ Emaciated appearance and failure to thrive
- ▪ Assessment findings dependent on the type and site of infection
- ▪ Signs of chronic otitis media and sepsis
- ▪ Signs of the usual childhood diseases such as chickenpox

TEST RESULTS

- ▪ Blood tests show severely diminished or absent T-cell number and function.

- Chest X-rays usually show bilateral pulmonary infiltrates.
- Lymph node biopsy shows an absence of lymphocytes.

TREATMENT

- Strict protective isolation (germ-free environment)
- Gene therapy (experimental)
- Immunoglobulin
- Antibiotic therapy
- Histocompatible bone marrow transplantation
- Fetal thymus and liver transplantation

  ▶ **COLLABORATION** *Transplant specialists along with hematologic, dermatologic, and gastroenterologic specialists may be necessary to help guide treatment. Infection control personnel may be consulted to reduce the patient's risk of infection. Other specialists, including neurologists and nephrologists, may be consulted for assistance depending on the involvement of the patient's organs and prognosis. The patient and his family may also benefit from supportive counseling and a referral for social services.*

KEY PATIENT OUTCOMES

The patient (or his parents) will:
- demonstrate age-appropriate skills and behaviors
- not experience chills, fever, and other signs of illness
- establish eye, physical, and verbal contact with the infant or child
- develop adequate coping mechanisms and support systems.

NURSING INTERVENTIONS

- Monitor respiratory status and skin integrity.
- Monitor for complications and response to treatments.
- Monitor closely for signs and symptoms of infection.

- If infection develops, provide prompt and aggressive drug therapy and supportive care, as ordered.
- Watch for adverse effects of drugs given.
- Monitor for signs and symptoms of transplant rejection.
- Avoid vaccinations, and give only irradiated blood products if a transfusion is ordered.
- Monitor growth and development and social interaction.

   ALERT *Although infants with SCID must remain in strict protective isolation, try to provide a stimulating atmosphere to promote growth and development.*
- Encourage parents to visit their child often, to hold him, and to bring him toys that can be easily sterilized.
- Maintain a normal day and night routine, and talk to the child as much as possible.
- If parents can't visit, call them often to report on the infant's condition.
- Provide emotional support for the family.
- Encourage the parents to seek genetic counseling.

PATIENT TEACHING

Be sure to cover:
- the disorder and its diagnosis and treatment
- the proper technique for strict protective isolation
- the signs and symptoms of infection and the need to notify a physician promptly
- drug administration, dosage, purpose, and adverse effects.

Life-threatening disorder

Sudden infant death syndrome

DESCRIPTION

- Sudden death of an infant younger than age 1 year without identifiable cause
- Occurs in approximately 2 out of every 1,000 live births; about 60% are males

■ Increasing incidence in non–breast-fed infants and infants who sleep on their stomachs
■ Slightly higher incidence in preterm neonates, Inuit neonates, disadvantaged Black neonates, neonates of mothers younger than age 20, neonates of multiple births, neonates of mothers who smoked during pregnancy, and neonates exposed to second-hand smoke
■ Most commonly occurs in fall and winter
■ Also known as *SIDS, crib death*, and *cot death*

   ALERT *SIDS occurs mostly between ages 2 and 4 months. Incidence declines rapidly between ages 4 and 12 months.*

PATHOPHYSIOLOGY

■ The infant may have damage to the respiratory control center in the brain from chronic hypoxemia.
■ The infant may not respond to increasing carbon dioxide levels; during an episode of apnea, carbon dioxide levels increase, but the child isn't stimulated to breathe; as apnea continues, high levels of carbon dioxide further suppress the ventilatory effort until the infant stops breathing.
■ The infant may have periods of sleep apnea and eventually die during one of these episodes.

CAUSES

■ Apnea theory
■ Hypoxia theory
■ Possibly viral
■ Risk factors: prone sleeping, loose bedding, overheating, exposure to second-hand smoke, preterm birth, low birth weight, male gender, and Black or Inuit race

ASSESSMENT FINDINGS

■ Occasionally, history of respiratory tract infection
■ Possible abnormal hepatic or pancreatic function

- Previous near-miss respiratory event in 60% of cases
- With infant wedged in a crib corner or with blankets wrapped around head, suffocation ruled out by autopsy as the cause of death
- With frothy, blood-tinged sputum found around infant's mouth or on crib sheets revealing a patent airway, aspiration of vomitus ruled out by autopsy as cause of death
- No crying or signs of disturbed sleep by infant
- Postmortem examination possibly showing:
  - Changes indicating chronic hypoxia, hypoxemia, and large airway obstruction
  - Bruising; possible fractured ribs
  - Blood in the infant's mouth, nose, or ears
  - Mottled complexion; extremely cyanotic lips and fingertips
  - Pooled blood in legs and feet
  - Diaper possibly wet and full of stool

TEST RESULTS

- The autopsy may show:
  - small or normal adrenal glands
  - enlarged thymus
  - petechiae over the visceral surfaces of the pleura, within the thymus, and in the epicardium
  - well preserved lymphoid structures
  - signs of chronic hypoxemia
  - increased pulmonary artery smooth muscle
  - edematous, congestive, and fully expanded lungs
  - stomach curd inside the trachea.

TREATMENT

- Emotional support for the family
- Prevention for any surviving infant found apneic and any sibling with apnea; assessment with home apnea monitor until the at-risk infant passes age of vulnerability

KEY PATIENT OUTCOMES

The family will:
- use available support systems to assist in coping
- share feelings about the event
- identify feelings of hopelessness about the current situation
- use effective coping strategies to ease spiritual discomfort.

NURSING INTERVENTIONS

- Make sure that both parents are present when the child's death is confirmed.
- Stay calm and allow the parents to express their feelings.
- Monitor the parents' reactions and coping mechanisms.
- Reassure the parents that they aren't to blame.
- Allow the parents to see the infant in a private room and to express their grief. Stay in the room with them, if appropriate.
- Offer to call clergy, friends, or relatives.
- Return the infant's belongings to the parents.
- Make sure that the parents receive the autopsy report promptly.
- Refer the parents and family to community and health care facility support services.
- Refer the family to a home health nurse for continued support, if indicated.
- Refer the parents to cardiopulmonary resuscitation classes, if appropriate.
- Advise the parents to contact the SIDS hotline (1 800-221-SIDS).
- Refer the parents to a local SIDS parents' group.

PATIENT TEACHING

Be sure to cover (with the parents):
- the need for an autopsy to confirm the diagnosis
- basic facts about SIDS

information to help parents cope with pregnancy and the first year of a new infant's life, if they decide to have another child.

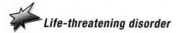

Life-threatening disorder

Tay-Sachs disease

DESCRIPTION

- Lipid storage disease that results from a congenital enzyme deficiency
- Leads to progressive mental and motor deterioration
- Always fatal, usually before age 5
- About 100 times more common (about 1 in 3,600 live births) in those with Ashkenazic Jewish ancestry than in the general population
- About 1 in 30 Ashkenazi Jews, French Canadians, and American Cajuns heterozygous carriers of the gene for this disorder
- Rare form occurring in people between ages 20 and 30
- No known cure

PATHOPHYSIOLOGY

- In this autosomal recessive disorder, the enzyme hexosaminidase A is absent or deficient.
- Without hexosaminidase A, lipid pigments (ganglioside GM2) accumulate and progressively destroy and demyelinate central nervous system cells.
- Juvenile form typically appears between ages 2 and 5 as a progressive deterioration of psychomotor skills and gait.

CAUSES

- Autosomal recessive disorder

ASSESSMENT FINDINGS

- Familial history of Tay-Sachs disease
- Normal appearance at birth (but with possible exaggerated Moro's reflex)
- Onset of clinical signs and symptoms between ages 5 and 6 months
- Progressive deterioration
- Psychomotor retardation
- Blindness
- Dementia
- In 3- to 6-month-old infant:
  - Apathetic appearance
  - Augmented response to loud sounds
  - Progressive weakness of the neck, trunk, arm, and leg muscles preventing child from sitting up or lifting head
  - Difficulty turning over
  - Inability to grasp objects
  - Progressive vision loss
- By age 18 months:
  - Possible seizures
  - Generalized paralysis
  - Spasticity
  - Blindness
  - Holding eyes wide open and rolling eyeballs
  - Pupils always dilated
  - Decerebrate rigidity
  - Complete vegetative state
  - Head circumference possibly showing enlargement
  - Pupils nonreactive to light
  - Ophthalmoscopic examination possibly showing optic nerve atrophy and a distinctive cherry red spot on the retina
- In a child who survives bouts of recurrent bronchopneumonia: possible ataxia and progressive motor retardation between ages 2 and 8 years

TEST RESULTS

- Serum analysis shows deficient hexosaminidase A.
- Amniocentesis or chorionic villus sampling allows prenatal diagnosis of hexosaminidase A deficiency.

TREATMENT

- Supportive care
- Suctioning
- Postural drainage to remove secretions
- Meticulous skin care
- Long-term care in special facility
- Tube feedings with nutritional supplements
- Activity as tolerated
- Active and passive range-of-motion exercises
- Mild laxatives
- Anticonvulsants

KEY PATIENT OUTCOMES

The patient (or his family) will:
- avoid complications
- maintain a patent airway
- express understanding of the disease process and treatment regimen
- seek outside sources to assist with coping and adjustment to the patient's situation.

NURSING INTERVENTIONS

- Monitor the patient, including vital signs; intake and output; respiratory, nutritional, and neurologic status; and response to treatment.
- Help the patient's family deal with progressive illness and death.
- Prevent skin breakdown.
- Provide adequate nutrition.
- Maintain a patent airway.

- Implement seizure precautions.
- Give drug treatments.
- Stress the importance of amniocentesis in future pregnancies.
- Refer the parents for genetic counseling.
- Refer the parents to the National Tay Sachs and Allied Diseases Association.
- Refer the parents for psychological counseling if indicated.
- Refer the siblings for screening to determine whether they're carriers.
- If the siblings are adult carriers, refer them for genetic counseling; stress that the disease isn't transmitted to offspring unless both parents are carriers.

PATIENT TEACHING

Be sure to cover:
- the disorder and its diagnosis and treatment
- how to perform suctioning when needed
- how to perform postural drainage
- how to give tube feedings
- need for proper skin care to prevent breakdown.

Tetralogy of Fallot

DESCRIPTION

- Combination of four heart defects: ventricular septal defect (VSD), right ventricular outflow tract obstruction (pulmonary stenosis), right ventricular hypertrophy, and overriding aorta (aorta positioned above the VSD) (see *Looking at tetralogy of Fallot*)
- Occurs equally in males and females and accounts for about 10% of all congenital heart diseases

FOCUS IN

LOOKING AT TETRALOGY OF FALLOT

This illustration shows the cardiac defects that create tetralogy of Fallot.

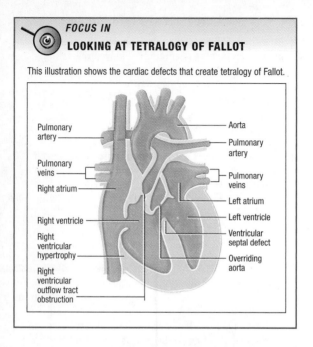

Pulmonary artery

Pulmonary veins

Right atrium

Right ventricle

Right ventricular hypertrophy

Right ventricular outflow tract obstruction

Aorta

Pulmonary artery

Pulmonary veins

Left atrium

Left ventricle

Ventricular septal defect

Overriding aorta

PATHOPHYSIOLOGY

- Blood shunts from right to left through the VSD, which permits unoxygenated blood to mix with oxygenated blood, resulting in cyanosis.
- VSD may (at times) coexist with other congenital heart defects, such as patent ductus arteriosus or atrial septal defect.

CAUSES

- Unknown
- Associated with maternal abuse of alcohol during pregnancy

ASSESSMENT FINDINGS

- Blue spells ("Tet spells"), which are characterized by dyspnea; deep, sighing respirations; bradycardia; fainting; seizures; and loss of consciousness
- Increasing dyspnea on exertion
- Growth retardation
- Eating difficulties
- Clubbing of fingers
- Cyanosis
- Loud systolic heart murmur (best heard along the left sternal border), which may diminish or obscure the pulmonic component of second heart sound
- Cardiac thrill at the left sternal border and an obvious right ventricular impulse
- Prominent inferior sternum

TEST RESULTS

- Arterial oxygen saturation is diminished.
- Blood tests show polycythemia (hematocrit may be more than 60%).
- Chest X-rays may show decreased pulmonary vascular marking, depending on the severity of the pulmonary obstruction, and a boot-shaped cardiac silhouette.
- Echocardiography identifies septal overriding of the aorta, the VSD, and pulmonic stenosis, and detects the hypertrophied walls of the right ventricle.
- Electrocardiogram shows right ventricular hypertrophy, right axis deviation and, possibly, right atrial hypertrophy.
- Cardiac catheterization confirms the diagnosis by showing pulmonic stenosis, the VSD, and the overriding aorta and rules out other cyanotic heart defects.

TREATMENT

- Prevention and treatment of complications

- During cyanotic spells, knee-chest position and administration of oxygen and morphine to improve oxygenation
- Beta-adrenergic blockers
- Prophylactic antibiotics
- Surgery: palliative for infants with potentially fatal hypoxic spells; goal to enhance blood flow to the lungs to reduce hypoxia; this is commonly accomplished by joining the subclavian artery to the pulmonary artery (Blalock-Taussig procedure)
- Complete corrective surgery relieving pulmonic stenosis and closing the VSD, directing left ventricular outflow to the aorta.

KEY PATIENT OUTCOMES

The patient (and his family) will:
- maintain hemodynamic stability
- foster improved cardiac blood flow
- express understanding of condition and treatment.

NURSING INTERVENTIONS

- Monitor vitals signs, oxygenation levels, and intake and output.
- Monitor for signs of blue spells.
- Monitor fluid status, enforcing fluid restrictions as appropriate.
- Provide postoperative care.
- Administer drug therapy.
- Explain the disorder and its treatment to the patient's parents. Inform them that their child will set his own exercise limits and will know when to rest.

PATIENT TEACHING

Be sure to cover:
- how to recognize serious hypoxic spells, which can cause dramatically increased cyanosis; deep, sighing respirations; and loss of consciousness

- preventing infective endocarditis and other infections, and keeping the child away from people with infections
- following good dental hygiene, and watching for ear, nose, and throat infections and dental caries, all of which require immediate treatment.

Thalassemia

DESCRIPTION

- Group of genetic disorders characterized by defective synthesis in one or more of the polypeptide chains needed for hemoglobin (Hb) production
- Most commonly occurs as a result of reduced or absent production of alpha or beta chains
- Affects Hb production and impairs red blood cell (RBC) synthesis
- Alpha-thalassemia more common in Blacks and Asians
- Beta-thalassemia more common in Mediterranean populations
- Beta-thalassemia classified three ways: major (also known as *Cooley's anemia*, *Mediterranean disease*, and *erythroblastic anemia*), intermedia, and minor

PATHOPHYSIOLOGY

- Total or partial deficiency of beta-polypeptide chain production impairs Hb synthesis and results in continual production of HbF, lasting even past the neonatal period.
- Normally, immunoglobulin synthesis switches from gamma- to beta-polypeptides at birth; this conversion doesn't happen in thalassemic infants as their RBCs are hypochromic and microcytic.

CAUSES

- Autosomal recessive disorder
- Thalassemia major and thalassemia intermedia: resulting from homozygous inheritance of the partially dominant autosomal gene responsible for this trait

■ Thalassemia minor: resulting from heterozygous inheritance of the same gene

ASSESSMENT FINDINGS

Thalassemia major

■ Healthy infant at birth; severe anemia, bone abnormalities, failure to thrive, and life-threatening complications developing during second 6 months of life
■ Pallor and jaundice (yellow skin and sclera) at ages 3 to 6 months
■ Splenomegaly or hepatomegaly with abdominal enlargement, frequent infections, bleeding tendencies (especially nosebleeds), anorexia
■ Small body and large head (characteristic features); possibly mental retardation
■ Features similar to Down syndrome in infants because of thickened bone at the base of the nose from bone marrow hyperactivity

Thalassemia intermedia

■ Some degree of anemia, jaundice, and splenomegaly
■ Possibly signs of hemosiderosis because of increased intestinal absorption of iron

Thalassemia minor

■ Mild anemia (usually produces no symptoms and is commonly overlooked; should be differentiated from iron deficiency anemia)

TEST RESULTS

■ Complete blood count shows decreased Hb level, hematocrit, and mean corpuscular volume.
■ Reticulocyte count is increased.
■ Serum iron level is normal or increased.
■ Total iron-binding capacity is normal.
■ Hb electrophoresis show decreased alpha- or beta-hemoglobulin chains.

FOCUS IN

SKULL CHANGES IN THALASSEMIA MAJOR

This illustration of an X-ray shows a characteristic skull abnormality in thalassemia major: diploetic fibers extend from internal lamina and resemble hair standing on end.

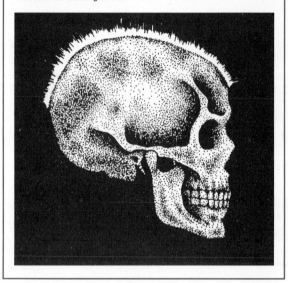

- In thalassemia major, X-rays of the skull and long bones show thinning and widening of the marrow space due to overactive bone marrow; long bones may exhibit areas of osteoporosis; phalanges may be deformed (rectangular or biconvex); bones of the skull and vertebrae may appear granular. (See *Skull changes in thalassemia major.*)

> **COLLABORATION** *The patient with thalassemia may require a referral to a dietitian to provide the parents with a diet that doesn't supply additional iron-rich foods. A hematologist may be consulted and genetic counseling may be recommended for the parents.*

TREATMENT

- No treatment for mild or moderate forms
- Iron supplements contraindicated in all forms
- Avoidance of iron-rich foods
- Avoidance of strenuous activities
- Transfusions of packed RBCs
- Surgery: splenectomy or bone marrow transplantation
- Drug therapy: deferoxamine (Desferal) for chelation therapy
- Referral to a hematologist
- Referral for genetic counseling

KEY PATIENT OUTCOMES

The patient will:
- develop no arrhythmias
- remain hemodynamically stable
- demonstrate age-appropriate skills and behaviors to the extent possible.

NURSING INTERVENTIONS

- Prepare for and administer multiple blood transfusions (every 3 to 4 weeks throughout the child's life).
- Administer chelating agents, such as Desferal, to remove excess iron from the system.
- Prepare the child for a possible splenectomy.
- Provide emotional support to help the patient and family cope with the chronic nature of the illness and need for lifelong transfusions.

PATIENT TEACHING

Be sure to cover:
- the disorder and its diagnosis and treatment
- the importance of good nutrition
- signs and symptoms of iron overload
- follow-up care

- with the parents of a young patient, various options for healthy physical and creative outlets. Such a child must avoid strenuous athletic activity. Reassure the parents that the child may be allowed to participate in less stressful activities.

Tonsillitis

DESCRIPTION

- Inflammation of the tonsils
- May be acute or chronic
- Typical viral infection: mild and of limited duration
- Commonly affects children between ages 5 and 10

PATHOPHYSIOLOGY

- Inflammatory response to cell damage by viruses or bacteria results in hyperemia and fluid exudation.

CAUSES

- Bacterial infection (group A beta-hemolytic streptococci)
- Tonsils tending to hypertrophy during childhood and atrophy after puberty
- Viral infection

ASSESSMENT FINDINGS

- Mild to severe sore throat
- Young child possibly stops eating
- Muscle and joint pain
- Chills
- Malaise
- Headache
- Pain, commonly referred to the ears
- Constant urge to swallow
- Constricted feeling in the back of the throat
- Fever
- Swollen, tender submandibular lymph nodes

- Generalized inflammation of pharyngeal wall
- Swollen tonsils projecting from between the pillars of the fauces and exuding white or yellow follicles
- Purulent drainage with application of pressure to tonsillar pillars
- Uvula possibly edematous and inflamed

TEST RESULTS

- Throat culture reveals infecting organism.
- Serum white blood cell count usually reveals leukocytosis.

TREATMENT

- Symptom relief
- Adequate fluid intake
- Rest periods as needed
- Aspirin or acetaminophen
- Antibiotics
- Possible tonsillectomy

KEY PATIENT OUTCOMES

The patient will:
- express feelings of increased comfort
- show no signs of aspiration
- maintain effective breathing pattern
- have balanced intake and output.

NURSING INTERVENTIONS

- Monitor hydration status and encourage oral fluids.
- Offer a child flavored drinks and ices.
- Provide humidification.
- Encourage gargling to soothe the throat and remove debris from tonsillar crypts.

After surgery
- Monitor vitals signs.

- Monitor respiratory status and maintain a patent airway.
- Prevent aspiration by side positioning.
- Keep suction equipment readily available.
- Provide water after gag reflex returns.
- Later, encourage nonirritating oral fluids.
- Avoid milk products and salty or irritating foods.
- Monitor pain status and provide analgesics for pain relief.
- Encourage deep-breathing exercises.
- Monitor for signs and symptoms of bleeding.

 ALERT *Immediately report excessive bleeding, increased pulse rate, or decreasing blood pressure.*

PATIENT TEACHING

Be sure to cover:
- the disorder and its diagnosis and treatment
- the importance of completing the entire course of antibiotics
- avoidance of irritants
- the need for soft foods for about 3 weeks after surgery to decrease risk of rebleeding
- drug administration, dosage, and possible adverse effects
- the possibility of throat discomfort and some bleeding after surgery
- expectation of a white scab to form in the throat 5 to 10 days after surgery
- the need to report bleeding, ear discomfort, or a fever that lasts 3 days or more.

 Life-threatening disorder

Tracheoesophageal fistula and esophageal atresia

DESCRIPTION

- Tracheoesophageal fistula: developmental anomaly characterized by an abnormal connection between the trachea and the esophagus; usually accompanies esophageal

FOCUS IN

TYPES OF
TRACHEOESOPHAGEAL ANOMALIES

Congenital malformations of the esophagus occur in about 1 in 4,000 live births. The American Academy of Pediatrics classifies the anatomic variations of tracheoesophageal anomalies according to type.

Type A
Esophageal atresia without fistula (7.7%)

Type B
Esophageal atresia with tracheoesophageal fistula to the proximal segment (0.8%)

Type C
Esophageal atresia with fistula to the distal segment (86.5%)

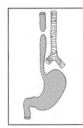

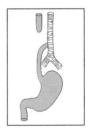

Type D
Esophageal atresia with fistula to both segments (0.7%)

Type E
Esophageal fistula without atresia (4.2%)

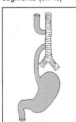

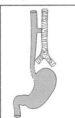

atresia, in which the esophagus is closed off at some point

■ Esophageal atresia: occurs in about 1 of 4,000 live births; approximately one-third of these neonates born prematurely

■ Numerous anatomic variations, most commonly, esophageal atresia with fistula to the distal segment (see *Types of tracheoesophageal anomalies*, page 230)

■ Two of the most serious surgical emergencies in neonates; requires immediate diagnosis and correction

PATHOPHYSIOLOGY

■ Tracheoesophageal fistula and esophageal atresia result from failure of the embryonic esophagus and trachea to develop and separate correctly.

■ Respiratory system development begins at about day 26 of gestation; abnormal development of the septum (during this time) may lead to tracheoesophageal fistula.

■ The most common abnormality is type C tracheoesophageal fistula with esophageal atresia, in which the upper section of the esophagus terminates in a blind pouch, and the lower section ascends from the stomach and connects with the trachea by a short fistulous tract.

■ In type A atresia, both esophageal segments are blind pouches, and neither connect to the airway.

■ In types B and D atresia, upper portion of the esophagus opens into the trachea; infants with this anomaly may experience life-threatening aspiration of saliva or food.

■ In type E (or H-type) tracheoesophageal fistula without atresia, the fistula may occur anywhere between the level of the cricoid cartilage and the mid-esophagus but is usually higher in the trachea than in the esophagus; such a fistula may be as small as a pinpoint.

CAUSES

■ Often found in infants with other anomalies, such as:
  – Congenital heart disease
  – Genitourinary abnormalities
  – Imperforate anus
  – Intestinal atresia

ASSESSMENT FINDINGS

■ Coughing and choking after eating
■ Respiratory distress
■ Drooling
■ Tracheoesophageal fistula:
  – Type B (proximal fistula) and Type D (fistula to both segments): immediate aspiration of saliva into the airway and bacterial pneumonitis
  – Type E (or H-type): repeated episodes of pneumonitis, pulmonary infection, and abdominal infection; choking followed by cyanosis
■ Esophageal atresia
  – Type A: normal swallowing, excessive drooling, possible respiratory distress
  – Type C: seemingly normal swallowing followed shortly afterward by coughing, struggling, cyanosis, lack of breathing

TEST RESULTS

■ Chest X-rays may show a dilated, air-filled upper esophageal pouch, pneumonia in the right upper lobe, or bilateral pneumonitis; both pneumonia and pneumonitis suggest aspiration.
■ Abdominal X-rays show gas in the bowel in a distal fistula (type C) but none in a proximal fistula (type B) or in atresia without fistula (type A).
■ Cinefluorography may define the tip of the upper pouch and differentiate between overflow aspiration from a blind end (atresia) and aspiration from passage of liquids through a tracheoesophageal fistula.
■ A size 6 or 8 French catheter passed through the nose meets an obstruction (esophageal atresia) about 4″ to 5″ (10 to 12.5 cm) distal to the nostrils; aspirate of gastric contents is less acidic than normal.

TREATMENT

■ I.V. fluids

- Supine position with the head low to facilitate drainage or with the head elevated to prevent aspiration
- After surgery: placement of a suction catheter in the upper esophageal pouch to control secretions and prevent aspiration
- Antibiotics for superimposed infection
- Tracheoesophageal fistula and esophageal atresia requiring surgical correction and are usually surgical emergencies (The type and timing of the surgical procedure depend on the nature of the anomaly, the patient's general condition, and the presence of coexisting congenital defects.)
- In premature neonates (nearly 33% of infants with this anomaly) who are poor surgical risks, correction of combined tracheoesophageal fistula and esophageal atresia occurring in two stages: first, gastrostomy (for gastric decompression, prevention of reflux, and feeding) and closure of the fistula; then, 1 to 2 months later, anastomosis of the esophagus
- Correction of esophageal atresia alone requiring anastomosis of the proximal and distal esophageal segments in one or two stages; end-to-end anastomosis commonly producing postoperative stricture; end-to-side anastomosis less likely to do so
- If the esophageal ends are widely separated, treatment possibly including a colonic interposition (grafting a piece of the colon) or elongation of the proximal segment of the esophagus by bougienage

KEY PATIENT OUTCOMES

The patient (and his parents or family) will:
- develop no respiratory complications
- remain hemodynamically stable
- express understanding of disorder and treatment.

NURSING INTERVENTIONS

- Monitor respiratory status and administer oxygen as needed.

- Perform pulmonary physiotherapy and suctioning, as needed.
- Provide a humid environment.
- Administer antibiotics and parenteral fluids.
- Monitor intake and output.
- Maintain gastrostomy tube feedings.
- After surgery, monitor the chest tubes and for signs of complications.
- Offer the parents support and guidance in dealing with their infant's acute illness. Encourage them to participate in care and to hold and touch the infant as much as possible to facilitate bonding.
- Instruct the parents that X-rays are required about 10 days after surgery, and again 1 and 3 months later, to evaluate the effectiveness of surgical repair.

PATIENT TEACHING

Be sure to cover:
- the disorder and its diagnosis and treatment
- feeding procedures
- recognizing and reporting complications
- proper positioning.

Transposition of the great vessels

DESCRIPTION

- Aorta rising from the right ventricle and the pulmonary artery from the left ventricle, producing two noncommunicating circulatory systems (see *A look at transposition of the great vessels*, page 234)

PATHOPHYSIOLOGY

- The transposed pulmonary artery carries oxygenated blood back to the lungs, rather than to the left side of the heart.
- The transposed aorta returns the unoxygenated blood to the systemic circulation, rather than to the lungs.

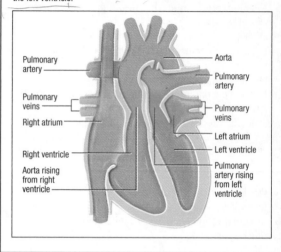

FOCUS IN

LOOKING AT TRANSPOSITION OF THE GREAT VESSELS

This illustration shows transposition of the great vessels, in which the aorta rises from the right ventricle, and the pulmonary artery rises from the left ventricle.

Pulmonary artery

Pulmonary veins

Right atrium

Right ventricle

Aorta rising from right ventricle

Aorta

Pulmonary artery

Pulmonary veins

Left atrium

Left ventricle

Pulmonary artery rising from left ventricle

■ Communication between the pulmonary and systemic circulation is necessary for survival; the presence of other congenital defects, such as atrial septal defect (ASD) or ventricular septal defect (VSD), is necessary to sustain life.

CAUSES

■ Unknown

ASSESSMENT FINDINGS

■ Cyanosis from birth and tachypnea (worsens with crying)
■ Gallop rhythm
■ Tachycardia

- Dyspnea
- Hepatomegaly
- Cardiomegaly
- Murmurs of ASD, VSD, or patent ductus arteriosus, loud second heart sound
- Diminished exercise tolerance
- Fatigue
- Clubbing

TEST RESULTS

- Chest X-rays reveal increased pulmonary vascular markings; they also show right atrial and ventricular enlargement, causing a characteristic oblong appearance to the heart.
- Electrocardiogram may indicate right axis deviation and right ventricular hypertrophy.
- Echocardiography demonstrates the reversed position of the aorta and pulmonary artery and detects other cardiac defects.
- Cardiac catheterization reveals decreased oxygen saturation in left ventricular blood and aortic blood; increased right atrial, right ventricular, and pulmonary artery oxygen saturation; right ventricular systolic pressure equal to systemic pressure; and transposed vessels and other heart defects (via dye injection).

TREATMENT

- Alprostadil (Prostin VR/Pediatric) to maintain patency of the ductus arteriosus
- Prophylactic antibiotics to prevent infective endocarditis
- Atrial balloon septostomy done during cardiac catheterization to enlarge the patent foramen ovale, which improves oxygenation by allowing greater mixing of the pulmonic and systemic circulations
- Corrective surgery to redirect blood flow by switching the position of the major blood vessels

KEY PATIENT OUTCOMES

The patient will:
- maintain hemodynamic stability
- improve oxygenation.

NURSING INTERVENTIONS

- Prepare the child for cardiac catheterization or surgery, explaining the heart defect and answering any questions.
- Monitor vital signs, pulse oximetry, and intake and output.
- Assess cardiovascular and respiratory statuses.
- Monitor fluid status, enforcing fluid restrictions as appropriate.
- Weigh the child daily.
- Weigh soiled diapers.
- Organize physical care and anticipate the need to reduce the child's oxygen demands.
- Give the child high-calorie foods that are easy to ingest and digest.
- Encourage parents to help their child assume new activity levels and independence.
- Offer emotional support.

PATIENT TEACHING

Be sure to cover (with the parents):
- the disorder and its diagnosis and treatment
- the importance of regular checkups to monitor cardiovascular status
- protecting the infant from infection and giving antibiotics.

Tricuspid atresia

DESCRIPTION

- Failure of the tricuspid valve to develop, preventing blood from entering the right ventricle from the right atrium

PATHOPHYSIOLOGY

- Deoxygenated blood shunts from the right atrium through an atrial septal defect or a patent foramen ovale to the left atrium, where it mixes with oxygenated blood.
- Mixed blood then passes to the left ventricle through a ventricular septal defect to the right ventricle, pulmonary artery, and lungs; or, mixed blood from the aorta refluxes back through a patent ductus arteriosus to the lungs.

CAUSES

- Unknown
- May be associated with pulmonic stenosis or transposition of the great vessels

ASSESSMENT FINDINGS

- Cyanosis
- Tachycardia
- Dyspnea
- Heart murmur

TEST RESULTS

- Chest X-rays show an enlarged right atrium and decreased pulmonary blood flow.
- Electrocardiogram indicates left-axis deviation and absent right ventricular forces.
- Echocardiography provides visualization of the defect and shunting.

TREATMENT

- Medications: alprostadil (Prostin VR/Pediatric) to maintain ductal patency
- Surgery: repair including a subclavian-to-pulmonary artery shunt to improve blood flow to the lungs, or the Fontan procedure, which restructures the right side of the heart

KEY PATIENT OUTCOMES

The patient will:
- maintain hemodynamic stability
- maintain adequate ventilation and oxygenation.

NURSING INTERVENTIONS

- Explain the heart defect and answer any questions.
- Monitor vital signs, pulse oximetry, and intake and output.
- Assess cardiovascular and respiratory statuses.
- Monitor fluid status, enforcing fluid restrictions as appropriate.
- Weigh the child daily.
- Weigh soiled diapers.
- Organize physical care and anticipate the need to reduce the child's oxygen demands.

PATIENT TEACHING

Be sure to cover (with the parents):
- the disorder and its diagnosis and treatment
- signs and symptoms that should be reported.

 Life-threatening disorder

Trisomy 18 syndrome

DESCRIPTION

- Second most common multiple malformation syndrome
- Full trisomy 18 in most affected infants: involves an extra (third) copy of chromosome 18 in each cell; partial trisomy 18 (with varying phenotypes) and translocation types also reported
- Intrauterine growth retardation, congenital heart defects, microcephaly, and other malformations occurring in most infants with this disorder
- Full trisomy 18 syndrome generally fatal or extremely poor prognosis (Thirty to 50% of infants die within the

first 2 months and 90% die within the first year; most surviving patients are profoundly mentally retarded.)
- Risk typically increasing with maternal age (mean maternal age 32½)
- Incidence ranging from 1 in 3,000 to 8,000 neonates, with three to four females affected for every male
- Also known as *Edwards' syndrome*

PATHOPHYSIOLOGY

- Most cases of trisomy 18 result from spontaneous meitotic nondisjunction, producing an extra copy of chromosome 18 in each cell.

CAUSES

- Chromosomal abnormality

ASSESSMENT FINDINGS

- Growth retardation, which begins in utero and remains significant after birth
- Initial hypotonia soon giving way to hypertonia
- Microcephaly and dolichocephaly
- Micrognathia
- Short, narrow nose with upturned nares
- Unilateral or bilateral cleft lip and palate
- Low-set, slightly pointed ears
- Short neck
- Conspicuous clenched hand with overlapping fingers (commonly seen on ultrasound)
- Cystic hygroma
- Choroid plexus cysts (also seen in some normal infants)

TEST RESULTS

- Karyotype, done either prenatally or on peripheral blood lymphocytes or skin fibroblasts in a neonate or an aborted fetus, confirms diagnosis.
- Results are abnormal (but not diagnostic) in multiple-marker maternal serum screening tests, involving differ-

ent combinations of alpha-fetoprotein, human chorionic gonadotropin, and unconjugated estriol.
■ Ultrasound commonly reveals variable abnormalities in the fetus.

TREATMENT

■ Emotional support for the family
■ Nutrition maintenance using gavage feedings

KEY PATIENT OUTCOMES

The patient will:
■ function at the highest level possible
■ appear comfortable.

NURSING INTERVENTIONS

■ Monitor intake and output.
■ Monitor growth.
■ Allow adequate time for the parents to bond with and hold their child.
■ Provide emotional support to the family.
■ Refer the parents of a child affected with trisomy 18 syndrome for genetic counseling.
■ Refer the parents to a social worker or grief counselor for additional support if needed.
■ Refer the parents to the Support Organization for Trisomy 18, 13, and Related Disorders (S.O.F.T.) national support program.

PATIENT TEACHING

Be sure to cover:
■ the disorder and its diagnosis and treatment
■ home care and feeding techniques.

Varicella

DESCRIPTION

- Acute, highly contagious viral infection
- Same virus that causes chickenpox, which is thought to become latent until the sixth decade of life or later, causing herpes zoster (shingles)
- Occurs through direct contact (primarily with respiratory secretions, less commonly with skin lesions) and indirect contact (airborne)
- Congenital varicella possible in infants whose mothers had acute infections in first or early second trimester
- Neonatal infection rare, probably due to transient maternal immunity
- Most commonly occurs in children ages 5 to 9, but may occur at any age
- Affects all races and both sexes equally
- Seasonal distribution varied; in temperate areas, incidence higher during late winter and spring
- Also known as *chickenpox*

PATHOPHYSIOLOGY

- Localized replication of the virus occurs (probably in the nasopharynx), leading to seeding of the reticuloendothelial system and development of viremia.
- Diffuse and scattered skin lesions result with vesicles involving the corium and dermis with degenerative changes (ballooning) and infection of localized blood vessels.
- Necrosis and epidermal hemorrhage result; vesicles eventually rupture and release fluid or are reabsorbed.
- Incubation period lasts 10 to 21 days.
- Infection is communicable from 48 hours before lesions erupt until after vesicles crust over.

CAUSES

- Varicella-zoster herpesvirus

ASSESSMENT FINDINGS

- Recent exposure to someone with chickenpox
- Malaise
- Pruritus
- Headache
- Anorexia
- Temperature 101° to 103° F (38.3° to 39.4° C)
- Crops of small, erythematous macules on the trunk or scalp
- Macules progressing to papules and then clear vesicles on an erythematous base (so-called dewdrops on rose petals)
- Vesicles becoming cloudy and breaking easily; then scabs forming
- Rash spreading to face and, rarely, to extremities
- Rash containing a combination of red papules, vesicles, and scabs in various stages
- Ulcers on mucous membranes of the mouth, conjunctivae, and genitalia

TEST RESULTS

- Virus is isolated from vesicular fluid within the first 3 to 4 days of the rash.
- Giemsa stain distinguishes the varicella zoster virus from the vaccinia variola virus.
- Serum samples contain antibodies 7 days after the onset of symptoms.
- Serologic testing differentiates rickettsial pox from varicella.

TREATMENT

- Strict isolation until all vesicles crust over; for congenital chickenpox, no isolation
- Increased fluid intake
- Rest periods when fatigued
- Antipruritics
- Antibiotics if complications develop, such as infections or pneumonia

- Analgesic and antipyretic
- Acyclovir (Zovirax)
- Varicella zoster immune globulin

KEY PATIENT OUTCOMES

The patient will:
- report or demonstrate an increased energy level
- exhibit improved or healed lesions or wounds
- interact with family and peers to decrease feelings of isolation
- express or demonstrate increased comfort.

NURSING INTERVENTIONS

- Monitor the patient for signs and symptoms of dehydration, signs and symptoms of infection, adverse drug reactions, and complications. Also monitor the patient's skin integrity and response to treatment.
- Observe an immunocompromised patient for manifestations of such complications as pneumonitis and meningitis, and report them immediately.
- Provide skin care comfort measures (calamine lotion, cornstarch, sponge baths, or showers).
- Administer varicella zoster immune globulin if ordered.
- Institute strict isolation measures until all skin lesions have crusted.
- Prevent exposure to pregnant women.

PATIENT TEACHING

Be sure to cover:
- the disorder and its diagnosis and treatment
- how to correctly apply topical antipruritic medications
- the importance of good hygiene and keeping the child's fingernails trimmed
- the need for the child to avoid scratching the lesions
- the parents' need to watch for and immediately report signs of complications (severe skin pain and burning that

may indicate a serious secondary infection and require prompt medical attention)

▨ the need for parents to refrain from giving the child aspirin because of its association with Reye's syndrome (an acute encephalopathy with cerebral cortex swelling but without inflammation, accompanied by impaired liver function and hyperammonemia)

▨ signs and symptoms of Reye's syndrome and the need to immediately report them to a physician.

Ventricular septal defect

DESCRIPTION

▨ Heart condition that allows blood to shunt between the left and right ventricles through an opening in the septum

▨ Most common congenital heart disorder

▨ Coexists with additional birth defects, especially Down syndrome and other autosomal trisomies, renal anomalies, and cardiac defects, such as patent ductus arteriosus and coarctation of the aorta

▨ Affects 2% to 7% of live births; slightly more common in females

▨ Also known as *VSD*

PATHOPHYSIOLOGY

▨ Ventricular septum fails to close completely by the 8th week of gestation, as it would normally.

▨ VSDs are located in the membranous or muscular portion of the ventricular septum and vary in size.

▨ Some defects close spontaneously; in other defects, the entire septum is absent, creating a single ventricle.

▨ Large VSD shunt eventually causes biventricular heart failure and cyanosis.

▨ VSD isn't readily apparent at birth because right and left ventricular pressures appear approximately equal, so blood doesn't shunt through the defect.

- As pulmonary vasculature relaxes (between 4 and 8 weeks after birth) right ventricular pressure decreases, allowing blood to shunt from the left to the right ventricle.

CAUSES

- Congenital defect

ASSESSMENT FINDINGS

- Dyspnea
- Cyanosis
- Slow weight gain
- Feeding difficulties
- Rapid grunting respirations
- Prominent anterior chest wall
- Clubbing
- With a large VSD, audible murmurs (at least a grade 3 pansystolic), loudest at the fourth intercostal space, usually with a thrill; pulmonic component of second heart sound (S_2) loud and widely split
- With fixed pulmonary hypertension, diastolic murmur possibly audible on auscultation, systolic murmur becoming quieter, and S_2 greatly accentuated
- Displacement of the point of maximal impulse to the left
- Typical murmur associated with a VSD, blowing or rumbling and varying in frequency
- In the neonate, moderately loud early systolic murmur along the lower left sternal border, possibly becoming louder and longer about the second or third day after birth
- In infants, murmur possibly loudest near the base of the heart, which may suggest pulmonary stenosis
- In small VSD, functional murmur or characteristic loud, harsh systolic murmur

TEST RESULTS

- Chest X-rays appear normal with small defects; with large VSDs, they show cardiomegaly, left atrial and left ventricular enlargement, and prominent pulmonary vascular markings.

■ Echocardiography may detect a large VSD and its location in the septum, estimate the size of a left-to-right shunt, suggest pulmonary hypertension, and identify associated lesions and complications.

■ Electrocardiogram is normal in children with small VSDs; in large VSDs, it shows left and right ventricular hypertrophy, suggesting pulmonary hypertension.

■ Cardiac catheterization determines the size and exact location of the VSD, calculates the degree of shunting by comparing the blood oxygen saturation in each ventricle, determines the extent of pulmonary hypertension, and detects associated defects.

TREATMENT

■ If the child has other defects and will benefit from delaying surgery, pulmonary artery banding to normalize pressures and flow distal to the band and prevent pulmonary vascular disease

■ Low-sodium diet

■ Fluid restriction

■ Activity as tolerated

■ Digoxin (Lanoxin)

■ Diuretics

■ Antibiotics

■ Surgery: for small defects, simple suture closure; for moderate to large defects, insertion of a patch graft using cardiopulmonary bypass

■ After surgery: analgesics, antibiotics, and vasopressors

KEY PATIENT OUTCOMES

The patient will:

■ maintain adequate ventilation

■ maintain hemodynamic stability

■ remain free from signs and symptoms of infection.

NURSING INTERVENTIONS

- Monitor the patient's vital signs, intake and output, and respiratory status.
- Monitor for signs of heart failure.
- After surgery, monitor cardiac rhythm, oxygenation, and hemodynamics.
- Provide emotional support.
- Give prescribed drugs.

PATIENT TEACHING

Be sure to cover:
- preventing complications until the child is scheduled for surgery or the defect closes
- watching for signs of heart failure, such as poor feeding, sweating, and heavy breathing
- drug administration, dosage, and possible adverse effects
- letting the child engage in normal activities
- the importance of prophylactic antibiotics before and after surgery.

Wilms' tumor

DESCRIPTION

- Malignant mixed tumor of the kidney
- Most common intra-abdominal tumor in children; average age at diagnosis is 2 to 4 years
- Usually appears on left kidney and is usually unilateral
- Remains encapsulated for a long time
- Excellent prognosis if metastasis hasn't occurred
- Also called *nephroblastoma*

PATHOPHYSIOLOGY

- Embryonal cancer of the kidney originates during fetal life.

- In early stages, the tumor is well encapsulated but may later spread into the lymph nodes, renal vein, or vena cava; the tumor may metastasize to the lungs or other sites.
- Staging
  - In stage I, the tumor is limited to one kidney.
  - In stage II, the tumor extends beyond the kidney but can be completely excised.
  - In stage III, the tumor has spread but is confined to the abdomen and lymph nodes.
  - In stage IV, the tumor has metastasized to the lung, liver, bone, and brain.
  - In stage V, the tumor involves both kidneys.

CAUSES

- Associated with several other congenital anomalies, including cryptorchidism and hypospadias
- Genetic inheritance

ASSESSMENT FINDINGS

- Nontender abdominal mass (most common), usually midline near the liver; commonly identified by the parent while bathing or dressing the child
- Enlarged abdomen
- High blood pressure
- Vomiting
- Hematuria
- Anemia
- Constipation

TEST RESULTS

- Abdominal ultrasound and computed tomography scan determine tumor size, location, and possible metastasis.
- Excretory urography assesses function of the normal kidney.

- Blood tests reveal polycythemia if tumor secretes erythropoietin.

TREATMENT

- Surgery: nephrectomy to remove the affected kidney and tumor in stage I and II
- Radiation: indicated with large tumors or those that weren't completely surgically resected
- Chemotherapy

KEY PATIENT OUTCOMES

The patient (or his family) will:
- avoid complications
- express understanding of the disease process and treatment regimen.

NURSING INTERVENTIONS

Preoperative
- Don't palpate the abdomen, and prevent others from doing so; it may disseminate cancer cells to other sites.
- Handle and bathe the child carefully.
- Loosen clothing near the abdomen.
- Prepare the family for a nephrectomy within 24 to 48 hours of diagnosis.

Postoperative
- Provide routine care as for a nephrectomy patient.
- Be aware that chemotherapy and radiation will follow.

PATIENT TEACHING

Be sure to cover:
- the disorder and its diagnosis and treatment
- the importance of handling the child carefully during bathing and dressing to avoid pressure on the abdominal area.

Part two

Treatments

Bowel resection

DESCRIPTION

■ Surgical procedure to remove a portion of the large intestine and connect, or resect, the healthy ends of the bowel
■ Preferred surgical technique for localized bowel cancer, but not for widespread carcinoma, which usually requires massive resection and a temporary or permanent colostomy or an ileostomy
■ Unlike the child undergoing total colectomy or more extensive surgery, the child undergoing simple resection and anastomosis usually retaining normal bowel function

PURPOSE

■ Helps to treat localized obstructive disorders, including diverticulosis, intestinal polyps, bowel adhesions, and malignant or benign intestinal lesions
■ Also performed to treat traumatic bowel injuries and ulcerative colitis that's refractory to medical therapy

PATIENT PREPARATION

■ Whenever the situation permits, arrange for the child and his parents to visit the health care facility before he's admitted for surgery.
■ Provide an age-appropriate explanation of why the surgery is being performed, and encourage the child and his parents to ask questions.
■ Reassure the child that he won't wake up during surgery, but that the physician knows how and when to wake him up afterward.
■ Administer antibiotics to reduce intestinal flora and a laxative or enemas to remove fecal contents.

PROCEDURE

- During surgery, the child is placed under general anesthesia.
- Through an abdominal incision, the surgeon removes, or resects, the diseased portion of the intestine and connects the healthy ends back together.
- In some cases, a temporary colostomy is created to spare the colon of its digestive function, allowing it to heal from the resection. A future surgery is performed to close the colostomy.
- In some cases, bowel resection may also be performed laparoscopically.

POSTPROCEDURE CARE

- For the first few days after surgery, monitor the child's intake, output, and daily weight.
- Maintain fluid and electrolyte balance through I.V. replacement therapy, and check regularly for signs of dehydration, such as decreased urine output and poor skin turgor.
- Keep the nasogastric (NG) tube patent

   ALERT *Warn the child that he should never attempt to reposition a dislodged tube himself.*
- Observe the child for signs of peritonitis or sepsis caused by leakage of bowel contents into the abdominal cavity. Sepsis may also result from wicking of colonic bacteria up the NG tube to the oral cavity and can be prevented with frequent mouth and tube care.
- Provide meticulous wound care, changing dressings when needed. Check dressings and drainage sites frequently for signs of infection (purulent drainage, foul odor) and fecal drainage.
- Watch for sudden fever, especially when accompanied by abdominal pain and tenderness.
- Regularly assess the child for postresection obstruction. Examine the abdomen for distention and rigidity, auscul-

tate for bowel sounds, and note the passage of any flatus
and stool.
■ After the child regains peristalsis and bowel function,
help him avoid constipation and straining during defecation. Encourage him to drink plenty of fluids, and administer a stool softener or other laxative, as ordered. Note
and record the frequency and amount of all bowel movements as well as characteristics of the stool.
■ Encourage regular coughing and deep breathing to prevent atelectasis; remind the child and his parents to splint
the incision site as necessary, and provide assistance as
needed.
■ Assess the child's pain and provide analgesics, as ordered.
■ Encourage the child and his parents to maintain the prescribed semibland diet until his bowel has healed completely (usually 4 to 8 weeks after surgery). Stress the
need to avoid carbonated beverages and gas-producing
foods.

Casting

DESCRIPTION

■ May be required for a fractured bone, weakness, paralysis, or spasticity
■ Also used after corrective orthopedic surgery
■ Possibly made of plaster or, more commonly, of synthetic
material, such as fiberglass or plastic; also made of poly-
ester and cotton impregnated with water-activated poly-
urethane resin

PURPOSE

■ To help correct, maintain, and support the body part in a
functional position

PATIENT PREPARATION

- To allay their fears, explain each step of the procedure to the child and his parents before the cast is applied.
- Cover the appropriate parts of the child's bedding and gown with a linen-saver pad.
- The skin that will be casted must be clean and dry.
- Assess the condition of the child's skin in the affected area, noting redness, contusions, or open wounds, to aid in evaluating complaints he may have after the cast is applied.
- To establish baseline measurements, assess the child's neurovascular status.
- Palpate the distal pulses and assess the color, temperature, and capillary refill of the appropriate fingers or toes.
- Inform the child and his parents that depending on which type of material is used, drying time for the cast may be as little as 7 minutes or as much as 72 hours.

PROCEDURE

- Explain each step of the procedure during application of the cast.
- If plaster is used, explain that the child will experience a sense of warmth when it's first applied. Tell him that the sensation of warmth will usually subside after 15 to 30 minutes.
- If a closed reduction is necessary, explain to the child that there will be some pain.
- Allow the parents to remain close to the child and hold his hand to help reduce anxiety as the physician applies the cast.
- As a plaster cast dries, the cast and the child will feel cold.

POSTPROCEDURE CARE

- Assess the casted area every 30 minutes for the first few hours, then every hour for 24 hours, then every 4 hours for an additional 48 hours.
- A child in a body cast must be turned every 2 hours to promote drying.
- Assess the child for pain, color, paresthesia, and paralysis, and check the pulse and capillary refill distal to the cast.
- Drainage from a wound under the cast should be noted.
- If there are any signs and symptoms of compromise in the affected area, notify the physician immediately. Also notify the physician if cracking or crumbling is noted in the cast.
- Pain that's nonspecific and unrelieved with analgesics and feelings of cast tightness must be reported to and evaluated by the physician.
- Assess for signs of skin breakdown, a common occurrence. The area around the cast edges will typically become pink and warm and swelling may also occur.
- Provide interventions to prevent further breakdown.
- Because cool air can relieve the itchiness that accompanies casting, instruct the parents to use a blow-dryer on a cool setting to blow cool air down into the cast.
- Advise against putting any object down the cast in an attempt to scratch.
- Explain to the child and his parents that the cast must be worn as recommended and shouldn't be removed.
- A plaster cast must be kept dry. Cover it with protective plastic during bathing. If soiled, a plaster cast may be cleaned with a damp cloth.
- If the child received a synthetic cast that may be immersed in water, instruct the child and his family to dry the cast following bathing or immersion by using a blow-dryer on cool setting.
- Don't use lotions or powders in or on a cast.

- Inform the child and his parents that there should be no weight bearing on the affected part until the cast has dried, and discourage overly rigorous activities to prevent dislodgment or malalignment of a fracture.
- Range-of-motion exercises should be used on non-affected extremities.
- After the cast is dry, rough areas may be cushioned with tape or elastic bandages.
- When the fracture is healed, prepare the child for cast removal with the cast cutter. Let him hear the noise and feel the vibrations and show him (on your body) how the cutter stops when it touches skin and won't, therefore, cut anything except the cast.
- Inform the child that his skin will look different after cast removal, especially if it has been in the cast for weeks. Reassure him that this is temporary, and apply baby oil, then gently wash the area to remove the dead skin.
- Instruct the child and his parents in an exercise regimen to help regain muscle strength and function following the injury.

Cleft lip and cleft palate repair

DESCRIPTION

- Occurs when the bone and tissue of the upper jaw and palate fail to fuse completely at the midline
- Cheiloplasty (cleft lip repair surgery) and palatoplasty (cleft palate repair surgery) are performed to correct these defects
- Defects being partial or complete, unilateral or bilateral, and possibly involving just the lip, just the palate, or both
- Defects that originate in the second month of pregnancy involve the front and sides of the face and the palatine shelves fusing imperfectly

■ Causes: congenital defects, prenatal exposure to teratogens, or a potential relation to another chromosomal abnormality.

PURPOSE

■ Minimize and reduce complications caused by cleft lip and cleft palate, such as: speech defects; dental and orthodontic problems; nasal defects; alterations in hearing; shock, guilt, and grief for the parents that may interfere with parent-child bonding; and increased risk of aspiration, upper respiratory infections, and otitis media

PATIENT PREPARATION

Cheiloplasty

■ Feed the infant slowly and in an upright position to decrease the risk of aspiration.
■ Special feeding devices may be used to reduce difficulty with feeding.
■ Burp the infant frequently during feeding to eliminate swallowed air and decrease the risk of emesis.
■ Use gavage feedings if oral feedings are unsuccessful.
■ Give a small amount of water after feedings to prevent formula from accumulating and becoming a medium for bacterial growth.
■ Give small, frequent feedings to promote adequate nutrition and prevent tiring.
■ Hold the infant while feeding.
■ Promote sucking between meals, which is important for speech development.

Palatoplasty

■ Be aware that the child must be weaned from the bottle or breast and able to drink from a cup before cleft palate surgery.

- Feed an infant with a cleft palate nipple or a Teflon implant to enhance nutritional intake.
- Teach the parents that the child is susceptible to pathogens and otitis media from the altered position of the eustachian tubes.

PROCEDURE

Cheiloplasty

- Cheiloplasty (cleft lip repair surgery) is performed most commonly by one of two procedures: the Tennison-Randall triangular flap (Z-plasty), or the Millard rotational advancement technique.
- The surgery is performed between birth and age 3 months to unite the lip and gum edges.
- Many surgeons delay lip repairs for 8 to 10 weeks to allow the infant to grow and mature, thereby minimizing surgical and anesthesia risks, ruling out associated congenital anomalies, and allowing time for parental bonding.
- Repair is performed in anticipation of tooth eruption, providing a route for adequate nutrition and sucking.
- If cleft lip is detected on sonogram while the infant is in utero, fetal repair may be possible.

Palatoplasty

- Palatoplasty (cleft palate repair surgery) is commonly scheduled between 12 and 18 months before speech patterns develop. However, the timing of repair is controversial and some surgeons will perform repairs on neonates.
- Some surgeons repair cleft palate in two steps, repairing the soft palate between ages 6 and 18 months and the hard palate as late as age 5.
- Make sure that the child is gaining weight and free from ear and respiratory infections before surgery.
- Surgery must be coupled with speech therapy.

POSTPROCEDURE CARE

Cheiloplasty
- Maintain a patent airway; edema or narrowing of a previously large airway may make the infant appear to be in distress.
- Observe for cyanosis to detect signs of respiratory compromise as the infant begins to breathe through his nose.
- Maintain an intact suture line; keep the infant's hands away from his mouth by using restraints (as ordered, per facility policy) or pinning his sleeves to his shirt.
- Suture care may include antibiotic ointment application after mouth care.
- Anticipate the infant's needs; this will help prevent crying.
- Give extra care and support because the infant's emotional needs can't be met by sucking.
- When feeding resumes, use a syringe with tubing to administer foods at the side of the mouth to prevent trauma to the suture line; never use a straw for feedings.
- Place the infant on his right side after feedings to prevent aspiration.
- Monitor for pain, and give pain medication as prescribed.

Palatoplasty
- Position the child on his abdomen or side to maintain a patent airway.
- Assess for signs of altered oxygenation to promote good respiration.
- Use a cup for feeding to prevent injury to the suture line; don't use a nipple or pacifier.
- Keep hard or pointed objects (oral thermometers, utensils, straws, frozen dessert sticks) away from the child's mouth to prevent trauma to the suture line.
- Use elbow restraints to keep the child's hands out of his mouth.
- Provide soft toys to prevent injury.
- Distract or hold the child to try to keep his tongue away from the roof of his mouth.

- Start the child on clear liquids and progress to a soft diet.
- Rinse the suture line by giving the child a sip of water after each feeding to prevent infection.
- Don't brush the child's teeth for 1 or 2 weeks after surgery.
- Help the parents deal with their feelings about the child's disability, and refer the parents to a social worker who can guide them to community resources, if needed.

Heart transplantation

DESCRIPTION

- Indications in children: cardiomyopathy and end-stage congenital heart disease
- Extensive cardiac evaluation performed first to determine if there are other medical or surgical options to treat the heart condition
- Remaining body systems assessed and evaluated to determine if other problems exist that may affect the success of the transplantation
- Eligible candidates placed on the United Network for Organ Sharing list to match a donor with the recipient

PURPOSE

- Serving as a treatment option for infants and children who have a limited life expectancy after other medical and surgical options have been explored to treat their worsening heart failure

PATIENT PREPARATION

- The child and his parents must be prepared thoroughly for this major procedure and must include a realistic representation of the procedure's risks and benefits.
- Include a brief visit to the coronary intensive care unit (CICU) and, if possible, the child should be introduced to the nurses who will be providing his care.

- Parents should be made aware of the visiting policies in the CICU and should be assisted in making arrangements to spend as much time with their child as possible.

PROCEDURE

- There are two surgical options for heart transplantation:
  - *Orthotopic procedure*, in which the diseased heart is removed in its entirety and a new, healthy heart from a donor (who has been declared brain dead) is implanted. Weight and blood type are factors used to match donor and recipient.
  - *Heterotopic procedure* (rarely performed in children), in which the patient's own heart is kept in place and a "piggyback" heart is implanted to serve as an additional pumping organ to assist the diseased heart.

POSTPROCEDURE CARE

- Monitor the child closely for signs of rejection, infection, and adverse reactions from immunosuppressive therapy.
- Monitor vital signs, intake and output, arterial blood gas levels, and laboratory values.
- Restrict fluids as ordered to prevent hypervolemia and heart strain.
- Provide adequate rest periods with gradual activity increases to further decrease the workload of the heart.
- Encourage compliance with the complex drug regimen required, especially in adolescents.
- Provide emotional support to the child and his family and offer resources for additional support.
- Help the parents (and the child, if age appropriate) come to terms with the reality that someone had to die for a heart to become available.
- The first 6 months to 1 year after the heart transplantation are the most intense and risky because complications are most common during this time and the family is adjusting to a totally new lifestyle requiring life-time management.

- The leading cause of demise after heart transplantation is organ rejection. Because life-long immunosuppressive therapy is required, infection is always a risk.

Heart valve replacement

DESCRIPTION

- Heart valve replacement with a prosthetic valve for a patient with heart valve narrowing (stenosis) and heart valve leaking (insufficiency)
- Valvular problems commonly caused by rheumatic fever and congenital heart defects; may also be caused by heart failure and infective endocarditis

PURPOSE

- To prevent the occurrence, or worsening, of heart failure in children with valvular stenosis or insufficiency and severe, unmanageable symptoms

PATIENT PREPARATION

- Whenever the situation permits, arrange for the child and his parents to visit the health care facility before he's admitted for surgery. This visit should include seeing and touching the equipment that will be used in the postoperative period.
- Provide an age-appropriate explanation of why the surgery is being performed, and encourage the child and his parents to ask questions.
- Reassure the child that he won't wake up during surgery, but that the physician knows how and when to wake him up afterward.
- Prepare the child for the equipment he'll wake up with; tell him that he'll be connected to a cardiac monitor, have I.V. lines and an indwelling urinary catheter, and will be connected to a machine that will help him breathe.

PROCEDURE

- A heart valve is replaced when the child's valve can't be repaired.
- The child's diseased valve is removed and replaced with a mechanical valve.
- Know that mechanical valves are strong and are designed to last a lifetime; they're made out of titanium, pyrolytic carbon, or Dacron.
- Another type of replacement valve is the biological valve, which is made of pig, cow, or human donor tissue; this type of valve isn't recommended for children because their durability is lower than mechanical valves.

POSTPROCEDURE CARE

- After surgery, monitor the child's vital signs, cardiac rhythms, and intake and output.
- Monitor arterial blood gas values, daily weight, blood chemistries, chest X-rays, and pulmonary artery catheter readings.
- Assess the chest tubes and urinary catheter output.
- Assess for signs of complications associated with surgery, anesthesia, and immobility, including infection, thrombus formation, and pneumonia.
- Use an age-appropriate pain scale to help provide optimal pain management.
- Turn the patient every 2 hours. Deep breathing and coughing should be encouraged. Incentive spirometry may be used.
- Encourage the child to talk about the experience; he may also express his feelings through art or play.
- The child's activity should be gradually increased. Nursing assessments should include the patient's tolerance of the activity.
- Because lifelong anticoagulant therapy will be necessary, teach the parents (and the child, if old enough) to recognize the signs and symptoms of bleeding, including

black, tarry stools (from GI bleeding); oral bleeding (a small, soft bristly toothbrush should be used to prevent this); and excessive bleeding from minor cuts and scrapes.

■ Stress to the child and his parents the importance of antibiotic therapy before dental work and other invasive procedures to prevent infective endocarditis. Children who undergo valve replacement will always need this type of prophylactic antibiotic therapy.

■ Teach the child and his parents the importance of good oral hygiene to reduce the risk of oral infection, which can lead to bacteremia.

■ Inform the child and his parents that clicking of the mechanical heart valve may be heard outside of the chest. Reinforce that this sound is normal.

Hemodialysis

DESCRIPTION

■ Involves the use of a machine to clean waste products from the bloodstream if the kidneys are severely damaged or have failed

■ Blood via tubes to an artificial kidney in the machine; waste products and excess fluid removed from the body

■ Purified blood then flowing back to the body through another set of tubes

PURPOSE

■ To clean waste products from the bloodstream if the kidneys are severely damaged or have failed

PATIENT PREPARATION

■ Weigh the child and assess his vital signs before beginning hemodialysis.

- Children on hemodialysis may have a double-lumen central catheter in place in their chest to serve as a site for blood removal.
- Children needing dialysis long-term may have a subcutaneous graft, anastomosing a vein and an artery (an AV graft). This reduces the risk of infection, but means that the child will need two venipunctures each time dialysis is performed. EMLA cream should be used to reduce the discomfort of this necessity.
- The thrill and bruit at the AV graft site must be evaluated.

PROCEDURE

- Hemodialysis separates solutes by differential diffusion through a cellophane membrane placed between the blood and the dialysate solution, in an external receptacle.
- If the child has a subcutaneous graft, check the blood access site every 2 hours for patency and signs of clotting; don't use the arm with this site for taking blood pressures, drawing blood, or giving I.V. therapy.
- During dialysis, monitor vital signs, clotting times, blood flow, the function of the vascular access site, and arterial and venous pressures.

  ALERT *To avoid septicemia from contamination, use strict aseptic technique during preparation of the machine.*

- Watch for complications, such as septicemia, embolism, hepatitis, and rapid fluid and electrolyte loss.
- Use standard precautions when handling blood and body fluids.
- Provide diversional activities for the child receiving hemodialysis to prevent boredom, such as games, drawing and coloring materials, and videos; encourage a family member to stay with the child.
- The procedure usually takes 4 to 6 hours (depending on the size of the child), and must be done 3 days per week.

POSTPROCEDURE CARE

■ After dialysis, monitor the child's vital signs and the vascular access site; weigh him and watch for signs of fluid and electrolyte imbalances.

■ Watch for complications, such as headache, vomiting, agitation, and twitching.

Kidney transplantation

DESCRIPTION

■ Involves replacing a child's diseased kidney with a healthy kidney from another person

■ Donor kidney possibly coming from a living donor or a cadaver donor

PURPOSE

■ To provide a method of necessary renal replacement in children with diseased kidneys and loss of renal function that offers the most opportunity for a normal life (Hemodialysis and peritoneal dialysis are other life-preserving treatments.)

PATIENT PREPARATION

■ Provide emotional support and guidance to the child and his parents. Prepare them for the procedure, including what will occur preoperatively, during the procedure, and postoperatively.

■ Arrange for the child and his parents to tour the intensive care unit and meet the nursing staff before the transplantation.

■ Administer immunosuppressive medications as ordered; a child who will have or has recently had a renal transplant will be taking immunosuppressive medications to decrease the risk of organ rejection.

■ Monitor for signs and symptoms of infection; while immunosuppressed, the child is at increased risk for infection. Explain to the child and his parents that he will be kept in temporary isolation after surgery.

PROCEDURE

■ With kidney transplantation, the donated organ is implanted in the iliac fossa. The organ's vessels are then connected to the internal iliac vein and internal iliac artery.
■ The diseased kidney is removed, and the renal artery and vein are ligated.
■ The renal artery of the donor kidney is sutured to the iliac artery and the renal vein is sutured to the iliac vein.
■ The ureter of the donor kidney is sutured to the bladder or the child's ureter.
■ Usually, children receiving a transplant receive only one kidney although, in some rare situations, a child may receive two kidneys from a cadaver donor.
■ The child is cared for by a transplant team who will usually keep the parents informed of the child's condition during surgery.
■ Surgery may take several hours, but depends on each individual case.

POSTPROCEDURE CARE

■ Take special precautions to reduce the risk of infection. For example, use strict sterile technique when changing the dressing and performing catheter care.
■ Limit the child's contact with staff, other patients, and visitors and have all people in the child's room wear surgical masks for the first 2 weeks after surgery.
■ Throughout the recovery period, watch for signs and symptoms of tissue rejection. Observe the transplantation site for redness, tenderness, and swelling.
■ Carefully monitor urine output; promptly report output of less than 100 ml/hr. A sudden decrease in urine out-

put could indicate thrombus formation at the renal artery anastomosis site.

■ Make sure that no one with any obvious infection takes care of the child.

■ Prepare the child (and his parents) for the possibility of continuing to need hemodialysis temporarily after the transplant because the transplanted kidney might not work effectively right away.

Lung transplantation

DESCRIPTION

■ Surgical procedure that replaces one or both of a child's diseased lungs with healthy lungs

■ Healthy lungs usually coming from a human donor who has been on life support and declared brain-dead

PURPOSE

■ To treat children with poor, life-threatening lung function (caused by a disease such as cystic fibrosis or infection) that isn't responsive to other therapies

PATIENT PREPARATION

■ A child must first undergo a thorough evaluation to ensure he's an appropriate candidate for transplantation. The transplant work-up involves an evaluation of all major organ functioning as well as a mental health evaluation.

■ Eligible candidates are placed on a nationwide waiting list.

■ Factors considered when a donor becomes available include the recipient's blood type, geographic distance between the donor and recipient, and the lung allocation score (a scoring system implemented in spring 2005 where donor lungs are allocated based on recipient need, not the amount of time the recipient spends on the waiting list).

■ Lung transplant must occur within 4 to 6 hours of the lungs being removed from the donor.

■ The child and his parents must be thoroughly prepared for this major procedure; provide an age-appropriate explanation of why the surgery is being performed, and encourage the child and his parents to ask questions.

■ Reassure the child that he won't wake up during surgery, but that the physician knows how and when to wake him up afterward.

■ Prepare the child for the equipment he'll wake up with; mention that he'll have I.V. lines, a·n indwelling urinary catheter, a heart monitor, chest tubes, and will be connected to a machine that will help him breathe.

■ Include a brief visit to the intensive care unit (ICU) and, if possible, the child should be introduced to the nurses who will be providing his care.

■ Parents should be made aware of the visiting policies in the ICU and should be assisted in making arrangements to spend as much time with their child as possible.

PROCEDURE

■ The child is placed under general anesthesia for the procedure and is sometimes connected to a heart-lung machine.

■ Prepare the family that the length of surgery varies and can take from 4 to 12 hours.

■ There are three main types of lung transplantations:
  – Single lung transplantation
    ▪ Involves one of the diseased lungs being replaced with a healthy, donor lung
    ▪ Typically done to treat a variety of lung diseases such as cystic fibrosis
    ▪ Incision made on the side of the chest
    ▪ Can provide approximately 50% to 90% of normal lung function

- Double lung transplantation
  - Involves both the diseased lungs being replaced with healthy donor lungs (usually from the same donor)
  - Children possibly waiting longer for this treatment because it takes more time to find an appropriate donor with two healthy lungs
  - Incision made across the middle of the chest
  - Typically done to treat lung infections
  - Can provide approximately 60% to 90% of normal lung function
- Heart-lung transplantation
  - Involves the heart and lungs being removed and replaced with the heart and lungs from a human donor
  - Rarest type of lung transplantation.

POSTPROCEDURE CARE

- Monitor the child closely for signs of rejection, infection, and adverse reactions to immunosuppressive therapy.
- Encourage compliance with the required complex drug regimen, especially in adolescents.
- Limit the child's contact with staff, other patients, and visitors and have all people in the child's room wear surgical masks for the first 2 weeks after surgery.
- Provide emotional support to the child and his family and offer resources for additional support.

Spinal fusion with instrumentation

DESCRIPTION

- Fusion surgically correcting curved vertebrae in children with scoliosis by using bone grafts (usually from the child's hip) to create a united (fused), straighter vertebral structure
- Spinal instrumentation involving use of internal metal rods, wires, and screws to help further straighten spinal curvature by holding the spine in place while the fusion heals

- Instrumentation remaining in the child's back and is *not* removed after the fusion has healed
- Used in children with scoliosis, a lateral curvature of the spine that occurs either in the thoracic or lumbar areas of the back (rarely in the cervical region), and usually becomes apparent at the onset of puberty
- Typically recommended for spinal curvature of 45 degrees or greater that has progressed despite more conservative therapies such as bracing

PURPOSE

- To stop the progression of, and provide stabilization to, curvatures of the spine in children with scoliosis

PATIENT PREPARATION

- Prepare the child for what to expect after surgery: the presence of various catheters and the use of certain body mechanics to restrict bending at the fusion site.
- Discuss postoperative recovery and rehabilitation with the child and his family.
- Reassure the child and his family that analgesics and muscle relaxants will be available during recovery.
- Explain that the child will return from surgery with a dressing over the incision and that he'll be kept on bed rest for the duration prescribed by the surgeon.
- Explain that he'll be turned often to prevent pressure ulcers and pulmonary complications.
- The preoperative workup should include laboratory tests, blood gas analysis, bleeding times, and X-rays.
- Just before surgery, perform a baseline assessment of motor function and sensation in the patient's lower trunk, legs, and feet. Carefully document the results for comparison with postoperative findings.

PROCEDURE

- The child is placed under general anesthesia for the procedure. He'll have a nasogastric tube and an indwelling urinary catheter inserted after the anesthesia takes effect.

- Types of spinal fusion surgeries:
  - Posterior
    - Performed through an incision made down the middle of the child's back; one or two metal rods keep the vertebrae in place and, commonly, a hip bone graft is placed along the spine to prevent further curvature
  - Anterior
    - Performed either through an incision on the side of the rib cage (for thoracic scoliosis) or across the lower rib cage and down the front of the abdomen (thoracic and lumbar scoliosis)
  - Anterior/posterior
    - Two-stage operation; one performed anteriorly and one posteriorly, usually 1 week apart.

POSTPROCEDURE CARE

- Assess motor and neurologic function in the child's trunk and lower extremities, and compare the results with baseline findings.
- Evaluate circulation in the patient's legs and feet and report any abnormalities.
- Give analgesics and muscle relaxants as ordered.
- Inspect the dressing frequently for bleeding or cerebrospinal fluid leakage, and report either immediately. The surgeon will probably perform the initial dressing change, and you may be asked to perform subsequent changes.
- The child will typically work with a physical therapist for mobility and strengthening exercises, and with the nurse for coughing and deep-breathing exercises.
- Peer support groups may be helpful after the child returns home.
- Contact sports aren't usually permitted for at least 6 months after surgery.

Tracheotomy

DESCRIPTION

- Surgical procedure that creates an opening in the anterior neck at the cricoid cartilage leading directly to the trachea; opening usually referred to as a *tracheostomy* (see *Tracheostomy tube placement*)
- Indicated for children requiring long-term ventilation or for those with epiglottiditis, croup, or foreign body aspiration
- May performed in emergency departments when endotracheal intubation isn't possible, in the field where immediate intervention is necessary, or in the more controlled setting of the operating room

PURPOSE

- To provide an airway for an intubated child who needs prolonged mechanical ventilation and to facilitate the removal of lower tracheobronchial secretions in a child who can't clear them
- To prevent an unconscious or paralyzed child from aspirating food or secretions and to bypass upper airway obstruction due to trauma, burns, epiglottiditis, or a tumor

PATIENT PREPARATION

- For an emergency tracheotomy, briefly explain the procedure to the child and his parents as time permits and quickly obtain supplies or a tracheotomy tray.
- For a scheduled tracheotomy, explain the procedure and the need for general anesthesia to the child and his family. If known, discuss whether the tracheostomy will be temporary or permanent. Discuss how the tracheostomy will look and feel.
- Choose a method of communication to be used after the procedure.

TRACHEOSTOMY TUBE PLACEMENT

This illustration shows a tracheostomy tube in place in the trachea. Note how the tied cloth tapes keep the tube securely in place.

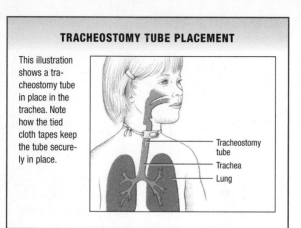

Tracheostomy tube

Trachea

Lung

- Introduce a child requiring a long-term or permanent tracheostomy to someone who has experienced the procedure and has adjusted well to tracheostomy care.
- Ensure that samples for arterial blood gas (ABG) analysis and other diagnostic tests have been collected and that the consent form is signed.

PROCEDURE

- A physician creates the surgical opening, then inserts a tracheostomy tube to permit access to the airway.
- A tracheostomy tube is inserted to keep the opening patent; the tube must be secured in place to prevent accidental extubation.
- Sterile gauze is placed between the skin and the tube to absorb drainage.

POSTPROCEDURE CARE

- After the procedure, monitor the child for complications, such as hemorrhage, infection, edema, decannulation (dislodgment of the tracheostomy tube), and tube obstruction.

- Auscultate the child's breath sounds every 2 hours and monitor respiratory status with ABG analysis. Note crackles, rhonchi, or diminished breath sounds.

- Turn the patient every 2 hours to prevent pooling tracheal secretions. As ordered, provide chest physiotherapy to help mobilize secretions, and note their quantity, consistency, color, and odor.

- To maintain patency, suction the tracheostomy tube as needed, using sterile technique.

- Provide stoma care per facility policy. The stoma can usually be gently cleaned with half-strength hydrogen peroxide to remove secretions. The skin around the stoma should be kept clean and dry. Monitor for signs of skin breakdown.

- Change the tracheostomy dressing when soiled or once per shift, using sterile technique, and check the color, odor, amount, and type of drainage. Also check for swelling, crepitus, erythema, and bleeding at the site and report excessive bleeding or unusual drainage immediately. Wear goggles, gloves, and a mask when changing tracheostomy tubes.

- Keep the tracheostomy tube ties secured tightly to help prevent accidental decannulation. Make sure there's enough room to slip a fingertip between the ties and the neck.

- Keep a sterile tracheostomy tube (with obturator) at the child's bedside and be prepared to replace an expelled or contaminated tube. Also keep available a sterile tracheostomy tube (with obturator) that's one size smaller than the tube currently being used, because it may be necessary if the trachea begins to close after tube expulsion, making insertion of the same size tube difficult.

- If the child is being discharged with suction equipment, make sure he and his family are knowledgeable and comfortable about using the equipment.

Traction

DESCRIPTION

- Involves the use of weights and pulleys to exert a pulling force and maintain a specified body part in correct alignment
- Weights, must hang freely; ropes, shouldn't have knots that could interfere with free movement

PURPOSE

- To stabilize or immobilize a certain body part, reduce muscle spasms, or realign fractures or joint dislocations

PATIENT PREPARATION

- Explain to the child and his parents what the child will see and feel before the traction is applied. Keep in mind that the sight and idea of a body part in skeletal traction can be frightening to a child (and his parents).
- Use dolls and toy traction devices to show the child what's about to happen, to help familiarize him with the equipment, and to reduce his fear.
- Involve the family as much as possible to reduce anxiety, encourage cooperation with the recommended treatment, and reduce the amount of disruption of the family structure.

PROCEDURE

- There are two basic types of traction that can be applied: skin and skeletal.
  - *Skin traction* is a non-invasive traction that's especially useful for a child who may not require continuous traction. It's applied by placing foam rubber straps against the affected part and then securing the straps with elastic bandages. Sometimes, the straps have an adhesive

TYPES OF SKIN TRACTION

This chart describes the various types of skin traction.

Traction	Purpose	Patient positioning
Buck's extension	Used for a fractured hip to prevent muscle spasms and dislocation	■ The child lies flat in bed. ■ Head of the bed is elevated only for activities of daily living.
Cervical traction	Used for neck strain and arthritic or degenerative conditions of the cervical vertebrae	■ The child lies flat in bed or with the head of the bed elevated 15 to 20 degrees.
Dunlop's traction	Used for a fractured humerus	■ The child lies flat in bed. ■ The child's arm is suspended horizontally.
Pelvic girdle	Used for muscle spasms, lower back pain, or a herniated disk	■ The child lies with head and knees raised to keep the hips flexed at a 45-degree angle.
Russell traction	Used for adolescents with a femur fracture or certain knee injuries	■ The child lies with the head of the bed elevated 30 to 45 degrees.
Bryant's traction	Used for children with a fractured femur who are younger than age 2 and weigh less than 31 lb (14 kg)	■ Hips are flexed at a 90-degree angle. ■ Buttocks are raised 1" (2.5 cm) above the mattress.

backing. If this type of strap is used, the nurse should protect the skin by first applying compound benzoin tincture or another skin protectant. (See *Types of skin traction*.)

– *Skeletal traction* exerts a greater force than skin traction by using wires or pins that are inserted into the bone, usually while the child is under anesthesia. Skeletal traction is continuous. (See *Types of skeletal traction*.)

TYPES OF SKELETAL TRACTION

This chart describes the different types of skeletal traction.

Traction	Purpose	Special considerations
Thomas leg splint with Pearson attachment	Used for bone alignment and as a more effective line of pull	■ The child is placed in the supine position with the knee flexed.
External fixation devices (Ilizarov)	Used to manage open fractures that have soft tissue damage, or to provide stability for severe comminuted fractures	■ The child is on bed rest (however, early mobility and active exercise of other joints are necessary).
Halo	Used to provide immobilization of the cervical spine and to support the neck following injury	■ Early ambulation is recommended. ■ The anterior metal bars maintain traction. ■ The posterior bars can be used to position the patient.
Skeletal tongs (Crutchfield, Vinke, Gardner-Wells)	Used to maintain alignment of the cervical spine, for immobilization, and for reduction of cervical roll fractures	■ The child is on bed rest. ■ Special frames may be used for turning.

POSTPROCEDURE CARE

- ■ Monitor the patient's vital signs, intake and output, and bowel elimination patterns.
- ■ Unless contraindicated, encourage increased fluids, protein, and fiber intake, as appropriate.
- ■ Maintain the traction system, and frequently check the ropes, pulleys, and weights for proper function. Ropes and pulleys should never rest on the floor.
- ■ The child should be kept in the center of the bed to maintain countertraction and prevent complications.

- Serial X-rays are done while the child is in traction to monitor progress and determine the need for changes in the direction and amount of traction pull.
- Traction can cause muscle spasms that may require analgesics or muscle relaxants.
- Frequently assess for signs of skin breakdown. Place sheepskin under the affected extremity to help alleviate pressure.
- Provide footplates for the affected side to prevent footdrop.
- Perform range-of-motion exercises on the unaffected extremity.
- Provide age-appropriate activities to help maintain the child's developmental level, prevent developmental delay, and alleviate boredom.
- For the patient in skeletal traction, assess the pin insertion sites for signs of infection or tenting (new skin that has attached to the insertion site, creating a tent-like configuration); tenting may cause the skin to tear, which can promote infection.
- Clean the area around the pin insertion sites frequently (a hydrogen peroxide solution is typically used), and cover the tips of the pins to prevent injury to the skin or other parts of the child's body. Notify the physician immediately if the pins become loose, and keep the child immobilized until the skeletal traction is assessed.
- Traction should be removed using two people.

Tympanoplasty ventilating tube insertion

DESCRIPTION

- Tympanoplasty ventilating tubes, or *pressure-equalizing tubes*, surgically inserted into the middle ear to create an artificial auditory canal that equalizes pressure on both sides of the tympanic membrane (see *Ventilating tube placement*)

VENTILATING TUBE PLACEMENT

This illustration shows where tubes are placed in the ear to equalize pressure on both sides of the tympanic membrane.

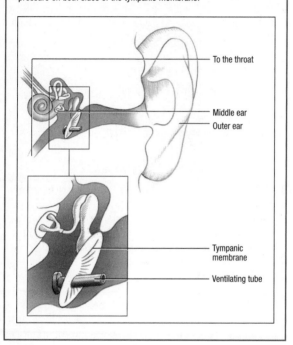

To the throat

Middle ear
Outer ear

Tympanic membrane

Ventilating tube

PURPOSE

- To treat ruptured eardrums, usually caused by repeated or complicated otitis media (middle ear) infections (Acute otitis media occurring as a result of pneumococci, beta-hemolytic streptococci, staphylococci, and gram-negative bacteria such as *Hemophilus influenzae;* chronic otitis media resulting from inadequate treatment of acute infection as well as by resistant strains of bacteria.)
- To allow air to get into the middle ear and allow fluids to drain out

PATIENT PREPARATION

■ Explain to the child and his parents that this is an outpatient procedure, so the child should be able to return home the same day.
■ Inform the child and his parents that the tubes will likely fall out in 6 to 18 months, but because they're so small they'll probably not be seen.

PROCEDURE

■ The child is usually placed under general anesthesia.
■ The surgeon makes an incision in the eardrum, drains any accumulated fluid, and inserts the tubes. Sutures aren't needed to hold the tubes in place.

POSTPROCEDURE CARE

■ Reinforce dressings, and observe for excessive bleeding form the ear canal.
■ Inform the child and his parents that the child may experience mild ear pain for a few hours after surgery, and that clear fluid may drain from the ear for about 24 hours.
■ Assess the child's hearing; he should notice immediate improvement.
■ After completing therapy for otitis media, evaluate the child. Make sure he's free from pain and fever, his hearing is completely restored, he understands the importance of completing his antibiotic therapy, and he understands how to prevent recurrence.
■ If needed, administered analgesics as ordered.
■ Warn the child against blowing his nose or getting his ear wet when bathing. Educate parents about the indications for and use of earplugs postoperatively for bathing and swimming (such as using Vaseline-coated cotton balls, ear putty, or specially made ear molds).

Urinary diversion surgery

DESCRIPTION

- Typically performed on a child who has undergone total or partial cystectomy
- May also be performed on a child with a congenital urinary tract defect or severe, unmanageable urinary tract infections that threaten renal function; injury to the ureters, bladder, or urethra; obstructive malignant tumors; or a neurogenic bladder

PURPOSE

- To provide an alternate route for urine excretion when a disorder or abnormality impedes normal flow through the bladder

PATIENT PREPARATION

- Provide an age-appropriate explanation of why the surgery is being performed, and encourage the child and his parents to ask questions.
- When the situation permits, arrange for the child and his parents to visit the health care facility before he's admitted for surgery.
- Prepare the child for the appearance and general location of the stoma. If he's scheduled for an ileal conduit, explain that the stoma will be located somewhere in the lower abdomen, probably below the waistline.
- Review the enterostomal therapist's explanation of the urine collection device that the child will use after surgery.

PROCEDURE

- Several types of urinary diversion surgery can be performed; however, the two most common procedures are the *ileal conduit* and *continent vesicostomy*.

■ In some cases, surgeons may perform a *continent* urinary diversion procedure, where the surgically constructed substitute bladder is attached to the urethra, thereby allowing the child to void spontaneously.

POSTPROCEDURE CARE

■ Carefully check and record the child's urine output; report any decrease, which could indicate obstruction from postoperative edema or ureteral stenosis.

■ Monitor the child for potential complications, including infection, impaired kidney drainage, and chemical imbalances.

■ Perform routine ostomy maintenance, if indicated. Make sure the collection device fits tightly around the stoma; allow no more than a ⅛″ margin of skin between the stoma and the device's faceplate.

> **ALERT** *To avoid irritating the patient's stoma, avoid touching it with adhesive solvent.*

■ Regularly check the appearance of the stoma and peristomal skin.

■ Instruct the child and his parents how to perform stoma care or ostomy self-catheterization.

■ Instruct the child and his parents to watch for and report signs and symptoms of complications, such as fever, chills, abdominal pain, and pus or blood in the urine.

■ Emphasize the importance of keeping all scheduled follow-up appointments with the physician and enterostomal therapist to evaluate stoma care and make any necessary changes in equipment.

■ Provide emotional support and refer the child and his parents to such support groups as the United Ostomy Association.

Valvuloplasty

DESCRIPTION

- Also called *balloon valvuloplasty;* involves opening narrowed (or stenosed) valves
- Used for aortic, mitral, and pulmonic stenosis
- May be performed in the cardiac catheterization laboratory and doesn't require open heart surgery; may take up to 4 hours

PURPOSE

- To improve valvular function by enlarging the orifice of a stenotic heart valve caused by a congential defect or rheumatic fever

PATIENT PREPARATION

- When the situation permits, arrange for the child and his parents to visit the health care facility before he's admitted for the procedure.
- Provide an age-appropriate explanation of why the procedure is being performed, and encourage the child and his parents to ask questions.
- Describe to the child and his parents the procedure room as well as the equipment that will be used during the procedure. Show the child where on his body the catheter will be inserted, using doll play to prepare him, as necessary.
- Tell the child that the lights in the room will be dimmed after the catheter is placed. Reassure him that you'll be right there with him and will talk to him throughout the procedure.
- Restrict food and fluid intake for at least 6 hours before the procedure, or as ordered.

PROCEDURE

■ In the cardiac catheterization laboratory, the physician inserts a thin, flexible, balloon-tipped catheter into the child's femoral artery and threads the catheter to the site of the narrowed heart valve.

■ After the catheter is in place, the physician (who's guided by X-ray on a video monitor) gently inflates the balloon repeatedly to a specified pressure and opens the valve narrowing.

■ The balloon is then deflated and removed along with the catheter.

■ The nurse should assess the child and prepare for complications of the procedure, such as:
  – worsening valvular insufficiency by misshaping the valve so that it doesn't close completely
  – severely damaging delicate valve leaflets, requiring immediate surgery to replace the valve (rare)
  – bleeding and hematoma at the arterial puncture site
  – myocardial infarction (rare), arrhythmias, myocardial ischemia, and circulatory defects distal to the catheter entry site.

POSTPROCEDURE CARE

■ Keep the affected extremity immobile for the prescribed amount of time to prevent hemorrhage.

■ Assess the cannulation site for bleeding or infection.

■ Monitor the effects of I.V. medications such as heparin.

■ Monitor peripheral pulses distal to the insertion site and the color, temperature, and capillary refill time of the extremity. If pulses are difficult to palpate, use a Doppler stethoscope and notify the physician if pulses are absent.

■ Monitor the child's temperature and report fever promptly.

■ Provide pain medication if needed, as ordered.

■ Encourage the child to talk about the experience; he may also express his feelings through art or play.

■ Inform the child and his parents that life-long follow-up is necessary due to possible recurrence of valve narrowing.

Ventriculoperitoneal shunt insertion

DESCRIPTION

■ Implanted in the child with hydrocephalus to prevent excess accumulation of cerebrospinal fluid (CSF) in the ventricles
■ Tubing diverting CSF from the ventricles into the peritoneal cavity, where it's reabsorbed

PURPOSE

■ To prevent accumulation of CSF in the ventricles

PATIENT PREPARATION

■ Provide an age-appropriate explanation of why the surgery is being performed, and encourage the child and his parents to ask questions.
■ Young children may have misconceptions about procedures involving general anesthesia; when explaining this procedure, make sure the child understands that he'll be given "a special medicine" to make sure he doesn't feel anything during the procedure. Tell the child that the medicine will give him a special kind of sleep that isn't like sleeping at night or nap time.
■ Monitor the child for signs of increased intracranial pressure (ICP).
■ Measure head circumference daily at the occipital frontal circumference; place the tape measure just above the top of the ears, around the midforehead, and around the most prominent part of the occiput.
■ Gently palpate fontanels and suture lines for signs of bulging, tenseness, and separation, which may indicate increased ICP or increasing ventricular size.

PROCEDURE

- The child is placed under general anesthesia.
- The surgeon places the shunt, which is a flexible, silicone rubber tube that connects the ventricles of the brain to the peritoneal cavity.
- As the child grows, shunt tubes may need to be replaced.

POSTPROCEDURE CARE

- Monitor the child for pain, and administer pain medications as ordered.
- Keep the child positioned flat and on the non-operative side.
- Check orders regarding allowable activities; the child may be allowed to sit up to reduce ICP.
- Follow the surgeon's orders and manufacturer's recommendations regarding pumping of the shunt (pressing on it to check for proper function); not all shunt devices require this step.
- Observe the child for signs of increased ICP, which may indicated an obstructed shunt.
- Monitor the child for abdominal distention, which may indicate distal catheter placement.
- Be alert for signs of CSF infection (fever, poor feeding, vomiting, decreased level of consciousness, seizures), which is the greatest postoperative risk.
- Administer antibiotics as ordered.
- Teach the parents how to change dressings and recognize shunt malfunctions.

Part three

Procedures

Cardiopulmonary resuscitation, child

DESCRIPTION

■ Cardiopulmonary resuscitation (CPR) in adults, children, and infants: based on the same principle of aiming to restore cardiopulmonary function by ventilating the lungs and pumping the victim's heart until natural function resumes

ALERT *For CPR purposes, the American Heart Association defines a patient by age. An infant is younger than age 1; a child is age 1 to onset of adolescence or puberty.*

■ Survival chances improving the sooner CPR begins and the faster advanced life support systems are implemented
■ When an infant or child is requiring CPR, likely suffering from hypoxia caused by respiratory difficulty or respiratory arrest
■ Most pediatric crises requiring CPR preventable, including motor vehicle accidents, drowning, burns, smoke inhalation, falls, poisoning, suffocation, and choking (usually from inhaling a plastic bag or small foreign bodies, such as toys or food)

EQUIPMENT

Hard surface (on which to place the patient) ◆ child-size bag-valve mask, if available

ESSENTIAL STEPS

■ Gently tap the apparently unconscious child's shoulder and ask if he's okay, calling his name if you know it.
■ If the child is conscious but has difficulty breathing, help him into a position that best eases his breathing.
■ Call for help to alert others and to enlist emergency assistance.
■ If you're alone and the child isn't breathing, perform CPR for five cycles (about 2 minutes), before calling for help. One cycle of CPR for the single rescuer is 30 compressions and two breaths.

- Place the child in a supine position on a firm, flat surface (usually the ground). The surface should provide the resistance needed for adequate compression of the heart.
- If you must turn the child from a prone position, support his head and neck and turn him as a unit to avoid twisting or turning the head or neck.

Establishing a patent airway

- Kneel beside the child's shoulder.
- Place one hand on the child's forehead and gently lift his chin with your other hand to open his airway (head tilt-chin lift maneuver).
- Avoid fingering the soft neck tissue to avoid obstructing the airway.
- Never let the child's mouth close completely.
- If you suspect a neck injury, use the jaw-thrust maneuver to open the child's airway to keep from moving the child's neck while you open his airway.
- To prepare for the maneuver, kneel beside the child's head.
- With your elbows on the ground, rest your thumbs at the corners of the child's mouth, and place two or three fingers of each hand under the lower jaw.
- Lift the jaw upward.
- While maintaining an open airway, place your ear near the child's mouth and nose to evaluate his breathing status.
- Look for chest movement, listen for exhaled air, and feel for exhaled air on your cheek.
- If the child is breathing, maintain an open airway and monitor respiration.

   ALERT *If you suspect that a mechanical airway blocks respiration (even if the child isn't conscious), attempt to clear the airway as you would in an adult, but with two exceptions: Don't use the blind finger-sweep maneuver, which could compound or re-lodge the obstruction, and adjust your technique to the child's size. Perform a finger-sweep maneuver only when you can see the object in the child's mouth.*

Restoring ventilation

- If the child isn't breathing, maintain the open airway position and take a breath.
- Then pinch the child's nostrils shut and cover the child's mouth with your mouth.
- Give two breaths that make the chest rise, pausing briefly after the first breath.
- While maintaining an open airway, take no more than 10 seconds to check breathing (rhythmic chest or abdominal movement, hearing exhaled breaths or feeling exhaled air on your cheek).
- If your first attempt at ventilation fails to restore the child's breathing, reposition the child's head to open the airway and try again.

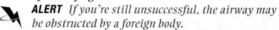 **ALERT** *If you're still unsuccessful, the airway may be obstructed by a foreign body.*

- Repeat the steps for establishing a patent airway.
- After you free the obstruction, check for breathing and pulse.
- If the child is breathing and there's no evidence of trauma, turn him onto his side or place him in the recovery position.
- If breathing and pulse are absent, proceed with chest compressions.

Restoring heartbeat and circulation

- Assess circulation by palpating the carotid artery for a pulse.
- Locate the carotid artery with two or three fingers of one hand. You'll need the other hand to maintain the head-tilt position that keeps the airway open.
- Place your fingers in the center of the child's neck on the side closest to you, and slide your fingers into the groove formed by the trachea and the sternocleidomastoid muscles.
- Palpate the artery for no more than 10 seconds to confirm the child's pulse status. The pulse should be greater than or equal to 60 beats/minute.
- If you feel the child's pulse and it's greater than or equal to 60 beats/minute, continue rescue breathing, giving

one breath every 3 seconds (20 breaths per minute) and recheck pulse every 2 minutes.

- If you can't feel a pulse or if the pulse is less than 60 beats/minute and there are signs of poor perfusion, begin cardiac compressions.
- Kneel next to the child's chest.
- Using the hand closest to his feet, locate the lower border of the rib cage on the side nearest you.
- Hold your middle and index fingers together, and move them up the rib cage to the notch where the ribs and sternum join.
- Put your middle finger on the notch and your index finger next to it.
- Lift your hand and place the heel just above the spot where the index finger was located.
- The heel of your hand should be aligned with the long axis of the sternum.
- Using the heel of one hand or with two hands, apply enough pressure to compress the child's chest downward approximately one-third to one-half the depth of the chest.
- Compressions should be hard and fast at a rate of 100 compressions/minute.
- After every 30 compressions, breathe two breaths into the child (for a single rescuer, 15 compressions and two breaths for two rescuers.
- If you can't detect a pulse, or if the pulse is less than 60 beats/minute and there are signs of poor perfusion, continue chest compressions and rescue breathing.
- If you can detect a pulse, check for spontaneous respirations.
- If not already done, phone 911 (call a code) and use an automated external defibrillator or defibrillator after five cycles of CPR.
- If the child begins breathing spontaneously, keep the airway open and place the child in a side-lying position to prevent aspiration.
- Monitor both the respirations and pulse.

NURSING CONSIDERATIONS

- A child's small airway can be easily blocked by his tongue. If this occurs, simply opening the airway may eliminate the obstruction.
- Take care to ensure smooth motions when performing cardiac compressions.
- Keep your fingers off, and the heel of your hand on, the child's chest at all times.
- Time your motions so that the compression and relaxation phases are equal to promote effective compressions.
- If the child has breathing difficulty and a parent is present, ask about whether the child recently had a fever or an upper respiratory tract infection.

   ALERT *If the child recently had a fever or an upper respiratory tract infection, suspect epiglottitis. In this instance, don't attempt to manipulate the airway because laryngospasm may occur and completely obstruct the airway. Allow the child to assume a comfortable position, and monitor his breathing until additional assistance arrives.*

- Persist in attempts to remove an obstruction. As hypoxia develops, the child's muscles will relax, allowing you to remove the foreign object.
- Make sure that someone communicates support and information to the parents during resuscitation efforts.
- Place a bag-valve mask, if available, over the child's nose and mouth when performing ventilations.

Cardiopulmonary resuscitation, infant

DESCRIPTION

- Objective of cardiopulmonary resuscitation (CPR) in an infant: same as in a child or adult, with varying techniques

EQUIPMENT

Hard surface (to place the infant on) ◆ infant-sized bag-valve mask, if available

ESSENTIAL STEPS

- Gently tap the foot of the apparently unconscious infant and call out his name.
- For a sudden, witnessed collapse, call for help or call emergency medical services. If you didn't witness the collapse, perform resuscitation measures for 2 minutes; then call for help. You may move an uninjured infant close to a telephone, if necessary.
- Place the infant supine on a hard surface.
- Open the airway using the head-tilt, chin-lift maneuver, unless contraindicated by trauma; don't hyperextend the infant's neck.
- Place your ear near the infant's mouth and nose to evaluate his breathing status. Look for chest movement, listen for exhaled air, and feel for exhaled air on your cheek.
- If the infant is breathing, maintain an open airway and monitor respirations.

Restoring ventilation

- If the infant isn't breathing, take a breath and tightly seal your mouth over the infant's nose and mouth.
- Give two breaths.
- If the infant's chest rises and falls, then the amount of air is probably adequate.
- Continue rescue breathing with one breath every 3 to 5 seconds (12 to 20 breaths per minute) if you can detect a pulse.
- Give each breath over 1 second.

Clearing the airway

- If you're unable to ventilate the infant, reposition the head and try again.
- To remove an airway obstruction, place the infant face-down on your forearm, with his head lower than his trunk.
- Support your forearm on your thigh.
- Give five blows between the infant's shoulder blades using the heel of your free hand.

■ If the airway remains obstructed, sandwich the infant between your hands and forearms and flip him over onto
his back.

    ALERT *Don't do a blind finger-sweep to find or re-
move an obstruction. In an infant, the maneuver
may push the object back into the airway and cause further obstruction. Only place your fingers in the infant's
mouth if you see an object to remove.*

■ Keeping the infant's head lower than his trunk, give five
midsternal chest thrusts, using your middle and ring fingers only, to raise the intrathoracic pressure enough to
force a cough that will expel the obstruction.

■ Remember to hold the infant's head firmly to avoid injury.

■ Repeat this sequence until the obstruction is dislodged
or the infant loses consciousness.

■ If the infant loses consciousness, start CPR. Every time
you open the airway to deliver breaths, check the mouth
and remove any object you see.

Restoring heartbeat and circulation

■ Assess the infant's pulse by palpating the brachial artery,
located inside his upper arm between the elbow and the
shoulder. Take no moe than 10 seconds to assess pulse.

■ If you find a pulse, continue rescue breathing but don't
initiate chest compressions.

■ Begin chest compressions if you find no pulse.

■ To locate the correct position on the infant's sternum for
chest compressions, draw an imaginary horizontal line
between the infant's nipples.

■ Place two fingers on the sternum, directly below — and
perpendicular to — the nipple line.

■ Use these two fingers to depress the sternum here $\frac{1}{3}''$ to
$\frac{1}{2}''$ the depth of the chest at least 100 compressions per
minute.

■ When two rescuers are present, use a 2-thumb encircling
technique to provide chest compressions. Use both
hands to encircle the infant's chest with both thumbs
together over the lower half of the sternum. Forcefully

compress the sternum with your thumbs as you squeeze the thorax with your fingers.

■ Supply two breaths after every 30 compressions or two ventilations for every 15 compressions if two rescuers are performing CPR.

■ Maintain this ratio whether you're the helper or the lone rescuer.

■ This ratio allows for about 100 compressions and 20 breaths per minute for an infant.

ALERT Be aware that, if available, you should use a bag-valve mask over the infant's nose and mouth when performing ventilations.

NURSING CONSIDERATIONS

■ An infant's airway can be easily blocked by his tongue. If this occurs, simply opening the airway may eliminate the obstruction.

■ Take care to ensure smooth motions when performing cardiac compressions.

■ Time your motions so that the compression and relaxation phases are equal to promote effective compressions.

■ If the infant has breathing difficulty and a parent is present, find out whether the infant recently had a fever or an upper respiratory tract infection.

ALERT If the infant recently had a fever or an upper respiratory tract infection, suspect epiglottitis. In this instance, don't attempt to manipulate the airway because laryngospasm may occur and completely obstruct the airway. Place the infant in a comfortable position, and monitor his breathing until additional assistance arrives.

■ Persist in attempts to remove an obstruction.

■ As hypoxia develops, the infant's muscles will relax, allowing you to remove the foreign object.

■ Make sure that someone communicates support and information to the parents during resuscitation efforts.

■ Place a bag-valve mask, if available, over the infant's nose and mouth when performing ventilations.

TYPES OF CASTS FOR CHILDREN

These illustrations show the types of casts commonly used for children.

FULL SPICA CAST

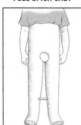

SINGLE SPICA CAST

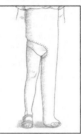

CYLINDER CAST

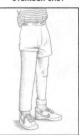

HIP SPICA CAST

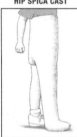

LONG LEG CAST

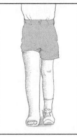

SHORT LEG CAST

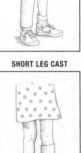

Cast care

DESCRIPTION

- Involves hard molds that encase a body part, usually an extremity, to provide immobilization of bones and surrounding tissue
- Used to treat injuries (including fractures), correct orthopedic conditions (such as deformities), or promote healing after general or plastic surgery, amputation, or nerve and vascular repair (see *Types of casts for children*)

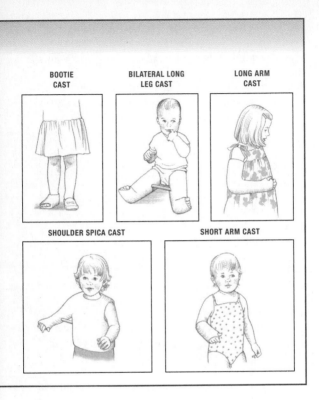

BOOTIE CAST

BILATERAL LONG LEG CAST

LONG ARM CAST

SHOULDER SPICA CAST

SHORT ARM CAST

- May be constructed of plaster, fiberglass, or other synthetic materials
- Fiberglass casts: lighter, stronger, and more resilient than plaster, but more difficult to mold because of rapid drying; can bear body weight immediately, if needed
- Cast applied and removed by physician; patient and equipment prepared by nurse who also assists during procedure

EQUIPMENT

Casting material ◆ plaster rolls ◆ tubular stockinette
◆ plaster splints (if necessary) ◆ bucket of water ◆ sink
equipped with plaster trap ◆ linen-saver pad ◆ sheet
◆ wadding ◆ cast stand ◆ sponge or felt padding (if necessary) ◆ cast scissors, cast saw, and cast spreader (if necessary, for removal) ◆ moleskin or adhesive tape (optional)

ESSENTIAL STEPS

- Explain the procedure to allay the child and his parents'
  fears.
- Cover the appropriate parts of the child's bedding and
  gown with a linen-saver pad.
- Assess the condition of the child's skin in the affected
  area, noting redness, contusions, or open wounds, to aid
  in evaluating complaints he may have after the cast is applied.
- To establish baseline measurements, assess the child's
  neurovascular status.
- Palpate the distal pulses and assess the color, temperature, and capillary refill of the appropriate fingers or toes.
- Support the limb in the prescribed position while the
  physician applies the tubular stockinette and sheet
  wadding.
- The stockinette, if used, should extend beyond the ends
  of the cast to pad the edges.

Preparing a fiberglass cast

- If using water-activated fiberglass, immerse the tape rolls
  in tepid water for 10 to 15 minutes to initiate the chemical reaction that causes the cast to harden.
- Open one roll at a time.

  ALERT *Avoid squeezing out excess water before application.*

- If you're using light-cured fiberglass, unroll the material
  more slowly.
- Light-cured fiberglass casting remains soft and malleable
  until it's exposed to ultraviolet light, which sets it.

HOW TO PETAL A CAST

Rough cast edges can be cushioned by petaling them with adhesive tape or moleskin. To do this, cut several 4″ × 2″ (10 × 5-cm) strips. Round off one end of each strip to keep it from curling. Then, making sure the rounded end of the strip is on the outside of the cast, tuck the straight end just inside the cast edge (as shown above right).

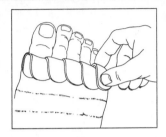

Smooth the moleskin with your finger until you're sure it's secured inside and out. Repeat the procedure, overlapping the moleskin pieces until you've covered the cast's edge (as shown below right).

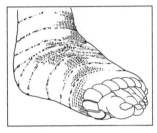

- As necessary, "petal" the cast's edges to reduce roughness and to cushion pressure points. (See *How to petal a cast.*)
- Use a cast stand or your palm to support the cast in the therapeutic position until it becomes firm (usually 6 to 8 minutes) to prevent indentations.
- Place the cast on a firm, smooth surface to continue drying.
- Place pillows under joints to maintain flexion, if necessary.
- To check circulation in the casted limb, palpate the distal pulse and assess the color, temperature, and capillary refill of the fingers or toes.
- Determine neurologic status by asking the child if he's experiencing paresthesia in the extremity or decreased motion of the extremity's uncovered joints.
- Assess the unaffected extremity and compare findings.

■ Elevate the limb above heart level with pillows or bath blankets, as ordered, to facilitate venous return and reduce edema.
■ The physician will send the child for X-rays to ensure proper positioning.

Removing a fiberglass cast

■ The physician usually removes the cast at the appropriate time, with a nurse assisting.
■ Tell the child that when the cast is removed, his casted limb will appear thinner and flabbier than the uncasted limb. The skin may also appear yellowish or gray from the accumulated dead skin and oils from the glands near the skin surface.
■ Apply baby oil, then gently wash the area to remove the dead skin.
■ Reassure the child and his parents that with exercise and good skin care, his limb will return to normal.

NURSING CONSIDERATIONS

■ Room temperature or slightly warmer water is best because it allows the cast to set in about 7 minutes without excessive exothermia; cold water retards the rate of setting and may be used to facilitate difficult molding.
■ During the drying period, the cast must be properly positioned to prevent a surface depression that could cause pressure areas or dependent edema.
■ After the cast dries completely, it looks white and shiny and no longer feels damp or soft.
■ Neurovascular status must be assessed, drainage monitored, and the condition of the cast checked periodically.
■ Care consists of monitoring for changes in the drainage pattern, preventing skin breakdown near the cast, and dealing with immobility.
■ Teaching must start right after the cast is applied and should continue until the child or a family member can care for the cast.
■ Tell the parents to notify the physician of pain, foul odor, drainage, or burning sensation under the child's cast.

- Warn the child and his parents not to get the cast wet, because moisture will weaken or ruin it.
- Urge the child and his parents not to insert anything into the cast to relieve itching because foreign matter can damage skin and cause infection.
- Never use the bed or a table to support the cast as it sets because molding can result, causing pressure necrosis of underlying tissue.
- Don't use rubber- or plastic-covered pillows before the cast hardens because they can trap heat under the cast.
- If a cast is applied after surgery or traumatic injury, remember that the most accurate way to assess for bleeding is to monitor vital signs.

ALERT *A visible blood spot on the cast can be misleading: One drop of blood can produce a circle 3"
(7.6 cm) in diameter.*

- Casts may need to be opened to assess underlying skin or pulses or to relieve pressure in a specific area.
- In a windowed cast, a specific area is cut out to allow inspection of underlying skin or to relieve pressure.
- A bivalved cast is split medially and laterally, creating anterior and posterior sections, and one section may be removed to relieve pressure while the other maintains immobilization.

Chest physiotherapy

DESCRIPTION

- Chest physiotherapy (CPT) techniques: postural drainage, chest percussion and vibration, and coughing and deep-breathing exercises
- Mobilizes and eliminates secretions, reexpands lung tissue, and promotes efficient use of respiratory muscles
- For the bedridden patient: helps to prevent or treat atelectasis and may also help prevent pneumonia — two respiratory complications that can seriously impede recovery
- Postural drainage: performed in conjunction with percussion and vibration, encouraging peripheral pulmonary

secretions to empty by gravity into the major bronchi or
trachea; accomplished by sequential repositioning of the
patient

- Lower and middle lobe bronchi usually emptying best
  with the patient in the head-down position; upper lobe
  bronchi, in the head-up position
- Percussing the chest with cupped hands (or special devices for percussing small areas): mechanically dislodges
  thick, tenacious secretions from the bronchial walls
- Vibration: can be used with percussion or as an alternative in a patient who's frail, in pain, or recovering from
  thoracic surgery or trauma
- Candidates for CPT: patients who expectorate large
  amounts of sputum, such as those with bronchiectasis
  and cystic fibrosis

EQUIPMENT

Stethoscope ◆ pillows ◆ tilt or postural drainage table (if
available) or adjustable hospital bed ◆ emesis basin ◆ facial
tissues ◆ suction equipment ◆ equipment for oral care
◆ trash bag ◆ optional: sterile specimen container, mechanical ventilator, supplemental oxygen, stuffed toy, straw,
soap bubbles, cotton balls, and tissues

ESSENTIAL STEPS

- Explain the procedure to the child and his parents, provide privacy, and wash your hands.
- Administer bronchodilators, if ordered, before CPT to enhance airway clearance.
- Auscultate the child's lungs to determine his baseline
  respiratory status.
- Position the child as ordered.

Performing postural drainage

- In *generalized* disease, drainage usually begins with the
  lower lobes, continues with the middle lobes, and ends
  with the upper lobes.

PERCUSSION DEVICES

Percussion is done to clear secretions from the airway. It can be performed by striking areas over the patient's lungs using either the hand (positioned as in the top illustration) or a percussion device (such as the one in the bottom illustration) that's used for infants.

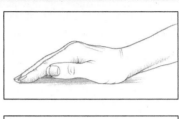

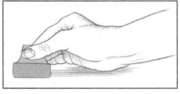

- In *localized* disease, drainage begins with the affected lobes and then proceeds to the other lobes to avoid spreading the disease to uninvolved areas.
- Encourage and assist the child to remain in each position for 10 to 15 minutes.

Performing percussion and vibration
- Perform percussion and vibration as ordered.
- For percussion, encourage the child to breathe slowly and deeply, using the diaphragm, to promote relaxation. Percuss each segment with a cupped hand or device (see *Percussion devices*) for 1 to 2 minutes. Listen for a hollow sound on percussion to verify correct performance of technique.
- To perform vibration, ask the child to inhale deeply, then exhale slowly. During exhalation, firmly press your hands against the chest wall. Tense the muscles of your arms and shoulders in an isometric contraction to send fine vibrations through the chest wall. Do this during 5 exhalations over each chest segment.

Performing coughing and deep breathing exercises
- After postural drainage, percussion, or vibration, encourage the child to breathe deeply to remove loosened secretions.
- Instruct him to inhale deeply through his nose and then exhale in three short huffs.
- Have him inhale deeply again and cough through a slightly open mouth (may be easier while sitting up).
- Give him a soft pillow or stuffed toy to hug while coughing to provide support.
- Three consecutive coughs are highly effective.
- An effective cough sounds deep, low, and hollow; an ineffective cough sounds high-pitched.
- Have the child perform exercises for about 1 minute and then rest for 2 minutes.
- Gradually progress to a 10-minute exercise period 4 times daily.
- Provide oral hygiene because secretions may have a foul taste or a stale odor.
- Auscultate the child's lungs to evaluate the effectiveness of therapy.

NURSING CONSIDERATIONS

- CPT is contraindicated in children who have pulmonary hemorrhage, pulmonary embolism, increased intracranial pressure, osteogenesis imperfecta, or minimal cardiac reserves.
- Perform percussion over the ribs only; don't percuss over the spine, sternum, liver, kidneys, or spleen to avoid injury to the spine or internal organs.
- Avoid percussing on bare skin; instead percuss over soft clothing (but not over buttons, snaps, or zippers) or place a thin towel over the chest wall.
- Encourage the child to perform deep-breathing exercises; use techniques to make this fun, such as having the child blow soap bubbles, blow through a straw, or blow cotton balls or tissues across a table.

- For optimal effectiveness and safety, modify CPT according to the child's condition. For example, initiate or increase the flow of supplemental oxygen, if indicated.
- Also, suction the patient who has an ineffective cough reflex.
- If the child tires quickly during therapy, shorten the sessions because fatigue leads to shallow respirations and increased hypoxia.
- Maintain adequate hydration in the child receiving CPT to prevent mucus dehydration and promote easier mobilization.
- Avoid performing postural drainage immediately before or within 1½ hours after meals to avoid nausea, vomiting, and aspiration of food or vomitus.
- Because chest percussion can induce bronchospasm, any adjunct treatment (for example, intermittent positive-pressure breathing, aerosol, or nebulizer therapy) should precede CPT.

Chest tube insertion and removal

DESCRIPTION

- Pleural space containing a thin layer of lubricating fluid that allows the visceral and parietal pleura to move without friction during respiration
- Excess fluid (hemothorax or pleural effusion), air (pneumothorax), or both in the pleural space changing intrapleural pressure and causing partial or complete lung collapse
- Allows drainage of air or fluid from the pleural space
- Usually performed by a physician with nurse assistance, and requires sterile technique
- Insertion sites varying; dependent on the child's condition and the physician's judgment
- After insertion, chest tubes connected to a thoracic drainage system that removes air and fluid from the pleural space, prevents backflow, and promotes lung reexpansion

EQUIPMENT

Two pairs of sterile gloves ◆ sterile drape ◆ povidone-
iodine solution ◆ vial of 1% lidocaine ◆ 10-ml syringe
◆ alcohol pad ◆ 22G 1″ needle ◆ 25G ⅜″ needle ◆ sterile scalpel (usually with #11 blade) ◆ sterile forceps ◆ two
rubber-tipped clamps for each chest tube ◆ sterile 4″ × 4″
gauze pads ◆ two sterile 4″ × 4″ drain dressings (gauze
pads with slit) ◆ 3″ or 4″ sturdy, elastic tape ◆ 1″ adhesive tape for connections ◆ chest tube of appropriate size
(#16 to #20 French catheter for air or serous fluid; #28 to
#40 French catheter for blood, pus, or thick fluid), with or
without a trocar ◆ sterile Kelly clamp ◆ suture material
(usually 2-0 silk with cutting needle) ◆ thoracic drainage
system sterile drainage tubing, 6′ (1.8 m) long, and connec-
tor ◆ sterile Y-connector (for two chest tubes on the same
side) ◆ petroleum gauze

ESSENTIAL STEPS

- Explain the procedure to the child and his parents, provide privacy, and wash your hands.
- Record baseline vital signs and respiratory assessment.
- If the child has *pneumothorax*, position him in high
  Fowler's, semi-Fowler's, or the supine position. The
  physician will insert the tube into the anterior chest at
  the midclavicular line in the second or third intercostal
  space.
- If the child has *hemothorax*, have him lean over the
  overbed table or straddle a chair with his arms dangling
  over the back. The physician will insert the tube into the
  fourth, fifth, or sixth intercostal space at the midaxillary
  line.
- For either pneumothorax or hemothorax, the child may
  lie on the unaffected side with arms extended over his
  head.
- When you've positioned the patient properly, place the
  chest tube tray on the overbed table.

- Open the equipment using sterile technique.
- The physician will prepare the insertion site by cleaning the area with povidone-iodine solution.
- Wipe the rubber stopper of the lidocaine vial with an alcohol pad.
- Invert the bottle and hold it for the physician to withdraw the anesthetic.
- After anesthetizing the site, he'll make a small incision, insert the chest tube, and connect it to the thoracic drainage system.
- As the physician is inserting the chest tube, reassure the child and assist the physician as needed.
- The physician may secure the tube to the skin with a suture.
- Open the packages containing the petroleum gauze, 4″ × 4″ drain dressings, and gauze pads, and put on sterile gloves.
- Place the petroleum gauze and two 4″ × 4″ drain dressings around the insertion site, one from the top and one from the bottom.
- Place several 4″ × 4″ gauze pads on top of the drain dressings.
- Tape the dressings, covering them completely.
- Securely tape the chest tube to the child's chest distal to the insertion site to prevent accidental tube dislodgment.
- Securely tape the junction of the chest tube and the drainage tube to prevent their separation.
- Make sure the tubing remains level with the child and that there are no dependent loops.
- Immediately after the drainage system is connected, tell the child to take a deep breath, hold it momentarily, and slowly exhale to assist drainage of the pleural space and lung reexpansion.
- A portable chest X-ray is done to check tube position.
- Check the child's vital signs every 15 minutes for 1 hour, then as indicated.
- Auscultate his lungs at least every 4 hours following the procedure to assess air exchange in the affected lung.

ALERT *Diminished or absent breath sounds indicate that the child's lung hasn't reexpanded.*

■ Monitor and record the drainage in the drainage collection chamber.

NURSING CONSIDERATIONS

■ Clamping the chest tube isn't recommended because of the risk of tension pneumothorax.

■ During patient transport, keep the thoracic drainage system below chest level.

ALERT *If the chest tube comes out, cover the site immediately with 4" × 4" gauze pads and tape in place. Stay with the child, and monitor his vital signs every 10 minutes. Look for signs and symptoms of tension pneumothorax (hypotension, distended jugular veins, absent breath sounds, tracheal shift, hypoxemia, weak and rapid pulse, dyspnea, tachypnea, diaphoresis, chest pain). Have another staff member notify the physician and gather the equipment needed to reinsert the tube.*

■ Place rubber-tipped clamps at the bedside.

■ If the drainage system cracks or a tube disconnects, clamp the chest tube as close to the insertion site as possible.

■ The tube may be clamped with large, smooth, rubber-tipped clamps for several hours before removal.

■ As an alternative to clamping the tube, submerge the distal end in a container of normal saline solution to create a temporary water seal while you replace the drainage system. Follow your facility's policy.

■ Look for signs and symptoms of respiratory distress, an indication that air or fluid remains trapped in the pleural space.

■ Chest tubes are usually removed within 7 days to prevent infection. (See *Removing a chest tube.*)

REMOVING A CHEST TUBE

After a child's lung has reexpanded, you may assist the physician in removing a chest tube. First, check vital signs and perform a respiratory assessment. After explaining the procedure to the patient's parents, give the child an analgesic as ordered 30 minutes before tube removal. Then follow these steps:

- Place the child in semi-Fowler's position or on his unaffected side.
- Place a linen-saver pad under the affected side.
- Put on clean gloves, remove chest tube dressings—being careful not to dislodge the chest tube, and discard soiled dressings.
- The physician holds the chest tube in place with sterile forceps and cuts the suture anchoring the tube.
- Make sure the chest tube is securely clamped, then instruct the patient to perform Valsalva's maneuver by exhaling fully and bearing down. Valsalva's maneuver effectively increases intrathoracic pressure.
- The physician holds an airtight dressing, usually petroleum gauze, so he can cover the insertion site immediately after removing the tube.
- After the tube is removed and the site is covered, secure the dressing with tape. Cover the dressing completely to make it as airtight as possible.
- Dispose of the chest tube, soiled gloves, and equipment according to your facility's policy.
- Check vital signs as ordered, and assess depth and quality of respirations. Assess carefully for signs and symptoms of pneumothorax, subcutaneous emphysema, or infection.

Colostomy and ileostomy care

DESCRIPTION

- With an ascending or transverse colostomy or an ileostomy: child must wear an external pouch to collect emerging fecal matter, which will be watery or pasty
- External pouch: helps to control odor and to protect the stoma and peristomal skin
- Most disposable pouching systems used for 2 to 7 days; some models lasting longer

- Pouching systems requiring immediate changing if leak develops
- Ileostomy pouch possibly needing to be emptied four or five times daily
- Pouching system needing to be changed when bowel is least active, usually between 2 and 4 hours after meals
- Selection requires considering which system provides the best adhesive seal and skin protection
- Selection also dependent on the stoma's location and structure, availability of supplies, wear time, consistency of effluent, personal preference, and finances

EQUIPMENT

Pouching system ◆ stoma measuring guide ◆ stoma paste (if drainage is watery to pasty or stoma secretes excess mucus) ◆ plastic bag ◆ water ◆ washcloth and towel ◆ closure clamp ◆ toilet or bedpan ◆ water or pouch cleaning solution ◆ gloves ◆ facial tissues ◆ optional: ostomy belt, paper tape, mild nonmoisturizing soap, liquid skin sealant, and pouch deodorant

ESSENTIAL STEPS

- Provide privacy and emotional support.

Fitting the pouch and skin barrier
- To fit a pouch with an attached skin barrier, use the stoma measuring guide.
- Select the opening size that matches the stoma.
- To fit an adhesive-backed pouch with a separate skin barrier, measure the stoma and select the opening that matches.
- Trace the selected size opening onto the paper back of the skin barrier's adhesive side and cut out the opening, as needed.
- If the pouch has precut openings, which can be handy for a round stoma, select an opening that's ⅛" larger than the stoma.

- If the pouch comes without an opening, cut the hole ⅛" wider than the measured tracing.
- The cut-to-fit system works best for an irregularly shaped stoma.
- Avoid fitting the pouch too tightly. A constrictive opening could injure the stoma or skin tissue without the child feeling a warning discomfort.
- Also avoid cutting the opening too big; it may expose the skin to fecal matter and moisture.
- The child with a descending or sigmoid colostomy who has formed stools and whose ostomy doesn't secrete much mucus may wear only a pouch. In this case, make sure the pouch opening closely matches the stoma size.
- Between 6 weeks and 1 year after surgery, the stoma will shrink to its permanent size. Pattern-making preparations will be necessary as the child gains weight, has additional surgery, or injures the stoma.

Applying or changing the pouch
- Collect all equipment.
- Wash your hands and provide privacy.
- Explain the procedure to the child and his parents. As you perform each step, explain what you're doing and why so the child and his parents learn to perform the procedure.
- Put on gloves.
- Remove and discard the old pouch.
- Wipe the stoma and peristomal skin gently with a facial tissue.
- Carefully wash the peristomal skin with mild soap and water and dry by patting gently; allow the skin to dry thoroughly.
- Inspect the peristomal skin and stoma.
- If applying a separate skin barrier, peel off the paper backing of the prepared skin barrier, center the barrier over the stoma, and press gently to ensure adhesion.
- You may want to outline the stoma on the back of the skin barrier (depending on the product) with a thin ring of stoma paste to provide extra skin protection (skip this

step if the patient has a sigmoid or descending colostomy, formed stools, and little mucus).

- Remove the paper backing from the adhesive side of the pouching system, center the pouch opening over the stoma, and press gently to secure.
- For a pouching system with flanges, align the lip of the pouch flange with the bottom edge of the skin barrier flange.
- Gently press around the circumference of the pouch flange, beginning at the bottom, until the pouch securely adheres to the barrier flange (the pouch will click into its secured position).
- Holding the barrier against the skin, gently pull on the pouch to confirm the seal.
- Have him stay still for about 5 minutes to improve adherence.
- Body warmth also helps improve adherence and soften a rigid skin barrier.
- Attach an ostomy belt to further secure the pouch, if desired. (Some pouches have belt loops, and others have plastic adapters for belts.)
- Leave some air in the pouch to allow drainage to fall to the bottom.
- Apply the closure clamp if necessary.
- If desired, apply paper tape to the pouch edges for additional security.

Emptying the pouch

- Put on gloves.
- Tilt the bottom of the pouch upward and remove the closure clamp.
- Turn up a cuff on the lower end of the pouch and allow it to drain into the toilet or bedpan.
- Wipe the bottom of the pouch and reapply the closure clamp.
- If desired, the bottom portion of the pouch can be rinsed with cool tap water.

 ALERT *Don't aim water up near the top of the pouch because this may loosen the seal on the skin.*

- A two-piece flanged system can also be emptied by unsnapping the pouch.
- Let the drainage flow into the toilet.
- Release flatus through the gas release valve if the pouch has one, or release flatus by tilting the pouch bottom upward, releasing the clamp, and expelling the flatus.
- To release flatus from a flanged system, loosen the seal between the flanges.

  ALERT *Never make a pinhole in a pouch to release gas. This destroys the odor-proof seal.*

- Remove gloves.

NURSING CONSIDERATIONS

- After performing and explaining each procedure, teach the patient and his family self-care.
- Use adhesive solvents and removers only after patch-testing the child's skin; some products may irritate the skin or produce hypersensitivity reactions.
- Consider using a liquid skin sealant, if available, to give skin tissue additional protection from drainage and adhesive irritants.
- Remove the pouching system if the child reports burning or itching or purulent drainage around the stoma.

  ALERT *Notify the physician or therapist of any skin irritation, breakdown, rash, or unusual appearance of the stoma or peristomal area.*

- Most pouches are odor-free; odor should only be evident when you empty the pouch or if it leaks.
- Before discharge, suggest that the patient avoid eating odor-causing foods, such as fish, eggs, onions, and garlic.
- Use commercial pouch deodorants if desired.
- If the child wears a reusable pouching system, suggest that the parents obtain two or more systems so he can wear one while the other dries after cleaning.
- With an ileostomy, provide a diet high in sodium and potassium; avoid highly seasoned foods.
- In a young child, protect the pouch from being pulled off by using one-piece shirt-and-pant outfits.

Drug administration, oral

DESCRIPTION

- Usually the safest, most convenient, and least expensive administration method; most drugs given orally in pediatric patients
- Available as tablets, enteric-coated tablets, capsules, syrups, elixirs, oils, liquids, suspensions, powders, and granules
- May require special preparation before administration, such as mixing with juice to make them more palatable; oils, powders, and granules typically requiring preparation
- Because a child responds to drugs more rapidly and unpredictably than an adult, pediatric drug administration requiring special care; such factors as age, weight, and body surface area may dramatically affect child's response
- Certain disorders possibly affecting a child's response to medication (for example, liver or kidney disorders can hinder the metabolism of some medications)
- Techniques possibly needing adjustment to account for the child's age, size, and developmental level (for example, a tablet for a young child may be crushed and mixed with a liquid for oral administration)

EQUIPMENT

Prescribed drug ◆ plastic disposable syringe, plastic medicine dropper, or spoon ◆ medication cup ◆ water, syrup, or jelly (for tablets) ◆ optional: fruit juice

ESSENTIAL STEPS

- Check the physician's order for the prescribed drug and dosage.
- Compare the order with the drug label, check the drug expiration date, and review the child's chart for any drug allergies.

- Carefully calculate the dosage. Double-check dosages with another nurse for potentially hazardous or lethal drugs, such as insulin, heparin, digoxin, epinephrine, and opioids. Check your facility's policy to learn which drugs must be calculated and checked by two nurses.
- Confirm the child's identity using two patient identifiers according to facility policy.

Giving an oral drug to an infant

- Use a plastic syringe without a needle or a drug-specific medicine dropper to measure the dose.
- If the drug comes in tablet form, first crush the tablet (if appropriate) and mix it with water or syrup. Then draw the mixture into the syringe or dropper.
- Pick up the infant, raising his head and shoulders or turning his head to one side to prevent aspiration.
- Hold the infant close to your body to help restrain him.
- Using your thumb, press down on the infant's chin to open his mouth.
- Slide the syringe or medicine dropper into the infant's mouth alongside his tongue. Release the drug slowly to let the infant swallow and to prevent choking. If appropriate, allow him to suck on the syringe as you expel the drug.
- If not contraindicated, give fruit juice after giving drugs.
- Place a particularly small or inactive infant on his side or back to decrease the risk of sudden infant death syndrome, as recommended by the American Academy of Pediatrics.
- Allow an active infant to assume a position that's comfortable for him; avoid forcing him into a side-lying position to prevent agitation.

Giving an oral drug to a toddler

- Use a plastic, disposable syringe or dropper to measure liquid drugs. Then transfer the fluid to a medication cup.
- Elevate the toddler's head and shoulders to prevent aspiration.

- If possible, ask him to help hold the cup to enlist his co-operation. Otherwise, hold the cup to the toddler's lips, or use a syringe or a spoon to administer the liquid. Make sure the toddler ingests the entire drug.
- If the drug is in tablet form, first crush the tablet, if appropriate, and mix it with water, syrup, or jelly.
- Use a spoon, syringe, or dropper to administer the drug.

Giving an oral drug to an older child

- If possible, let the child choose the liquid drug mixer and a beverage to drink after taking the drug.
- If appropriate, allow him to choose where he'll take the drug, for example, sitting in bed or sitting on a parent's lap.
- If the drug comes in tablet or capsule form, and if the child is old enough (between ages 4 and 6), teach him how to swallow the solid drug. (If he knows how to do this, review the procedure with him for safety's sake.) Tell him to place the pill on the back of his tongue and to swallow it immediately by drinking water or juice. Focus most of your explanation on the water or juice to draw the child's attention away from the pill. Make sure the child drinks enough water or juice to keep the pill from lodging in his esophagus. Afterward, look inside the child's mouth to confirm that he swallowed the pill.
- If the child can't swallow the pill whole, crush it (if appropriate) and mix it with water, syrup, or jelly. Alternatively, after checking with the child's physician, order the drug in liquid form.

NURSING CONSIDERATIONS

- Consult the parents for tips on successfully giving drugs to their child. If possible, have a parent administer a prescribed oral drug while you supervise.
- Allow the child to play with an empty medication cup and to pretend to give the drug to a doll.
- When giving a drug to an older child, be honest. Reassure him that distaste or discomfort will be brief.

- If the prescribed drug comes only in tablet form, consult the pharmacist (or an appropriate drug reference book) to make sure crushing the tablet won't invalidate its effectiveness.
- Avoid adding the drug to a large amount of liquid such as the child's milk or formula because the child may not drink the entire amount, resulting in an inaccurate dose of the drug.

   ALERT *Because infants and toddlers can't tell you what effects they're experiencing from a drug, you must be alert for signs of an adverse reaction. Compile a list of appropriate emergency drugs, calculating the dosages to the patient's weight. Post the list near the patient's bed for reference in an emergency.*

- If you have any doubt about proper drug dosage, always consult the physician who ordered the drug and double-check information in a reliable drug reference.
- Advise the patient and his family that his drugs must be taken as prescribed.
- For home administration, teach the patient and his family about the proper dosage and administration of all prescribed medications.

Hip-spica cast care

DESCRIPTION

- Used to immobilize a child's legs after orthopedic surgery to correct a fracture or deformity, and sometimes used to treat an orthopedic deformity that doesn't require surgery
- Poses several challenges regarding care, including protecting the cast from urine and feces, keeping the cast dry, ensuring proper blood supply to the legs, and teaching the child and his parents how to care for the cast at home
- Infants usually more adaptable to the cast than older children; but both needing encouragement, support, and diversionary activity during their prolonged immobilization

UNDERSTANDING THE HIP-SPICA CAST

As you talk with parents about their child's hip-spica cast, describe how it will extend from the child's lower rib margin (or sometimes from the nipple line) down to the tips of the toes on the affected side and to the knee on the opposite, unaffected side. Mention that it expands at the waist to allow the child to eat comfortably. A stabilizer bar positioned between the legs keeps the hips in slight abduction and separates the legs.

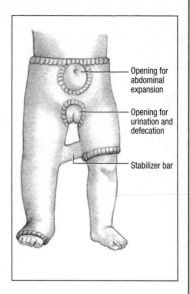

Opening for abdominal expansion

Opening for urination and defecation

Stabilizer bar

EQUIPMENT

Waterproof adhesive tape ◆ moleskin or plastic petals ◆ cast cutter or saw ◆ scissors ◆ nonabrasive cleaner ◆ blow-dryer ◆ optional: disposable diaper or perineal pad

ESSENTIAL STEPS

- Before the physician applies the cast, describe the procedure to the child and his parents.
- For children ages 3 to 12, illustrate your explanation. Draw a picture, present a diagram, or use a doll with a cast or elastic gauze dressing wrapped around its trunk and limbs. (See *Understanding the hip-spica cast*.)
- After the physician constructs the cast, keep all but the perineal area uncovered. Provide privacy by draping a small cover over this opening.

- Turn the patient every 1 to 2 hours to speed drying time. Be sure to turn the child to his unaffected side to prevent adding pressure to the affected side (seek assistance before turning an older child, if needed).
- After the cast dries, inspect the inside edges of the cast for stray pieces of casting material that can irritate the skin.
- Cut several petal-shaped pieces of moleskin and place them, overlapping, around the open edges of the cast to protect the child's skin. Use waterproof adhesive tape around the perineal area.
- Give the child a sponge bath to remove any cast fragments from his skin.
- Assess the child's legs for coldness, swelling, cyanosis, or mottling. Also assess pulse strength, toe movement, sensation (numbness, tingling, or burning), and capillary refill. Perform these circulatory assessments every 1 to 2 hours while the cast is wet and every 2 to 4 hours after the cast dries.
- If the cast is applied after surgery, remember that the most accurate way to assess for bleeding is to monitor vital signs.

  ALERT *A visible blood spot on the cast can be misleading: One drop of blood can produce a circle 3" (7.6 cm) in diameter.*
- Check the child's exposed skin for redness or irritation, and assess for pain or discomfort caused by hot spots (pressure-sensitive areas under the cast). Also be alert for a foul odor. These signs and symptoms suggest a pressure ulcer or infection.
- Encourage the child's family to visit and participate in his care and recreation. This increases the child's sense of security and enhances the parents' sense of participation and control.

NURSING CONSIDERATIONS

- When turning the patient, don't use the stabilizer bar between his legs for leverage because excessive pressure on this bar may disrupt the cast.

- Handle a damp cast only with your palms to avoid misshaping the cast material.
- A traditional hip-spica cast requires 24 to 48 hours to dry. However, a hip-spica cast made from newer, quick-drying substances takes only 8 to 10 hours to dry. If made of fiberglass, it will dry in less than 1 hour.
- If the child is incontinent (or isn't toilet trained), protect the cast from soiling by tucking a folded disposable diaper or perineal pad around the perineal edges of the cast. Then apply a second diaper to the child, over the top of the cast, to hold the first diaper in place. Also, tuck plastic petals into the cast to channel urine and feces into a bedpan. If the cast still becomes soiled, wipe it with a nonabrasive cleaner and a damp sponge or cloth. Then air-dry it with a blow-dryer set on "cool."
- Frequent turnings, range-of-motion exercises, incentive spirometry, and adequate hydration and nutrition can minimize complications, such as constipation, urinary stasis, renal calculi, skin breakdown, respiratory compromise, and contractures.
- Keep a cast cutter or saw available at all times to remove the cast quickly in case of an emergency.
- Teach the patient and his family how to care for the cast. Give them the opportunity to demonstrate their understanding. Include instructions for checking circulatory status, recognizing signs of circulatory impairment, and notifying the physician.
- Demonstrate how to turn the child, apply moleskin, clean the cast, and ensure adequate nourishment.
- To relieve itching, advise the child and his parents to set a handheld blow-dryer on "cool" and blow air under the cast. Warn them not to insert any object (such as a ruler, coat hanger, or knitting needle) into the cast to relieve itching by scratching because these objects could disrupt the suture line, break adjacent skin, and introduce infection.
- Teach the parents to treat dry, scaly skin around the cast by washing the child's skin frequently.

- Be vigilant in ensuring that small objects or food particles don't become lodged under the cast and cause skin breakdown and infection.
- During mealtimes, position older children on their abdomens to promote safer eating and swallowing.
- Before removing the cast, reassure the parents and the child that the noisy sawing process is painless. Explain how the saw works and that it will stop automatically after it cuts the cast.

I.V. therapy

DESCRIPTION

- May be prescribed to administer medications or to correct a fluid deficit, improve serum electrolyte balance, or provide nourishment
- Primary nursing concerns related to pediatric I.V. therapy: correlating the I.V. site and equipment with the reason for therapy and the child's age, size, and activity level (for example, a foot or scalp vein I.V. site may be used for infants, whereas a peripheral hand or wrist vein may be more suitable for ambulatory older children)
- During I.V. therapy: nurse must continually assess the child and the infusion to prevent fluid overload and other complications

EQUIPMENT

Prescribed I.V. fluid ◆ volume-control set with microdrip tubing ◆ infusion pump ◆ I.V. pole ◆ normal saline solution or sterile dextrose 5% in water (D_5W) for injection ◆ antiseptic solution ◆ alcohol pads ◆ 3-ml syringe ◆ child-size butterfly needle or I.V. catheter ◆ tourniquet ◆ ½″ or 1″ sterile tape ◆ gloves ◆ optional: arm board, insulated foam or medicine cup, luer-lock cap, air eliminator I.V. filter

ESSENTIAL STEPS

Preparing the equipment

■ Gather the I.V. equipment, check the expiration date on the I.V. fluid, and inspect the I.V. container (an I.V. bag for leakage, a bottle for cracks) and tubing (for defects or cracks).

■ Open the wrappings on the I.V. solution and the volume-control tubing set. Close all clamps on the tubing set; then insert the tip of the tubing set into the entry port of the I.V. bag or bottle. (If you're using an I.V. bag, be sure to hold the bag upright when attaching the tubing. This will keep the sterile air inside the bag from escaping and making the fluid level difficult to read.)

■ Hang the bottle or bag from the I.V. pole. Open the clamp between the bag and the volume-control set and allow 30 to 50 ml of solution to flow into the calibrated chamber. Close the clamp.

■ Squeeze the drip chamber located below the calibrated chamber or volume-control set to create a vacuum, allowing it to fill halfway with solution. Then release the clamp below the drip chamber so that fluid flows into the remaining tubing, removing any air. After the tubing fills, close the clamp.

■ If you're using an infusion pump, attach the I.V. tubing to the infusion cassette, and insert the cassette into the infusion pump. Prime the cassette tubing according to the manufacturer's instructions.

■ To minimize the risk of infection, maintain sterility at the tip of the I.V. tubing until you connect it to the I.V. needle.

■ Cut as many strips of ½″ or 1″ tape as you'll need to secure the I.V. line. Prepare a syringe with 3 ml of flush solution — either the normal saline solution or D_5W.

Inserting the I.V. catheter

■ Confirm the child's identity using two patient identifiers according to facility policy.

■ Ask the child or his parents whether he's allergic to any type of tape.

FOCUS IN

COMMON PEDIATRIC I.V. SITES

Below are the most common sites for I.V. therapy in infants and children. Peripheral hand, wrist, or foot veins are typically used with older children, whereas scalp veins are used with an infant.

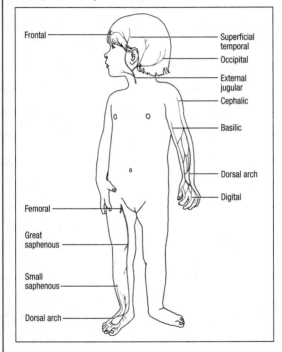

- Explain the reason for the I.V. therapy. Reassure the parents, and enlist their assistance in explaining the procedure to the child in terms he can understand.
- Have a staff member available to help the child remain still, if necessary, during the procedure.
- Wash your hands and put on gloves.
- Select the insertion site for the butterfly needle or catheter. (See *Common pediatric I.V. sites.*)

- Aim for the most distal site possible, and avoid placing the I.V. line in the patient's dominant arm or in areas of flexion if possible. Avoid previously used or sclerotic veins.
- To locate an appropriate scalp vein, carefully palpate the site for arterial pulsations. If you feel these pulsations, select another site.
- To find an appropriate peripheral site, apply a tourniquet to the patient's arm or leg and palpate a suitable vein.
- If you're inserting a butterfly needle, flush the tubing connected to the butterfly with D_5W or normal saline solution.
- Clean the insertion site.
- Insert the I.V. needle into the vein. Watch for blood to flow backward through the catheter or butterfly tubing, which confirms that the needle is in the vein.
- Loosen the tourniquet, and attach the I.V. tubing to the hub of the needle or catheter. Begin the infusion.
- Secure the device by applying a piece of ½" tape over the hub.
- Place a piece of tape, adhesive side up, underneath and perpendicular to the device. Lift the ends of the tape and crisscross them over the device.
- Further secure and protect the I.V. line as needed.

  ALERT *Remember to use only sterile tape under the transparent dressing.*

- Adjust the infusion's flow, as ordered, by using the clamp on the I.V. volume-control tubing or by setting the infusion rate on the infusion pump.

NURSING CONSIDERATIONS

- Assess the I.V. site frequently for signs of infiltration, and check the I.V. bottle or bag for the amount of solution infused.
- Change the I.V. dressing every 24 hours, according to your facility's policy, or as needed to prevent infection.
- Change the I.V. tubing every 48 to 72 hours and the I.V. solution bottle or bag every 24 hours.
- Label the I.V. bottle or bag, tubing, and volume control set with the time and date of change.

- Record the date and time of the I.V. infusion, the insertion site, and the type and size of I.V. needle or catheter.
- Change the I.V. insertion site every 72 hours, if possible, to minimize the risk of infection.
- Try not to select an I.V. site that impairs the child's ability to seek comfort (for example, avoid placing the I.V. needle or catheter in his right arm if the infant sucks his right thumb).
- Forewarn parents if you'll start the I.V. infusion in a scalp vein. Also tell them that you may have to shave hair from a small section of the infant's head.
- Ask an older child to participate in selecting the I.V. site, if possible, to give him a sense of control.
- If the child is mobile, aim for an I.V. site on the upper extremity so that he can still get out of bed.
- Evaluate the need for restraints after inserting the I.V. line and apply, if ordered. Follow your facility's restraint use policy.
- Whenever possible, use a catheter instead of a needle. A flexible catheter is less likely to perforate the vein wall.
- You may apply an antimicrobial ointment over the I.V. site to prevent infection.
- To promote compliance and reduce discomfort associated with catheter insertion, consider using a transdermal anesthetic cream.
- After inserting the I.V. needle or catheter, reward preschool and school-age children. Popular rewards are colorful stickers to wear on clothes or on the I.V. dressing.
- Watch for complications of I.V. therapy, including infection, fluid overload, electrolyte imbalance, infiltration, and circulatory impairment.

Metered-dose inhaler

DESCRIPTION

- Uses pressurized air to produce a mist containing tiny droplets of drug
- Delivers topical medications to the respiratory tract, producing local and systemic effects

- Mucosal lining of respiratory tract absorbs inhalant almost immediately
- Travels deep into the lungs

EQUIPMENT

Child's drug record and chart ◆ metered-dose inhaler
◆ prescribed drug ◆ normal saline solution (or another appropriate solution) for gargling ◆ emesis basin (optional)

ESSENTIAL STEPS

- Verify the physician's order.
- Wash your hands.
- Check the label on the inhaler against the drug record.
- Verify the expiration date.
- Confirm the child's identity using two patient identifiers according to facility policy.
- Explain the procedure to the child and his parents, and teach them how to use the inhaler so treatments can continue after discharge.
- Shake the inhaler bottle to mix the drug and aerosol propellant.
- Remove the mouthpiece and cap.
- Some metered-dose inhalers have a spacer built into the inhaler. Pull the spacer away from the section holding the drug canister until it clicks into place.
- Insert the metal stem on the bottle into the small hole on the flattened portion of the mouthpiece and turn the bottle upside down.
- Have the child exhale; then place the mouthpiece in his mouth and close his lips around it.
- As you firmly push the bottle down against the mouthpiece, ask the child to inhale slowly until his lungs feel full. This draws the medication into his lungs.
- Compress the bottle against the mouthpiece once.
- Remove the mouthpiece from the child's mouth.
- Tell him to hold his breath for several seconds, and then have him exhale slowly through pursed lips.

- Offer normal saline solution (or other appropriate solution) to gargle with, to remove drug from the mouth and the back of the throat.
- Rinse the mouthpiece thoroughly with warm water.

NURSING CONSIDERATIONS

- Know that the lungs retain about 10% of the inhalant; most of the remainder is exhaled.
- Store the medication cartridge below 120° F (48.9° C).
- Spacer inhalers may be recommended for children; a spacer attachment is an extension to the inhaler's mouthpiece, which provides more dead-air space for mixing the medication (some inhalers have built-in spacers).
- Dosages are usually set in numbers of puffs or inhalations. Instruct the child and his parents on the correct prescribed dosage.
- Explain that overdosage — which is common — can cause medication to lose its effectiveness.
- Tell the child and his parents to record the following: date and time of each inhalation and the response to treatment.
- Inform the child and his parents of possible adverse reactions.
- If more than one inhalation is ordered, advise waiting at least 2 minutes before repeating the procedure.
- If the child is also using a steroid inhaler, instruct use of the bronchodilator first and then waiting 5 minutes before using the steroid. This allows the bronchodilator to open the air passages for maximum effectiveness.

Mist tent therapy

DESCRIPTION

- Houses a nebulizer that transforms distilled water into mist
- Also known as a *croupette* for infants or a *cool-humidity tent* for children

- Benefits children by providing a cool, moist environment that eases breathing and helps to decrease respiratory tract edema, liquefy secretions, and reduce fever
- Oxygen may be administered with mist
- Commonly used in treating croup and such infections or inflammations as bronchiolitis and pneumonia

EQUIPMENT

Mist tent frame and plastic tenting ◆ bed sheets ◆ plastic sheet or linen-saver pad ◆ two bath blankets ◆ nebulizer with water reservoir and filter ◆ oxygen flowmeter and oxygen analyzer, if ordered ◆ sterile distilled water ◆ optional: stockinette cap or booties, infant seat

ESSENTIAL STEPS

Preparing the equipment

- Review your facility's policy to determine who sets up a mist tent (in some facilities the nurse sets up the tent; in others a respiratory therapist may do so).
- Wash your hands and place the tent frame and the plastic tenting at the head of the child's crib or bed.
- Cover the mattress with a bed sheet, cover the bed sheet with a plastic sheet or linen-saver pad (tucked under the mattress), and cover these layers with a bath blanket.
- Fill the reservoir of the nebulizer with sterile distilled water and make sure the inlet for air contains a clean filter.
- If the child will have oxygen in the tent, make sure the oxygen flowmeter connects to the tent, and turn the flowmeter to the desired setting.
- Wait 2 minutes after the mist begins filling the tent before placing the child in it.

Implementing the mist tent

- Carefully explain the mist tent's purpose to the child and his parents in terms they can understand to alleviate anxiety and promote cooperation (for example, compare the mist tent with a vaporizer for parents; compare the tent with a teepee or a spaceship cabin for children).

■ Elevate the head of the bed to a position that enhances child comfort.

■ If the patient is an infant, consider placing him in an infant seat because the more upright position will help him to mobilize secretions.

■ If the child will be in the room alone, position him on his side to prevent him from aspirating mucus from liquefied secretions and productive coughing.

■ Use a stockinette cap, booties, and the other bath blanket, as needed, to keep the child from becoming chilled as the mist condenses inside the tent.

■ Change the child's bed sheets and clothing as they dampen, and check his temperature frequently to detect impending hypothermia.

■ Monitor the child frequently for a change in condition, keeping in mind that the mist may make observation difficult.

■ If secretions coat the inside of the tent, wipe the tent down with a hospital-approved cleaner such as soap and water.

■ Clean the reservoir with sterile water to prevent bacterial growth.

ALERT *Because the tent alone won't stop an infant or a small child from falling out of bed, raise the side rails according to your facility's policy. Check on the patient frequently; if possible, place him near the nurses' station.*

NURSING CONSIDERATIONS

■ Allow the child to have toys in the mist tent to provide distraction.

■ Encourage parents to stay with the child. If he grows irritable and uncooperative while in the tent, take him out and let his parents comfort him. Inform the parents that excessive irritability causes labored breathing and increases oxygen consumption. Return the child to the tent when he calms down.

■ To amuse infants, string plastic toys across the top bar of the tent.

■ Discourage cloth or stuffed toys in the tent because these objects absorb moisture and supply a medium for bacterial growth.

■ To prevent a fire, forbid toys or games that may spark or trigger an electric shock, such as battery-operated toys.

■ Remove the electric call light, and give older children a hand bell instead.

■ Prohibit smoking by anyone near the mist tent to minimize the risk of a fire or an explosion (especially if the patient is receiving oxygen).

■ If the child is receiving oxygen, analyze the percentage at least every 4 hours.

■ For bathing, remove the child from the tent to prevent hypothermia.

Oxygen administration

DESCRIPTION

■ Used for hypoxemia resulting from a respiratory or cardiac emergency or an increase in metabolic function

■ In respiratory emergency, enables reduction of ventilatory effort by boosting alveolar oxygen levels

■ In a cardiac emergency, helps to meet the increased myocardial workload as the heart tries to compensate for hypoxemia

■ When metabolic demand is high, supplies the body with enough oxygen to meet its cellular needs

■ Usually required for a child who has a partial pressure of arterial oxygen less than 60 mm Hg or an oxygen saturation range of 89% to 92%

■ Useful in the patient with a reduced blood oxygen-carrying capacity (such as with carbon monoxide poisoning or sickle cell crisis)

- Effectiveness determined by arterial blood gas (ABG) analysis, oximetry monitoring, and clinical examinations
- Administered through an endotracheal or tracheostomy tube during mechanical ventilation or via an anesthesia bag and mask; for a child breathing on his own, delivered via nasal cannula, an oxygen hood or tent, or mask
- Most appropriate method of administration dependent on such factors as disease, physical condition, and age

EQUIPMENT

Oxygen source (wall unit, cylinder, liquid tank, or concentrator) ◆ flowmeter ◆ adapter, if using a wall unit, or a pressure-reduction gauge, if using a cylinder ◆ sterile humidity bottle and adapters ◆ sterile distilled water ◆ "Oxygen Precaution" signs ◆ appropriate oxygen delivery system (nasal cannula, simple mask, partial rebreather mask, or nonrebreather mask for low-flow and variable oxygen concentrations, Venturi mask, aerosol mask) ◆ T tube ◆ tracheostomy collar ◆ tent or oxygen hood for high-flow and specific oxygen concentrations ◆ small-diameter and large-diameter connection tubing ◆ flashlight (for nasal cannula) ◆ water-soluble lubricant ◆ gauze pads ◆ tape (for oxygen masks) ◆ jet adapter for Venturi mask (if adding humidity) ◆ oxygen analyzer (optional)

ESSENTIAL STEPS

- A respiratory therapist usually sets up, maintains, and manages the equipment, but you should have a working knowledge of the oxygen system being used.
- Oxygen is a drug and should be administered only in the prescribed dosage.
- Confirm the child's identity using two patient identifiers according to facility policy
- Check the oxygen outlet port to verify flow.
- Pinch the tubing near the prongs to ensure that an audible alarm will sound if the oxygen flow stops.
- Assess the child's condition; verify open airway.

- Explain the procedure to the child and his parents.
- Perform a safety check of the patient's room to be sure it's safe for oxygen use.
- Whenever possible, replace electric devices with nonelectric ones.

> **ALERT** *For a child in an oxygen tent, remove all toys that may produce a spark. Oxygen supports combustion, and the smallest spark can cause a fire.*

- Place an "Oxygen Precaution" sign over the child's bed and on the door to his room.
- Fit the oxygen delivery device to the child.
- Monitor his response to oxygen therapy.
- Check his ABG values during initial adjustments of oxygen flow.
- When stable, use pulse oximetry instead.
- Check the child frequently for signs of hypoxia.
- Observe the child's skin integrity to prevent skin breakdown.
- Wipe moisture from the child's face and mask.
- Watch for signs of oxygen toxicity.
- Remind the child to cough and deep-breathe frequently.
- Measure ABG values repeatedly to determine whether high oxygen concentrations are still necessary.

NURSING CONSIDERATIONS

- Monitor or measure ABG values 20 to 30 minutes after adjusting the oxygen flow.
- Monitor the child for adverse response to a change in oxygen flow.
- Evaluate the child and his family's ability and motivation to administer oxygen therapy at home.
- Teach the child and his family about the proper use and care of equipment and supplies.
- Document the date and time of oxygen administration, type of delivery device, oxygen flow rate, vital signs, lung sounds, skin color, respiratory effort, and any teaching performed.

Pulse oximetry

DESCRIPTION

- Used intermittently or continuously to noninvasively monitor arterial oxygen saturation (Sao_2)
- Photodetector slipped over finger measures the transmitted light as it passes through the vascular bed, detecting the relative amount of color absorbed by arterial blood, and calculating the exact mixed venous oxygen saturation without interference from surrounding venous blood, skin, connective tissue, or bone
- With an ear probe, works by monitoring transmission of light waves through the vascular bed of a child's earlobe; results possibly inaccurate if the child's earlobe is poorly perfused

EQUIPMENT

Oximeter ◆ finger or ear probe ◆ alcohol pads ◆ nail polish remover, if necessary

ESSENTIAL STEPS

- Explain the procedure to the child and his parents.
- Put the probe on the parent or nurse so the child can see that it's painless.

For pulse oximetry using a finger probe

- Select a finger (usually index finger) for the test.
- Remove nail polish from the test finger if applicable.
- Place the transducer (photodetector) probe over the child's finger so light beams and sensors oppose each other.
- Trim long fingernails or position the probe perpendicular to the finger.
- Position the child's hand at heart level.
  - **ALERT** *If testing a small infant, wrap the probe around the foot so the light beams and detectors op-*

pose each other. For a large infant, use a probe that fits on the great toe and secure it to the foot.

- Turn on the power switch. If the device is working properly, a beep will sound, a display will light momentarily, and the pulse searchlight will flash.
- After 4 to 6 heartbeats, the pulse amplitude indicator will begin tracking the pulse.

Using an ear probe

- Using an alcohol pad, massage the child's earlobe for 10 to 20 seconds.
- Mild erythema indicates adequate vascularization.
- Securely attach the ear probe to the child's earlobe or pinna.
- Use the ear probe stabilizer for prolonged or exercise testing.

    ALERT *Periodically rotate sites for probe placement to prevent skin breakdown under the probe.*

- After a few seconds, a saturation reading and pulse waveform will appear on the oximeter's screen.
- Leave the ear probe in place for 3 or more minutes.
- After the procedure, remove the probe, turn off and unplug the unit, and clean the probe by gently rubbing it with an alcohol pad.

NURSING CONSIDERATIONS

- The pulse rate on the pulse oximeter should correspond to the child's actual pulse. If it doesn't, assess the child, check the oximeter, and reposition the probe.
- Factors that interfere with accuracy include:
  - elevated bilirubin level
  - elevated carboxyhemoglobin or methemoglobin levels
  - lipid emulsions and dyes
  - excessive light
  - excessive patient movement
  - excessive ear pigment
  - hypothermia
  - hypotension
  - vasoconstriction.

- Use the bridge of the nose if the child has compromised circulation in his extremities.
- If Sao_2 is used to guide weaning the patient from forced inspiratory oxygen, obtain arterial blood gas analysis occasionally to correlate pulse oximetry readings with Sao_2 levels in the blood.
- If an automatic blood pressure cuff is used on the same extremity used for measuring Sao_2, the cuff will interfere with Sao_2 readings during inflation.
- If light is a problem, cover the probes.
- If patient movement is a problem, move the probe or select a different probe.
- If ear pigment is a problem, reposition the probe, revascularize the site, or use a finger probe.
- An ideal Sao_2 level for a child is greater than 92%.
- Lower levels may indicate hypoxemia that warrants intervention.
- You may need to resuscitate the child immediately.
- Notify the physician of any significant change in the child's condition.

Tracheostomy care

DESCRIPTION

- Required to ensure airway patency by keeping the tube free of mucus buildup, maintaining mucous membrane and skin integrity, preventing infection, and providing psychological support
- Three types of tracheostomy tubes: uncuffed, cuffed, or fenestrated; selection dependent on the child's condition and the physician's preference
  - *Uncuffed plastic* or *metal tube* — allows air to flow freely around the tracheostomy tube and through the larynx, reducing the risk of tracheal damage
  - *Plastic cuffed tube (disposable)* — the cuff and tube won't separate inside trachea because the cuff is bonded to the tube; doesn't require periodic deflating to lower pressure because cuff pressure is low and evenly

distributed against the tracheal wall; reduces the risk of tracheal damage
- *Plastic fenestrated tube* — permits speech through the upper airway when the external opening is capped and the cuff is deflated; also allows easy removal of the inner cannula for cleaning, but it may become occluded

EQUIPMENT

Aseptic stoma and outer-cannula care
Waterproof trash bag ◆ two sterile solution containers ◆ sterile normal saline solution ◆ hydrogen peroxide ◆ sterile cotton-tipped applicators ◆ sterile 4″ × 4″ gauze pads ◆ sterile gloves ◆ prepackaged sterile tracheostomy dressing (or 4″ × 4″ gauze pad) ◆ supplies for suctioning and mouth care ◆ water-soluble lubricant or topical antibiotic cream ◆ materials as needed for cuff procedures and for changing tracheostomy ties (see below)

Aseptic inner-cannula care
All of the preceding equipment plus a prepackaged commercial tracheostomy care set, or sterile forceps ◆ sterile nylon brush ◆ sterile 6″ (15-cm) pipe cleaners ◆ clean gloves ◆ a third sterile solution container ◆ disposable temporary inner cannula (for a child on a ventilator)

Changing tracheostomy ties
30″ (76.2-cm) length of tracheostomy twill tape ◆ bandage scissors ◆ sterile gloves ◆ hemostat

Emergency tracheostomy tube replacement
Sterile tracheal dilator or sterile hemostat ◆ sterile obturator that fits the tracheostomy tube ◆ extra, appropriate-sized, sterile tracheostomy tube and obturator ◆ suction equipment and supplies

Cuff procedure
5- or 10-ml syringe ◆ padded hemostat ◆ stethoscope

ESSENTIAL STEPS

- Prepare the equipment properly as follows:
  - Wash your hands, and assemble all equipment and supplies in the child's room.
  - Check the expiration date on each sterile package and inspect for tears.
  - Place the open waterproof trash bag next to you so that you can avoid reaching across the sterile field or the child's stoma when discarding soiled items.
  - Establish a sterile field near the child's bed and place equipment and supplies on it.
  - Pour normal saline solution, hydrogen peroxide, or a mixture of equal parts of both solutions into one of the sterile solution containers; pour normal saline solution into the second sterile container for rinsing.
  - For inner-cannula care, use a third sterile solution container to hold the gauze pads and cotton-tipped applicators saturated with cleaning solution.
  - If replacing the disposable inner cannula, open the package containing the new inner cannula while maintaining sterile technique.
  - Obtain or prepare new tracheostomy ties, if indicated.
  - Keep supplies in full view for easy emergency access. Consider taping a wrapped, sterile tracheostomy tube to the head of the bed for emergencies.
- Assess the child's condition to determine need for care.
- Explain the procedure to the child and his parents, even if he's unresponsive. Provide privacy.
- Place the child in semi-Fowler's position, unless contraindicated, to decrease abdominal pressure on the diaphragm and promote lung expansion.
- Remove any humidification or ventilation device.
- Using sterile technique, suction the entire length of the tracheostomy tube to clear the airway of any secretions that may hinder oxygenation.
- Reconnect the patient to the humidifier or ventilator, if necessary.

Cleaning a stoma and outer cannula

■ Put on sterile gloves if you aren't already wearing them.

■ With your dominant hand, saturate a sterile gauze pad or cotton-tipped applicator with the cleaning solution.

■ Squeeze out the excess liquid to prevent accidental aspiration.

■ Wipe the patient's neck under the tracheostomy tube flanges and twill tapes.

■ Saturate a second pad or applicator, and wipe until the skin surrounding the tracheostomy is cleaned. Use additional pads or cotton-tipped applicators to clean the stoma site and the tube's flanges.

> **ALERT** *Wipe only once with each pad or applicator, and then discard it to prevent contamination of a clean area with a soiled pad or applicator.*

■ Rinse debris and peroxide (if used) with one or more sterile 4″ × 4″ gauze pads dampened in normal saline solution.

■ Dry the area thoroughly with additional sterile gauze pads; then apply a new sterile tracheostomy dressing.

■ Remove and discard your gloves.

Cleaning a nondisposable inner cannula

■ Put on sterile gloves. Using your nondominant hand, remove and discard the patient's tracheostomy dressing.

■ With the same hand, disconnect the ventilator or humidification device, and unlock the tracheostomy tube's inner cannula by rotating it counterclockwise.

■ Place the inner cannula in the container of hydrogen peroxide.

■ Working quickly, use your dominant hand to scrub the cannula with the sterile nylon brush.

■ If the brush doesn't slide easily into the cannula, use a sterile pipe cleaner.

■ Immerse the cannula in the container of normal saline solution, and agitate it for about 10 seconds to rinse it.

■ Inspect the cannula for cleanliness. Repeat the cleaning process if necessary.

■ If it's clean, tap it gently against the inside edge of the sterile container to remove excess liquid and prevent aspiration.

 ALERT *Don't dry the outer surface; a thin film of moisture acts as a lubricant during insertion.*

■ Reinsert the inner cannula into the patient's tracheostomy tube.

■ Lock it in place make sure it's positioned securely. Reconnect the mechanical ventilator. Apply a new sterile tracheostomy dressing.

■ If the patient can't tolerate being disconnected from the ventilator for the time it takes to clean the inner cannula, replace the existing inner cannula with a clean one and reattach the mechanical ventilator. Then clean the cannula just removed from him, and store it in a sterile container for the next time.

Caring for a disposable inner cannula

■ Put on clean gloves. Using your dominant hand, remove the inner cannula.

■ After evaluating the secretions in the cannula, discard it properly.

■ Pick up the new inner cannula, touching only the outer locking portion. Insert the cannula into the tracheostomy and, following the manufacturer's instructions, lock it securely.

Changing tracheostomy ties

■ Get help from another nurse or a respiratory therapist to avoid accidental tube expulsion. Patient movement or coughing can dislodge the tube.

■ Wash your hands and put on sterile gloves if you aren't already wearing them.

■ If you aren't using commercially packaged tracheostomy ties, prepare new ties from a 30″ (76.2-cm) length of twill tape by folding one end back 1″ (2.5 cm) on itself; then, with bandage scissors, cutting a ½″ (1.3-cm) slit down the center of the tape from the folded edge.

■ Prepare the other end of the tape the same way.

- Holding both ends together, cut the resulting circle of tape so one piece is approximately 10″ (25 cm) long and the other is about 20″ (51 cm) long.
- Assist the child into semi-Fowler's position if possible.
- After your assistant puts on gloves, instruct her to hold the tracheostomy tube in place to prevent its expulsion during replacement of the ties. (If performed without assistance, fasten the clean ties in place before removing the old ties to prevent tube expulsion).
- With the assistant's gloved fingers holding the tracheostomy tube in place, cut the soiled tracheostomy ties with the bandage scissors or untie them and discard.

   ALERT *Be careful not to cut the tube of the pilot balloon.*

- Thread the slit end of one new tie a short distance through the eye of one tracheostomy tube flange from the underside; use the hemostat, if needed, to pull the tie through. Thread the other end of the tie completely through the slit end and pull it taut so it loops firmly through the flange. This avoids knots that can cause throat discomfort, tissue irritation, pressure, and necrosis.
- Fasten the second tie to the opposite flange in the same manner.
- Instruct the child to flex his neck while you bring the ties around to the side, and tie them together with a square knot. Flexion produces the same neck circumference as coughing and helps prevent an overly tight tie.
- Have your assistant place one finger under the tapes as you tie them to ensure they're tight enough to avoid slippage but loose enough to prevent choking or jugular vein constriction.
- Placing the closure on the side allows easy access and prevents pressure necrosis at the back of the neck when the patient is recumbent.
- After securing the ties, cut off the excess tape with the scissors and have your assistant release the tracheostomy tube.
- Make sure the child is comfortable and can reach the call button easily.

ALERT *Check tracheostomy-tie tension frequently on children with traumatic injury, radical neck dissection, or cardiac failure because neck diameter can increase from swelling and cause constriction; also check neonatal or restless children frequently because ties can loosen and cause tube dislodgment.*

Concluding tracheostomy care

- Replace any humidification device.
- Provide oral care as needed because the oral cavity can become dry and malodorous or develop sores from encrusted secretions.
- Observe soiled dressings and any suctioned secretions for amount, color, consistency, and odor.
- Properly clean or dispose of all equipment, supplies, solutions, and trash, according to your facility's policy, then remove and discard your gloves.
- Make sure that the child is comfortable and that he can easily reach the call button.
- Make sure all necessary supplies are readily available at the bedside.
- Repeat the procedure at least once every 8 hours or as needed.
- Change the dressing as often as necessary regardless of whether you also perform the entire cleaning procedure. A wet dressing with exudate or secretions predisposes the patient to skin excoriation, breakdown, and infection.

NURSING CONSIDERATIONS

- If the child is being discharged with a tracheostomy, start self-care teaching with the child and his parents as soon as they are receptive.
- Teach the child, if appropriate, and his parents, how to change and clean the tube.
- If the child is being discharged with suction equipment, make sure that he and his parents feel knowledgeable and comfortable about using the equipment.
- Keep appropriate equipment at the patient's bedside for immediate use in an emergency.

■ Consult the physician about first-aid measures you can use for your tracheostomy patient should an emergency occur.

ALERT *Follow your facility's policy if a tracheostomy tube is expelled or if the outer cannula becomes blocked. If the patient's breathing is obstructed, call the appropriate code and provide manual resuscitation with a handheld resuscitation bag or reconnect the patient to the ventilator. Don't remove the tracheostomy tube; the airway may close completely. Use caution when reinserting, to avoid tracheal trauma, perforation, compression, and asphyxiation.*

■ Don't change tracheostomy ties unnecessarily during the immediate postoperative period before the stoma track is well formed (usually 4 days) to avoid accidental dislodgment and expulsion of the tube. Unless secretions or drainage is a problem, ties can be changed once a day.

■ Don't change a single-cannula tracheostomy tube or the outer cannula of a double-cannula tube. Because of the risk of tracheal complications, the physician usually changes the cannula; the frequency depends on the child's condition.

■ If the child's neck or stoma is excoriated or infected, apply a water-soluble lubricant or topical antibiotic cream as ordered. Don't use a powder or an oil-based substance on or around a stoma; aspiration can cause infection and abscess.

■ Replace all equipment regularly (including solutions) to reduce the risk of nosocomial infections.

Urine collection

DESCRIPTION

■ Allows screening for urinary tract infection and renal disorders, evaluation of treatment, and detection of systemic and metabolic disorders

■ Provides a simple, effective alternative by offering minimal risk of specimen contamination without resorting to catheterization or suprapubic aspiration

- Contraindicated in a patient with extremely sensitive or excoriated perineal skin, due to collection bag being secured with adhesive flaps
- Alternative methods of collecting urine from small children: use of an inside-out disposable diaper or a test tube

EQUIPMENT

Pediatric urine collection bag (individually packaged) ◆ urine specimen container ◆ label ◆ laboratory request form ◆ two disposable diapers of appropriate size ◆ scissors ◆ gloves ◆ washcloth ◆ soap ◆ water ◆ towel ◆ bowl ◆ linen-saver pad

ESSENTIAL STEPS

- Explain the procedure to the child and his parents.
- Provide privacy, especially if the patient is beyond infancy.
- Confirm the child's identity using two patient identifiers according to facility policy.

Collecting a random specimen

- Wash your hands.
- Place the child on a linen-saver pad.
- Clean the perineal area with soap, water, and a washcloth, working from the urinary meatus outward to prevent contamination of the urine specimen. Wipe gently to prevent tissue trauma and stimulation of urination.
- Separate the labia of the female patient and retract the foreskin of the uncircumcised male patient to expose the urinary meatus.
- Thoroughly rinse the area with clear water and dry with a towel. Don't use powders, lotions, or cream because these counteract the adhesive.
- Place the patient in the frog position, with his legs separated and knees flexed. If necessary, have the child's parent hold him while you apply the collection bag.
- Remove the protective coverings from the collection bag's adhesive flaps.

- For the female patient, first separate the labia and gently press the bag's lower rim to the perineum. Then, working upward toward the pubis, attach the rest of the adhesive rim inside the labia majora.
- For the male patient, place the bag over the penis and scrotum, and press the adhesive rim to the skin.
- After the bag is attached, gently pull it through the slit in the diaper to prevent compression of the bag by the diaper and to allow observation of the specimen immediately after the patient voids. Then fasten the diaper on the patient.
- When urine appears in the bag, put on gloves and gently remove the diaper and the bag. Hold the bag's bottom port over the collection container, remove the tab from the port, and let the urine flow into the container.
- Measure the output if necessary.
- Label the specimen and attach the laboratory request form to the container. Send it directly to the laboratory.
- Remove and discard gloves.
- Put the second diaper on the child, and make sure he's comfortable.

NURSING CONSIDERATIONS

- Avoid forcing fluids to prevent dilution of the specimen, which can alter test results.
- Obtain a first-voided morning specimen if possible.
- To collect a urine specimen from an infant or a young child with extremely sensitive or excoriated perineal skin, use the inside-out disposable diaper method. Place cotton balls in the perineal area of the diaper to absorb urine. After he has voided, remove the diaper and squeeze urine from the cotton balls into a specimen cup. Alternatively, tape a test tube to a male patient's penis to collect urine.

Part four

Diagnostic tests

Arterial blood gas analysis

PURPOSE

■ To evaluate the efficiency of pulmonary gas exchange
■ To assess the integrity of the ventilatory control system
■ To determine the acid-base level of the blood (see *Understanding acid-base disorders*)
■ To monitor respiratory therapy

PATIENT PREPARATION

■ Explain that arterial blood gas analysis evaluates how well the lungs are delivering oxygen to the blood and eliminating carbon dioxide.
■ If the blood sample will be drawn from an arterial catheter, reassure the child that he won't feel pain.
■ If the sample will be taken via arterial puncture, keep in mind that this is typically more painful than a venous puncture. Be honest and explain that it will hurt for a few seconds.
■ Allow the parents to comfort the child during the blood drawing to reassure the child.
■ Explain that only a small amount of blood will be taken, and that the child's body will quickly make new blood to replace it.
■ Inform the child and his parents that he need not restrict food and fluids.
■ Instruct the child to breathe normally during the test.

PROCEDURE

■ Wait at least 20 minutes before drawing arterial blood when starting, changing, or discontinuing oxygen therapy; after initiating or changing mechanical ventilation settings; or after extubation.
■ Use a heparinized blood gas syringe to draw the sample.
■ Confirm the child's identity by checking two patient identifiers.

UNDERSTANDING ACID-BASE DISORDERS

Acid-base disorders may have several causes and signs and symptoms, as outlined in this chart, along with arterial blood gas (ABG) analysis findings for each disorder.

Disorder and ABG findings	Possible causes	Signs and symptoms
Respiratory acidosis (excess carbon dioxide [CO_2] retention) pH < 7.35 Bicarbonate (HCO_3^-) > 26 mEq/L (if compensating) Partial pressure of arterial carbon dioxide ($Paco_2$) > 45 mm Hg	■ Central nervous system depression from drugs, injury, or disease ■ Asphyxia ■ Hypoventilation from pulmonary, cardiac, musculoskeletal, or neuromuscular disease	Diaphoresis, headache, tachycardia, confusion, restlessness, apprehension, flushed face
Respiratory alkalosis (excess CO_2 excretion) pH > 7.45 HCO_3^- < 22 mEq/L (if compensating) $Paco_2$ < 35 mm Hg	■ Hyperventilation from anxiety, pain, or improper ventilator settings ■ Respiratory stimulation from drugs, disease, hypoxia, fever, or high room temperature ■ Gram-negative bacteremia ■ HCO_3^- depletion from diarrhea	Rapid, deep respirations; paresthesia; lightheadedness; twitching; anxiety; fear
Metabolic acidosis (HCO_3^- loss, acid retention) pH < 7.35 HCO_3^- < 22 mEq/L $Paco_2$ < 35 mm Hg (if compensating)	■ Excessive production of organic acids from hepatic disease, endocrine disorders, shock, or drug intoxication ■ Inadequate excretion of acids from renal disease	Rapid, deep breathing; fruity breath; fatigue; headache; lethargy; drowsiness; nausea; vomiting; coma (if severe); abdominal pain

(continued)

UNDERSTANDING ACID-BASE DISORDERS *(continued)*

Disorder and ABG findings	Possible causes	Signs and symptoms
Metabolic alkalosis (HCO_3^- retention, acid loss) pH > 7.45 HCO_3^- > 26 mEq/L $Paco_2$ > 45 mm Hg (if compensating)	■ Loss of hydrochloric acid from prolonged vomiting or gastric suctioning ■ Loss of potassium from increased renal excretion (as in diuretic therapy) or steroids ■ Excessive alkali ingestion	Slow, shallow breathing; hypertonic muscles; restlessness; twitching; confusion; irritability; apathy; tetany; seizures; coma (if severe)

- Perform an arterial puncture or draw blood from an arterial line.
- Eliminate air from the sample, place it on ice immediately, and prepare to transport it for analysis.
- Comfort the child and apply a bandage as soon as the sample has been drawn.
- Before sending the sample to the laboratory, note on the laboratory request whether the child was breathing room air or receiving oxygen therapy when the sample was collected.
- Note the flow rate of oxygen therapy and the delivery method. If the child is on a ventilator, note the fraction of inspired oxygen, tidal volume mode, respiratory rate, and positive end-expiratory pressure.

POSTPROCEDURE CARE

- After applying pressure to the puncture site for 3 to 5 minutes or until bleeding has stopped, tape a gauze pad firmly over it.
- If the puncture site is on the arm, don't tape the entire circumference; this may restrict circulation.

- If the child is receiving anticoagulants or has a coagu-lopathy, apply pressure to the puncture site longer than 5 minutes if necessary.
- Monitor the child's vital signs and observe him for signs of circulatory impairment, such as swelling, discoloration, pain, numbness, and tingling in the bandaged arm or leg.

NORMAL RESULTS

- Pao_2: 80 to 100 mm Hg (SI, 10.6 to 13.3 kPa)
- $Paco_2$: 30 to 40 mm Hg (SI, 4.0 to 5.3 kPa)
- pH: 7.32 to 7.42 (SI, 7.32 to 7.42)
- O_2CT: 15% to 22% (SI, 6.6 to 9.7 mmol/L)
- Sao_2: 94% to 100% (SI, 0.94 to 1)
- HCO_3^-: 22 to 26 mEq/L (SI, 22 to 26 mmol/L)

ABNORMAL RESULTS

- Low Pao_2, O_2CT, and Sao_2 levels and a high $Paco_2$ level, possibly resulting from conditions that impair respiratory function, such as respiratory muscle weakness or paralysis, respiratory center inhibition (from head injury, brain tumor, or drug abuse), and airway obstruction (possibly from mucus plugs or a tumor)
- Low readings possibly resulting from bronchiole obstruction caused by asthma, from an abnormal ventilation-perfusion ratio caused by partially blocked alveoli or pulmonary capillaries, or from alveoli that are damaged or filled with fluid because of disease, hemorrhage, or near-drowning
- When inspired air containing insufficient oxygen, Pao_2, O_2CT, and Sao_2 levels decrease but $Paco_2$ level may be normal; findings common in pneumothorax, impaired diffusion between alveoli and blood, or an arteriovenous shunt that permits blood to bypass the lungs
- Low O_2CT — with normal Pao_2, Sao_2 and, possibly, $Paco_2$ values — possibly resulting from severe anemia, decreased blood volume, and reduced hemoglobin oxygen-carrying capacity

Arteriogram

PURPOSE

- To radiographically examine the target circulation (kidneys, heart, lungs) after injection of a radiopaque contrast medium into an artery (also called *angiogram*)
- To repair certain blood vessels (can be used in conjunction with balloon angioplasty)
- To evaluate circulation abnormalities
- To distinguish benign and malignant neoplasms
- To evaluate the presence and degree of arterial disease

PATIENT PREPARATION

- Make sure that the consent form is signed by the child's parents or legal guardians.
- Note and report all allergies.
- Check the child's history for hypersensitivity to iodine, seafood, or iodinated contrast media.
- Check for and report a history of anticoagulation.
- Check for and report a history of renal insufficiency.
- Note and inform the physician of abnormal laboratory results.
- Instruct the child to fast for 8 hours before the test.
- Stop heparin infusion 3 to 4 hours before the test, if applicable.
- Tell the child that he will need to lie still during the test.
- Explain the need to use a local anesthetic.
- Warn the child that nausea, warmth, or burning may occur with the contrast injection.

PROCEDURE

- The child is placed in a supine position on a radiographic table.
- The access site is prepared and draped and a local anesthetic is injected.

- The artery is punctured with the appropriate needle and catheterized under fluoroscopic guidance.
- Catheter placement is verified by fluoroscopy, and a contrast medium is injected.
- A series of radiographs is taken and reviewed.
- The child's vital signs and neurologic status are monitored continuously.
- The catheter is removed, firm pressure is applied to the access site until bleeding stops, and a pressure dressing is applied.

POSTPROCEDURE CARE

- Monitor the puncture site for bleeding or hematoma formation.
- If active bleeding or expanding hematoma occurs, apply firm pressure to the puncture site and inform the physician immediately.
- Ensure adequate hydration.
- Provide analgesia as needed and as ordered.
- Monitor the child's vital signs, along with intake and output.
- Monitor the neurovascular status of the extremity distal to the access site.
- Inform the physician immediately if distal pulses are absent.

NORMAL RESULTS

- Varying according to the target circulation
- Normal vasculature

ABNORMAL RESULTS

- Varying according to the target circulation
- Vessel displacement possibly suggesting a tumor

Arthrography

PURPOSE

- To outline joint contour and soft-tissue structures
- To evaluate persistent unexplained joint discomfort or pain
- To identify acute or chronic abnormalities of the joint capsule or supporting ligaments of the knee, shoulder, ankle, hip, or wrist
- To detect internal joint derangements
- To locate synovial cysts
- To evaluate damage from recurrent dislocations

PATIENT PREPARATION

- Make sure that the consent form is signed by the child's parents or legal guardians.
- Note and report all allergies.
- Explain the purpose of the study, how it's done, who will perform the study, and where it will take place.
- Inform the child and his parents that he need not restrict food and fluids.
- Warn the child that a tingling sensation, burning, or pressure in the joint may occur with the contrast injection.
- Explain to the child that some swelling, discomfort, or crepitant noises may occur in the joint after the study and that these usually disappear after 1 or 2 days. Tell the child and his parents to contact the physician if symptoms persist.
- Inform the child and his parents that the study takes about 45 minutes.

PROCEDURE

- The skin is cleaned around the puncture site with an antiseptic solution and injected with a local anesthetic.
- A needle is then inserted into the joint space.

- Fluid may be aspirated and sent to the laboratory for analysis.
- When fluoroscopic examination shows correct needle placement, a contrast medium is injected into the joint space.
- The needle is removed, and the puncture site is covered with a sterile dressing.
- The joint is put through its range of motion to distribute the contrast medium within the joint space.
- A series of radiographs is rapidly taken before the joint tissue can absorb the contrast medium.

POSTPROCEDURE CARE

- Emphasize the need to rest the joint for 6 to 12 hours.
- Wrap the knee in an elastic bandage for several days if a knee arthrography was performed.
- Apply ice to the joint for swelling.
- Give the child an analgesic as ordered.
- Ask the child and his parents to report signs and symptoms of infection.

NORMAL RESULTS

- Knee arthrogram showing a characteristic wedge-shaped shadow pointed toward the interior of the joint, indicating a normal medial meniscus
- Shoulder arthrogram showing the bicipital tendon sheath, redundant inferior joint capsule, and intact subscapular bursa

ABNORMAL RESULTS

- Structural abnormalities of the knee commonly suggesting tears and lacerations of the meniscus
- Extrameniscal lesions possibly suggesting osteochondral fractures, cartilaginous abnormalities, synovial abnormalities, cruciate ligament tears, and joint capsule and collateral ligament disruptions

- Shoulder abnormalities possibly suggesting adhesive capsulitis, bicipital tenosynovitis or rupture, and rotator cuff tears

Bone marrow aspiration and biopsy

PURPOSE

- To diagnose thrombocytopenia, leukemias, granulomas, anemias, and primary and metastatic tumors
- To determine causes of infection
- To help stage diseases such as with Hodgkin's disease
- To evaluate chemotherapy
- To monitor myelosuppression

PATIENT PREPARATION

- Make sure that the consent form is signed by the child's parents or legal guardians.
- Note and report all allergies.
- Explain that collection of a blood sample is necessary before the biopsy for laboratory testing.
- Explain to the child that he'll feel pressure on insertion of the biopsy needle and a brief, pulling pain on removal of the marrow.
- Explain which bone site (sternum, anterior or posterior iliac crest, vertebral spinous process, rib, or tibia) will receive the test.
- If age appropriate, allow the child to "perform" the procedure on a doll (use correct positioning, a syringe, and a bandage) to enhance the child's understanding of the procedure and help ease his fears.
- Give a mild sedative 1 hour before the test, as ordered.
- Provide analgesics as ordered.
- Explain that the test usually takes about 20 minutes.
- Explain that the puncture site may remain tender for a few weeks.

PROCEDURE

■ The child is positioned and instructed to remain as still as possible. Allowing a parent to be present to comfort the child may be helpful.

Aspiration biopsy (removal of a fluid specimen from bone marrow)

■ The biopsy site is prepared and draped and a local anesthetic is injected. The marrow aspiration needle is inserted through the skin, subcutaneous tissue, and bone cortex, using a twisting motion.

■ The stylet is removed from the aspiration needle, and a 10- to 20-ml syringe is attached. From 0.2 to 0.5 ml of marrow is aspirated and the needle is withdrawn.

■ If the aspiration specimen is inadequate, the needle may be repositioned within the marrow cavity or removed and reinserted in another anesthetized site. If the second attempt fails, a needle biopsy may be necessary.

Needle biopsy (removal of a core of marrow cells)

■ The biopsy site is prepared and draped. The skin is marked at the site with an indelible pencil or marking pen. A local anesthetic is injected intradermally, subcutaneously, and at the surface of the bone.

■ The biopsy needle is inserted into the periosteum and the needle guard set as indicated. Rotating the inner needle alternately clockwise and counterclockwise directs the needle into the marrow cavity.

■ A tissue plug is removed and the needle assembly withdrawn. The marrow is expelled into a labeled bottle containing a special fixative.

POSTPROCEDURE CARE

■ While the marrow slides are being prepared, apply pressure to the biopsy site until bleeding stops.

■ Clean the biopsy site and apply a sterile dressing.

■ Monitor the child's vital signs and the biopsy site for signs and symptoms of infection.

NORMAL RESULTS

- Yellow marrow containing fat cells and connective tissue
- Red marrow containing hematopoietic cells, fat cells, and connective tissue
- Iron stain, which measures hemosiderin (storage iron), having a +2 level
- Negative Sudan black B stain (shows granulocytes)
- Negative periodic acid–Schiff (PAS) stain (detects glycogen reactions)

ABNORMAL RESULTS

- Decreased hemosiderin levels in an iron stain possibly indicating a true iron deficiency
- Increased hemosiderin levels possibly suggesting other types of anemias or blood disorders
- Positive stain differentiating acute myelogenous leukemia from acute lymphoblastic leukemia (negative stain)
- Positive stain possibly suggesting granulation in myeloblasts
- Positive PAS stain possibly suggesting acute or chronic lymphocytic leukemia, amyloidosis, thalassemia, lymphoma, infectious mononucleosis, iron deficiency anemia, or sideroblastic anemia

Bronchoscopy

PURPOSE

- To allow visual examination of tumors, obstructions, secretions, or foreign bodies in the tracheobronchial tree
- To diagnose bronchogenic carcinoma, tuberculosis, interstitial pulmonary disease, and fungal or parasitic pulmonary infections
- To obtain specimens for microbiological and cytologic examination
- To locate bleeding sites in the tracheobronchial tree

■ To remove foreign bodies, malignant or benign tumors, mucus plugs, and excessive secretions from the tracheo-bronchial tree

PATIENT PREPARATION

■ Make sure that a consent form is signed by the child's parents or legal guardians.
■ Note and report all allergies.
■ Instruct the child and his parents that he must fast for 6 to 12 hours before the test.
■ Obtain results of preprocedure studies; report abnormal results.
■ Obtain the child's baseline vital signs.
■ Administer an I.V. sedative as ordered.
■ Explain to the child and his parents that the test takes 45 to 60 minutes.
■ Explain to the child and his parents that blocking of the airway won't occur and that hoarseness, loss of voice, hemoptysis, and a sore throat may occur.

PROCEDURE

■ Position the child properly.
■ Give supplemental oxygen by nasal cannula if ordered.
■ Monitor the child's pulse oximetry, vital signs, and cardiac rhythm.
■ A local anesthetic is sprayed into the mouth and throat to suppress the gag reflex.
■ The bronchoscope is inserted through the mouth or nose; a bite block is placed in the mouth if using the oral approach.
■ When the bronchoscope is just above the vocal cords, about 3 to 4 ml of 2% to 4% lidocaine is flushed through the inner channel of the scope to the vocal cords to anesthetize deeper areas.
■ A fiber-optic camera is used to take photographs for documentation.
■ Tissue specimens are obtained from suspect areas.

- A suction apparatus may remove foreign bodies or mucus plugs.
- Bronchoalveolar lavage may remove thickened secretions or may diagnose infectious causes of infiltrates.
- Specimens are prepared properly and immediately sent to the laboratory.

POSTPROCEDURE CARE

- Position a conscious child in semi-Fowler's position.
- Position an unconscious child on one side, with the head of the bed slightly elevated, to prevent aspiration.
- Instruct the child to spit out saliva rather than swallow it.
- Observe for bleeding.
- Resume the child's usual diet, beginning with sips of clear liquid or ice chips, when the gag reflex returns.
- Provide lozenges or a soothing liquid gargle to ease discomfort when the gag reflex returns.
- Check the follow-up chest X-ray for pneumothorax.
- Monitor the child's vital signs, sputum characteristics, and respiratory status.

NORMAL RESULTS

- Bronchi appearing structurally similar to the trachea
- Right bronchus slightly larger and more vertical than the left
- Smaller segmental bronchi branching off from the main bronchi

ABNORMAL RESULTS

- Structural abnormalities of the bronchial wall indicating inflammation, ulceration, tumors, and enlargement of submucosal lymph nodes
- Structural abnormalities of endotracheal origin suggesting stenosis, compression, ectasia, and diverticula
- Structural abnormalities of the trachea or bronchi suggesting calculi, foreign bodies, masses, and paralyzed vocal cords

- Tissue and cell study abnormalities suggesting interstitial pulmonary disease, infection, carcinoma, and tuberculosis

Cardiac catheterization

PURPOSE

- To evaluate valvular insufficiency or stenosis, septal defects, congenital anomalies, myocardial function, myocardial blood supply, and cardiac wall motion
- To aid in diagnosing left ventricular enlargement, aortic root enlargement, ventricular aneurysms, and intracardiac shunts

PATIENT PREPARATION

- Make sure that the consent form is signed by the child's parents or legal guardians.
- Notify the physician of hypersensitivity to shellfish, iodine, or contrast media.
- Stop anticoagulants, as ordered, to reduce complications of bleeding.
- Restrict food and fluids for at least 6 hours before the test.
- Describe to the child and his parents the procedure room as well as the equipment that will be used during the procedure. Show the child where on his body the catheter will be inserted, using a doll to prepare him (if age appropriate and as necessary).
- Tell the child that the lights in the room will be dimmed after the catheter is placed. Reassure him that you'll be right there with him and will talk to him throughout the procedure.
- Tell the child that he may feel warm after the contrast medium is injected.
- Inform the child and his parents that the test will take 1 to 2 hours.

■ Assess the child's color, temperature of his extremities, and pedal pulses.

PROCEDURE

■ The child is placed supine on a table and his heart rate and rhythm, respiratory status, and blood pressure are monitored throughout the procedure.
■ An I.V. line is started, if not already in place, and a local anesthetic is injected at the insertion site.
■ A small incision is made into the artery or vein, depending on whether the test is for the left or right.
■ The catheter is passed through the sheath into the vessel and guided using fluoroscopy.
■ In right-sided heart catheterization, the catheter is inserted into the antecubital or femoral vein and advanced through the vena cava into the right side of the heart and into the pulmonary artery.
■ In left-sided heart catheterization, the catheter is inserted into the brachial or femoral artery and advanced retrograde through the aorta into the coronary artery ostium and left ventricle.
■ When the catheter is in place, contrast medium is injected to make visible the cardiac vessels and structures.
■ After the catheter is removed, direct pressure is applied to the incision site until bleeding stops, and a sterile dressing is applied.

POSTPROCEDURE CARE

■ Reinforce the dressing as needed.
■ Monitor the site for bleeding and hematoma formation.
■ Enforce bed rest for 8 hours.
■ If the femoral route was used for catheter insertion, keep the leg straight at the hip for 6 to 8 hours.
■ If the antecubital fossa route was used, keep the arm straight at the elbow for at least 3 hours.
■ Resume medications and give analgesics, as ordered.
■ Encourage fluid intake.

- Monitor the child's vital signs, intake and output, cardiac rhythm, neurologic and respiratory status, and peripheral vascular status distal to the puncture site.
- Check the catheter insertion site and dressings for signs and symptoms of infection.
- If cardiac catheterization was done on an outpatient basis, instruct the parents to:
  - Keep the insertion site covered with an adhesive bandage for several days after the procedure.
  - Keep the site clean and dry; give only sponge baths until the site is healed.
  - Observe the site for redness, swelling, drainage, and bleeding.
  - Monitor the child's temperature and report fever promptly.
  - Have the child avoid strenuous exercise.
  - Administer acetaminophen or ibuprofen as needed for discomfort or pain.
  - Keep follow-up appointments.

NORMAL RESULTS

- No abnormalities of heart valves, chamber size, pressures, configuration, wall motion or thickness, and blood flow
- Coronary arteries having smooth and regular outline

ABNORMAL RESULTS

- Coronary artery narrowing greater than 70% suggesting significant coronary artery disease
- Narrowing of the left main coronary artery and occlusion or narrowing high in the left anterior descending artery suggesting the need for revascularization surgery
- Impaired wall motion suggesting myocardial incompetence
- Pressure gradient indicating valvular heart disease
- Retrograde flow of the contrast medium across a valve during systole indicating valvular incompetence

Computed tomography

PURPOSE

- To produce cross-sectional images of various layers of tissue generating images not readily seen on standard X-rays

PATIENT PREPARATION

- Make sure that the consent form is signed by the child's parents or legal guardians.
- Note and report all allergies.
- Check the child's history for hypersensitivity to shellfish, iodine, or iodinated contrast media, and document such reactions on his chart.
- Show the child a picture of the computed tomography (CT) machine to help alleviate his fears. (It may be necessary to premedicate the child.)
- Explain that the child won't be able to eat or drink for 4 hours before the scan (depending on age).
- The specific type of CT scan dictates the need for an oral or I.V. contrast medium.
- Explain to the child that he may experience discomfort from the needle puncture and a warm or flushed feeling from an I.V. contrast medium, if used.
- Instruct the child to remain still during the test because movement can limit the accuracy of results.
- Tell the child that he may hear a clicking noise as the scanner moves around his head but that the machine won't touch him.
- Tell the child he may experience minimal discomfort because of lying still.
- Tell the child to immediately report feelings of nausea, vomiting, dizziness, headache, itching, or hives.
- Inform the child and his parents that the study takes from 5 minutes to 1 hour depending on the type of CT scan and his ability to remain still.

■ A CT scan usually isn't recommended during pregnancy because of potential risk to the fetus.

PROCEDURE

■ The child is positioned on an adjustable table inside a scanning gantry.
■ A series of transverse radiographs is taken and recorded.
■ The information is reconstructed by a computer and selected images are photographed.
■ After the images are reviewed, I.V. contrast enhancement may be ordered.
■ Additional images are obtained after I.V. contrast injection.
■ The child is observed carefully for adverse reactions to the contrast medium.

POSTPROCEDURE CARE

■ Normal diet and activities may resume, unless otherwise ordered.
■ Encourage the child to drink fluids after the scan (dye is excreted by the kidneys).

NORMAL RESULTS

■ Specific type of CT scan dictating normal findings
■ Tissue densities appearing as black, white, or shades of gray on the CT image
■ Bone having densest tissue, appearing white
■ Cerebrospinal fluid having the least dense, appearing black

ABNORMAL RESULTS

Abdomen and pelvis
■ Primary and metastatic neoplasms, abscesses, cysts, and obstructive disease from a tumor or calculi

Bone
- Primary bone tumors, soft-tissue tumors, skeletal metastasis, bone fractures, and joint abnormalities (hard to detect by other methods)

Brain
- Cerebral atrophy, cerebral edema, arteriovenous malformation, intracranial tumors, intracranial hematoma, infarction, edema, and congenital anomalies such as hydrocephalus (indicated by enlargement of the fourth ventricle in children)

Ear
- Tympanosclerosis and osseous changes of the external auditory canal and middle and inner ear structures
- Cochlear abnormalities

Kidneys
- Renal masses, renal cysts, solid tumors, vascular tumors, adrenal tumors, obstructions, calculi, polycystic kidney disease, congenital anomalies, and abnormal accumulations of fluid around the kidneys

Liver and biliary tract
- Small lesions, hepatic abscesses, hepatic cysts, hepatic hematoma, subcapsular hematomas, nonobstructive jaundice, obstructive jaundice, dilation (of the common hepatic duct, common bile duct, and gallbladder), and obstructions

Pancreas
- Pseudocysts (unilocal or multilocal), acute pancreatitis (either edematous [interstitial] or necrotizing [hemorrhagic]), abscesses (within or outside the pancreas), and chronic pancreatitis

Spine
- Spinal lesions, tumors, neurinomas (schwannomas), meningiomas, degenerative processes and structural

changes, a herniated nucleus pulposus, cervical spondylosis, lumbar stenosis, facet disorders, paraspinal cysts, vascular malformations, and congenital spinal malformations

Thorax

■ Tumors, nodules, cysts, aortic aneurysms, enlarged lymph nodes, pleural effusion, and accumulations of blood, fluid, or fat

Echocardiography

PURPOSE

■ To diagnose and evaluate valvular abnormalities
■ To measure and evaluate the size of the heart's chambers and valves
■ To help diagnose cardiomyopathies and atrial tumors
■ To evaluate cardiac function or wall motion after myocardial infarction (rare in children)
■ To detect pericardial effusion or mural thrombi

PATIENT PREPARATION

■ Make sure that the consent form is signed by the child's parents or legal guardians.
■ Tell the child that he may be asked to breathe in and out slowly or to hold his breath while changes in heart function are recorded.
■ Stress the importance of holding still during the test because movement may distort results. Assist as necessary.
■ Administer mild sedation if needed, as ordered. Use distractions, such as a videotape, to help calm the child.
■ Explain that the procedure is painless.
■ Explain to the child and his parents that the test takes 15 to 30 minutes.

PROCEDURE

- The child is placed in the supine position, and conductive gel is applied to the third or fourth intercostal space to the left of the sternum. The transducer is placed directly over it.
- The transducer is systematically angled to direct ultrasonic waves at specific parts of the heart.
- During the test, the oscilloscope screen is observed; significant findings are recorded on a strip chart recorder or on a videotape recorder.
- For a left lateral view, the child is placed on his left side.
- Doppler echocardiography may also be used. Color flow simulates red blood cell flow through the heart valves. The sound of blood flow may also be used to assess heart sounds and murmurs as they relate to cardiac hemodynamics.

POSTPROCEDURE CARE

- Remove the conductive gel from the child's skin.

NORMAL RESULTS

- For the mitral valve, anterior and posterior mitral valve leaflets separating in early diastole and attaining maximum excursion rapidly, then moving toward each other during ventricular diastole; after atrial contraction, the mitral valve leaflets coming together and remaining together during ventricular systole
- For the aortic valve, aortic valve cusps moving anteriorly during systole and posteriorly during diastole
- For the tricuspid valve, motion resembling that of the mitral valve
- For the pulmonic valve, movement being posterior during atrial systole and during ventricular systole; in right ventricular ejection, cusp moving anteriorly, attaining its most anterior position during diastole

---

TRANSESOPHAGEAL ECHOCARDIOGRAPHY

Transesophageal echocardiography combines ultrasound with endoscopy. It's an alternative method for detecting cardiovascular problems in children and is used when the transthoracic approach isn't possible or would be difficult.

During the procedure, the transducer is passed into the esophagus to an area behind the atria. The procedure is more complicated than the transthoracic approach and may require intubation to preserve the airway in young children.

- For the ventricular cavities, left ventricular cavity normally appearing as an echo-free space between the interventricular septum and the posterior left ventricular wall
- The right ventricular cavity normally appearing as an echo-free space between the anterior chest wall and the interventricular septum

ABNORMAL RESULTS

- In mitral stenosis, the valve narrowing abnormally because of the leaflets' thickening and disordered motion; during diastole, both mitral valve leaflets moving anteriorly instead of posteriorly
- In mitral valve prolapse, one or both leaflets ballooning into the left atrium during systole
- In aortic insufficiency, leaflet fluttering of the aortic valve during diastole
- In stenosis, the aortic valve thickening and generating more echoes
- In bacterial endocarditis, valve motion being disrupted and fuzzy echoes usually appearing on or near the valve
- Large chamber size possibly indicating cardiomyopathy, valvular disorders, or heart failure
- Small chamber possibly indicating restrictive pericarditis
- Hypertrophic cardiomyopathy identified by systolic anterior motion of the mitral valve and asymmetrical septal hypertrophy

- Myocardial ischemia or infarction possibly causing absent or paradoxical motion in ventricular walls
- Pericardial effusion suggested when fluid accumulates in the pericardial space, causing an abnormal echo-free space to appear
- In large effusions, pressure exerted by excess fluid restricting pericardial motion — may be better viewed by performing transesophageal ultrasound (see *Transesophageal echocardiography*, page 369)

Electrocardiography

PURPOSE

- To identify conduction abnormalities, cardiac arrhythmias, myocardial ischemia or myocardial infarction (rare in children), injury, necrosis, bundle-branch block, fascicular blocks, and chamber enlargement
- To document pacemaker performance

PATIENT PREPARATION

- Explain the test to the child and his parents, stressing that the test is painless.
- Describe the equipment that will be used for the test; show the child a picture or, if possible, the actual equipment.
- Explain to the patient the need to lie still, relax, and breathe normally during the procedure. He may sit on his parent's lap if necessary.
- Explain that the child may have to lie on his left side, inhale and exhale slowly, or hold his breath at intervals during the test.
- Note current cardiac drug therapy on the test request form as well as other pertinent clinical information such as the presence of a pacemaker.
- Explain that the test is painless and takes 5 to 10 minutes.

PROCEDURE

- Confirm the child's identity by checking two patient identifiers.
- Place the child in a supine or semi-Fowler's position.
- Expose the chest, ankles, and wrists.
- Place electrodes on the inner aspect of the wrists, on the medial aspect of the lower legs, and on the chest.
- After all the electrodes are in place, connect the lead wires.
- Press the START button and input any required information.
- Make sure that all leads are represented in the tracing. If not, determine which electrode is not attached properly, reattach it, and restart the tracing.
- All recording and other nearby electrical equipment should be properly grounded.
- Make sure that electrodes are firmly attached.

POSTPROCEDURE CARE

- Disconnect the equipment, remove the electrodes, and remove the gel with a moist cloth towel.

NORMAL RESULTS

- Cardiac rate appearing within normal limits for child's age
- Cardiac rhythm showing normal sinus rhythm
- P wave preceding each QRS complex
- PR, QRS, and QT intervals varying according to child's age
- T wave appearing rounded and smooth and positive in leads I, II, V_3, V_4, V_5, and V_6

ABNORMAL RESULTS

- Heart rate below (bradycardia) or above (tachycardia) the normal limits for the child's age (see *Normal heart rates*, page 372)

NORMAL HEART RATES

Age	Awake (beats/ minute)	Asleep (beats/ minute)	Exercise or fever (beats/ minute)
Neonate	100 to 160	80 to 140	< 220
1 week to 3 months	100 to 220	80 to 200	< 220
3 months to 2 years	80 to 150	70 to 120	< 200
2 to 10 years	70 to 110	60 to 90	< 200
> 10 years	55 to 100	50 to 90	< 200

- Missing P waves possibly indicating atrioventricular (AV) block, atrial arrhythmia, or junctional rhythm
- Short PR interval possibly indicating a junctional arrhythmia; a prolonged PR interval possibly indicating an AV block
- Prolonged QRS complex possibly indicating intraventricular conduction defects; missing QRS complexes possibly indicating an AV block or ventricular asystole
- ST-segment elevation of 0.2 mV or more above the baseline possibly indicating myocardial injury; ST-segment depression possibly indicating myocardial ischemia or injury
- T wave inversion in leads I, II, and V_3 to V_6 possibly indicating myocardial ischemia; peaked T waves possibly indicating hyperkalemia or myocardial ischemia; variations in T wave amplitude possibly indicating electrolyte imbalances
- Prolonged QT interval possibly suggesting life-threatening ventricular arrhythmias

Electroencephalography

PURPOSE

- To determine the presence and type of epilepsy
- To aid in the diagnosis of intracranial lesions
- To evaluate brain activity in metabolic disease, head injury, meningitis, encephalitis, and psychological disorders
- To help confirm brain death

PATIENT PREPARATION

- Make sure that the consent form is signed by the child's parents or legal guardians.
- Note and report all allergies.
- Wash and dry the child's hair to remove hairsprays, creams, or oils.
- Withhold tranquilizers, barbiturates, and other sedatives for 24 to 48 hours before the test.
- Minimize sleep (4 to 5 hours) the night before the study.
- If a sleep EEG is ordered, give a sedative to promote sleep during the test.
- Make sure that the child continues to eat and drink before the test because fasting may cause hypoglycemia, which could alter the test results.
- Make sure that the child doesn't drink anything with caffeine on the morning of the test because of caffeine's stimulating effect.
- Reassure the child that he won't feel anything during the test.
- Tell the child that he needs to remain still during the test; any movement will create interference and alter the EEG recording.
- Infants and very young children may require sedation to prevent crying and restlessness, but sedatives may alter test results.
- Inform the child and his parents that the test that takes about 1 hour.

PROCEDURE

- The child is positioned, and electrodes are attached to the scalp.
- During recording, the child is carefully observed and movements, such as blinking, swallowing, or talking, are noted; these movements can cause artifact.

POSTPROCEDURE CARE

- Help the child remove electrode paste from his hair.
- Monitor the child for seizures and maintain seizure precautions.
- Provide a safe environment.
- Drug therapy may resume.
- If brain death is confirmed, provide emotional support to the family.

NORMAL RESULTS

- Alpha waves occurring at frequencies of 8 to 13 cycles/second in a regular rhythm
- Alpha waves presenting only in the waking state when the child's eyes are closed but he's mentally alert and usually disappearing with visual activity or mental concentration
- Alpha waves decreasing by apprehension or anxiety and most prominent in the occipital leads
- Beta waves (13 to 30 cycles/second) indicating normal activity when the child appears alert with his eyes open; appearing most readily in the frontal and central regions of the brain
- Theta waves (4 to 7 cycles/second) most common in children and young adults
- Delta waves (fewer than 4 cycles/second) visible in deep sleep stages and in serious brain dysfunction

ABNORMAL RESULTS

- Spikes and waves at a frequency of 3 cycles/second suggesting absence seizures
- Multiple, high-voltage, spiked waves in both hemispheres suggesting generalized tonic-clonic seizures
- Spiked waves in the affected temporal region suggesting temporal lobe epilepsy
- Localized, spiked discharges suggesting focal seizures
- Slow waves (usually delta waves but possibly unilateral beta waves) suggesting intracranial lesions
- Focal abnormalities in the injured area suggesting vascular lesions
- Generalized, diffuse, and slow brain waves suggesting metabolic or inflammatory disorders or increased intracranial pressure
- An absent EEG pattern or a flat tracing (except for artifacts) possibly indicating brain death

Electromyography

PURPOSE

- To differentiate among primary muscle disorders, such as muscular dystrophy, and certain metabolic disorders
- To identify diseases characterized by central neuronal degeneration
- To aid in diagnosing neuromuscular disorders
- To aid in diagnosing radiculomyopathies

PATIENT PREPARATION

- Make sure that the consent form is signed by the child's parents or legal guardians.
- Note and report all allergies.
- Check for and note drugs that may interfere with test results (cholinergics, anticholinergics, anticoagulants, and skeletal muscle relaxants).

- Tell the child and his parents that he need not restrict food and fluids before the test, but that it may be necessary to restrict cola for 2 to 3 hours beforehand.
- Prepare the child for insertion of the needle and the feeling in the muscle when the electrical impulses are sent through. Explain that it will feel like a hard hit to the "funny bone," and that residual bruising may occur.
- Explain that the child may be asked to voluntarily contract the muscle; help him practice the different positions or movements.
- Use deep-breathing exercises and play preparation to help lessen the fear and anxiety the child may experience.
- Reassure the child that his parents may stay with him during the procedure.
- Inform the child and his parents that the test takes at least 1 hour.

PROCEDURE

- The child is positioned in a way that relaxes the muscle to be tested.
- Needle electrodes are quickly inserted into the selected muscle.
- A metal plate lies under the child to serve as a reference electrode.
- The resulting electrical signal is recorded during rest and contraction, amplified 1 million times, and displayed on an oscilloscope or computer screen.
- Lead wires are usually attached to an audio-amplifier so that voltage fluctuations within the muscle are audible.

POSTPROCEDURE CARE

- Apply warm compresses and give analgesics for discomfort.
- Resume medications that were withheld before the test.

- Monitor the site for bleeding and signs and symptoms of infection.
- Monitor the child's pain level and response to the analgesics.

NORMAL RESULTS

- At rest, muscle exhibiting minimal electrical activity
- During voluntary contraction, electrical activity increasing markedly
- Sustained contraction, or one of increasing strength, producing a rapid "train" of motor unit potentials

ABNORMAL RESULTS

- Short (low-amplitude) motor unit potentials, with frequent, irregular discharges suggesting possible primary muscle disease such as muscular dystrophy
- Isolated and irregular motor unit potentials with increased amplitude and duration suggesting possible disorders such as peripheral nerve disorders
- Initially normal motor unit potentials that progressively diminish in amplitude with continuing contractions suggesting possible myasthenia gravis

Evoked potentials

PURPOSE

- To aid in the diagnosis of nervous system lesions and abnormalities
- To monitor spinal cord function during spinal surgery
- To assess neurologic function
- To evaluate neurologic function in infants
- To monitor comatose or anesthetized patients

PATIENT PREPARATION

- Make sure that the consent form is signed by the child's parents or legal guardians.
- Note and report all allergies.
- Provide reassurance to the child that the electrodes won't hurt, but that he may feel a small shock when somatosensory evoked responses occur.
- Encourage the child to relax because tension can affect the test results.
- Inform the child and his parents that the test takes 45 to 60 minutes.

PROCEDURE

- The child is positioned in a reclining or straight-backed chair or on a bed.
- The child is asked to relax and remain still.
- Depending on the specific type of evoked potential study, electrodes may be attached.
- Visual evoked potentials, produced by exposing the eye to a rapidly reversing checkerboard pattern, help evaluate demyelinating disease, such as multiple sclerosis (MS), traumatic injury, and puzzling visual complaints.
- Somatosensory evoked potentials, produced by electrically stimulating a peripheral sensory nerve, help diagnose peripheral nerve disease and locate brain and spinal cord lesions.
- Auditory brain stem evoked potentials, produced by delivering clicks to the ear, are used in locating auditory lesions and evaluating brain stem integrity and in assessing brain stem integrity when cranial nerve testing is inconclusive or can't be performed.
- A computer amplifies and averages the brain's response to each stimulus and plots the results as a waveform.

POSTPROCEDURE CARE

- Monitor the child's response to testing.

NORMAL RESULTS

- In visual evoked potential testing, the most significant wave on the waveform appearing as P100, a positive wave appearing about 100 msec after applying the pattern-shift stimulus
- Normal results varying greatly among laboratories and patients
- In somatosensory evoked potential testing, the waveforms varying, depending on locations of the stimulating and recording electrodes

ABNORMAL RESULTS

- In visual evoked potential testing, abnormal (extended) P100 latencies confined to one eye suggesting a visual pathway lesion anterior to the optic chiasm; bilateral abnormal P100 latencies suggesting MS
- In somatosensory evoked potential testing, changes in the electrical waveforms possibly indicating damaged or degenerated nerve pathways to the brain from the eyes, ears, or limbs; absence of activity in a pathway possibly meaning complete loss of nerve function in that pathway
- Other changes possibly providing evidence of the type and location of nerve damage
- Abnormal upper-limb interwave latencies suggesting possible cervical spondylosis, intracerebral lesions, or sensorimotor neuropathies
- Abnormalities in the lower limb suggesting peripheral nerve and root lesions such as those in Guillain-Barré syndrome

Exercise electrocardiography (stress testing)

PURPOSE

- To determine functional capacity of the heart
- To screen for asymptomatic coronary artery disease (CAD)

- To diagnose the cause of chest pain
- To help set limitations for an exercise program
- To identify cardiac arrhythmias that develop during physical exercise
- To evaluate the effectiveness of antiarrhythmic or anti-anginal therapy
- To evaluate myocardial perfusion

PATIENT PREPARATION

- Make sure that the consent form is signed by the child's parents or legal guardians.
- Note and report all allergies.
- Check the child's history for a recent physical examination (within 1 week) and for baseline 12-lead electrocardiogram (ECG) results.
- Instruct the child not to eat or to drink caffeinated beverages before the test.
- Continue medications the child is currently taking unless the physician directs otherwise.
- Describe the equipment that will be used for the test; show the child a picture or, if possible, the actual equipment.
- Warn the child that he might feel fatigued, slightly breathless, and sweaty during the test.
- Provide reassurance that testing will stop if the child experiences significant symptoms such as chest pain.
- Instruct the child to wear comfortable socks and shoes and loose, lightweight shorts or pants during the procedure.
- Inform the child and his parents that the test takes about 30 minutes.

PROCEDURE

- Baseline ECG and blood pressure readings are taken.
- ECG and blood pressure readings are taken while the child walks on a treadmill or pedals a stationary bicycle.

- Unless complications develop, the test continues until the child reaches the target heart rate (determined by an established protocol — usually 85% of the maximum predicted heart rate for the child's age and gender).
- The cardiac monitor is observed continuously for changes in the heart's electrical activity.
- The rhythm strip is checked at preset intervals for arrhythmias, premature ventricular contractions, and ST-segment and T-wave changes.
- Blood pressure is monitored at predetermined intervals (usually at the end of each test level).
- The test is stopped immediately if the ECG shows significant arrhythmias or an increase in ectopy, if systolic blood pressure falls below the resting level, if the heart rate falls 10 beats/minute or more below the resting level, or if the child becomes exhausted or experiences severe symptoms such as chest pain.
- Stop the test if the child has persistent ST-segment elevation, possibly indicating myocardial injury.

POSTPROCEDURE CARE

- Assist the child to a chair and continue monitoring his heart rate and blood pressure for 10 to 15 minutes or until the ECG returns to the baseline.
- Remove the electrodes and clean the application sites.
- Have the child resume a normal diet and activities.
- Monitor the child's vital signs, ECG, heart sounds, and anginal symptoms.

NORMAL RESULTS

- Heart rate increasing in direct proportion to the workload and metabolic oxygen demand
- Systolic blood pressure increasing as workload increases
- Child attaining the endurance levels appropriate for his age and the exercise protocol

ABNORMAL RESULTS

- T-wave inversion or ST-segment depression possibly signifying ischemia
- Exercise-induced hypotension, an ST-segment depression of 2 mm or more, and downsloping ST segments possibly indicating significant CAD
- ST-segment elevation possibly indicating myocardial injury

Lumbar puncture

PURPOSE

- To measure cerebrospinal fluid (CSF) pressure
- To aid in the diagnosis of viral or bacterial meningitis, subarachnoid or intracranial hemorrhage, tumors and brain abscesses, and neurosyphilis and chronic central nervous system infections

PATIENT PREPARATION

- Make sure that the consent form is signed by the child's parents or legal guardians.
- Note and report all allergies.
- Inform the child and his parents that there are no food or fluid restrictions.
- Instruct the child to empty his bladder and bowels before the procedure.
- Explain the importance of remaining still throughout the procedure.
- Inform the child and his parents that the test takes at least 15 minutes.
- Explain that headache is the most common adverse effect.

PROCEDURE

- Confirm the child's identity by checking two patient identifiers.
- Position the child on his side at the edge of the bed with his knees drawn up to his abdomen and his chin tucked against his chest (the fetal position), or position the child sitting while leaning over a bedside table. (See *Lumbar puncture positioning*, page 384.)
- If the child is in a supine position, provide pillows to support the spine on a horizontal plane.
- Gently hold even a cooperative child during the procedure to prevent injury from unexpected or involuntary movement.
- The skin site is prepared and draped.
- A local anesthetic is injected.
- Monitor the child's vital signs and neurologic status throughout the procedure.
- The spinal needle is inserted in the midline between the spinous processes of the vertebrae (usually between L3 and L4 or L4 and L5).
- The stylet is removed from the needle; CSF will drip out of the needle if properly positioned.
- A stopcock and manometer are attached to the needle to measure the initial (opening) CSF pressure.
- Specimens are collected and placed in the appropriate containers.
- The needle is removed and a small sterile dressing is applied.

ALERT *During lumbar puncture, observe the child closely for signs of an adverse reaction (elevated pulse rate, pallor, or clammy skin).*

POSTPROCEDURE CARE

- Keep the child in a reclined position for up to 12 hours after the procedure to avoid the discomfort of potential postprocedure spinal headache.

LUMBAR PUNCTURE POSITIONING

When positioning a child for a lumbar puncture, follow these steps:
- Have the child lie on his side at the edge of the bed, with his chin tucked to his chest and his knees drawn up to his abdomen.
- Make sure that the child's spine is curved and his back is at the edge of the bed (as shown below); this position widens the spaces between the vertebrae, easing needle insertion.
- To help the child maintain this position, place one of your hands behind his neck; place the other hand behind his knees, and pull gently.

POSITIONING A YOUNG CHILD

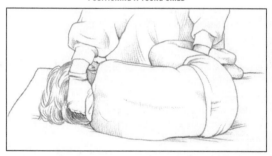

- Hold the child firmly in this position throughout the procedure to prevent accidental needle displacement. (Typically, the physician inserts the needle between L3 and L4.)
- The sitting position may be used for infants. However, because the flexed position may interfere with the infant's breathing, monitor his color and respiratory status closely during the procedure.

POSITIONING AN INFANT

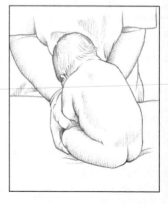

- Inform the child that he can turn from side to side.
- Encourage the child to drink increased amounts of fluid with a straw to replace the CSF removed during the procedure. Drinking with a straw allows the patient to keep his head flat.
- Give analgesics as ordered.
- Monitor the child's vital signs, neurologic status, and intake and output. Assess for numbness, tingling, and decreased movement of the extremities; pain at the injection site; drainage of blood or CSF at the injection site; and an inability to void.
- Monitor the puncture site for redness, swelling, and drainage.

NORMAL RESULTS

- Pressure: 50 to 180 mm H_2O
- Appearance: clear, colorless
- Protein: 10 to 30 mg/dl (SI, 100 to 300 mg/L)
  – Neonates: 15 to 100 mg/dl (SI, 150 to 1,000 mg/dl)
- Gamma globulin: 3% to 12% of total protein
- Glucose: 40 to 80 mg/dl
  – Neonates (0 to 14 days): 60 to 80 mg/dl
- Cell count: 0 to 5 white blood cells; no red blood cells (RBCs)
- Venereal Disease Research Laboratory (VDRL) test: nonreactive
- Chloride: 115 to 130 mEq/L
- Gram stain: no organisms

ABNORMAL RESULTS

- Increased intracranial pressure (ICP), indicating tumor, hemorrhage, or edema caused by trauma
- Decreased ICP, indicating spinal subarachnoid obstruction
- Cloudy appearance, suggesting infection
- Yellow or bloody appearance, suggesting intracranial hemorrhage or spinal cord obstruction

- Brown or orange appearance, indicating increased protein level or RBC breakdown
- Increased protein, suggesting tumor, trauma, diabetes mellitus, or blood in CSF
- Decreased protein, indicating rapid CSF production
- Increased gamma globulin, associated with demyelinating disease or Guillain-Barré syndrome
- Increased glucose, suggesting hyperglycemia
- Decreased glucose, which could result from hypoglycemia, infection, or meningitis
- Increased cell count, indicating meningitis, tumor, abscess, or demyelinating disease
- Presence of RBCs from hemorrhage
- Positive VDRL test result, indicating neurosyphilis
- Decreased chloride, pointing to infected meninges
- Gram-positive or gram-negative organisms, indicating bacterial meningitis

Magnetic resonance imaging

PURPOSE

- Powerful magnetic field and radio-frequency waves used to produce computerized images of internal organs and tissues not readily visible on standard X-rays

PATIENT PREPARATION

- Make sure that the consent form is signed by the child's parents or legal guardians.
- Note and report all allergies. Be sure to assess for a history of iodine or seafood allergies before the procedure if a contrast medium is to be used.
- Children requiring life-support equipment, including ventilators, require special preparation; contact magnetic resonance imaging (MRI) staff ahead of time.
- Explain to the child and his parents that there's no exposure to radiation during MRI.

- Tell the parents that, because no radiation is used, they may read or talk to their child in the imaging room during the procedure.
- Inform the parents that a young child will need to be sedated because of the need to remain motionless during the procedure.
- Tell the parents and child that he may eat or drink as usual before and after the procedure; no food or fluid restrictions are necessary before MRI.
- A claustrophobic child may require sedation or an open MRI to reduce anxiety.
- Because no metal can go in the scanner, assist the child in removing hair clips, jewelry, and other metal items as necessary.
- Advise the child that he'll be asked to remain still during the procedure.
- Prepare the child for the movements and the loud, clicking noises made by the scanner; reassure him that the machine won't touch him.
- Inform the child and his parents that the test takes about 30 to 90 minutes.

PROCEDURE

- If the child will receive a contrast medium, an I.V. line is started and the medium is administered before the procedure.
- The child is checked for metal objects at the scanner room door.
- The child is placed in the supine position on a padded scanning table.
- The table is positioned in the opening of the scanning gantry.
- A call bell or intercom is used to maintain verbal contact.
- The child may wear earplugs if needed.
- Varying radio-frequency waves are directed at the area being scanned.
- A computer reconstructs information as images on a television screen.

POSTPROCEDURE CARE

- Tell the child to resume his normal activities unless otherwise indicated.
- Monitor the child's vital signs.
- Watch for orthostatic hypotension.

NORMAL RESULTS

Bone and soft tissue
- No evidence of pathology in bone, muscles, and joints

Ear
- Cranial nerves and auditory bones appearing normal

Neurologic system
- Appearance of brain and spinal cord structures defined and distinct

Urinary tract
- Visualization of soft tissue structures of the kidneys
- Visualization of blood vessels

ABNORMAL RESULTS

Bone and soft tissue
- Structural abnormalities suggesting possible primary and metastatic tumors and various disorders of the bone, muscles, and joints

Ear
- Structural abnormalities suggesting possible disorders, such as viral labyrinthitis, increased intracranial pressure, or paragangliomas

Neurologic system

■ Structural changes that increase tissue water content suggesting possible cerebral edema, demyelinating disease, and pontine and cerebellar tumors
■ Changes in normal anatomy suggesting possible tumors

Urinary tract

■ Tumors, strictures, stenosis, thrombosis, malformations, abscess, inflammation, edema, fluid collection, bleeding, hemorrhage, or organ atrophy

Myelography

PURPOSE

■ To demonstrate lesions partially or totally blocking cerebrospinal fluid (CSF) flow in the subarachnoid space (tumors and herniated intervertebral disks)
■ To detect arachnoiditis, spinal nerve root injury, or tumors in the posterior fossa of the skull

PATIENT PREPARATION

■ Make sure that the consent form is signed by the child's parents or legal guardians.
■ Check the child's history for hypersensitivity to iodine and iodine-containing substances, such as shellfish and contrast media.
■ Enforce restriction of food and fluids for 8 hours before the test.
■ Notify the radiologist if the child has a history of epilepsy or of antidepressant or phenothiazine use.
■ Give the child a sedative and an anticholinergic, as ordered.
■ Explain to the child that when the contrast medium is injected, he may feel a burning sensation, warmth, headache, salty taste, or nausea and vomiting.

PROCEDURE

- The child is positioned on his side at the edge of the table with his knees drawn up to his abdomen and his chin on his chest.
- The child may receive a cisternal puncture if a lumbar deformity or infection at the puncture site is present.
- A lumbar puncture is performed.
- Fluoroscopy verifies proper needle position in the subarachnoid space.
- Some CSF may be removed for routine laboratory analysis.
- The child is then placed in the prone position.
- The contrast medium is injected.
- If a subarachnoid space obstruction blocks the upward flow of the contrast medium, a cisternal puncture may be performed.
- The flow of the contrast medium is studied with fluoroscopy; X-rays are taken.
- The contrast medium is withdrawn, if oil-based, and the needle is removed.
- The puncture site is cleaned and a small dressing applied.
- If a spinal tumor is confirmed, the child may go directly to the operating room.

POSTPROCEDURE CARE

- If the child received an oil-based contrast medium, keep him flat in bed for 8 to 12 hours.
- If the test involved a water-based contrast, make sure that the large dye load doesn't reach the surface of the brain; to prevent this, keep the child's head elevated 60 degrees for 6 to 8 hours after the procedure.
- Encourage the child to drink fluids to assist the kidneys in eliminating the contrast medium.
- Notify the physician if the child fails to void within 8 hours.
- Instruct the child to resume his usual diet and activities the day after the test.

- Monitor the child's vital signs, intake and output, and neurological status.
- Observe the puncture site; watch for bleeding and infection.
- Monitor the child for seizure activity.
- If radicular pain, fever, back pain, or signs and symptoms of meningeal irritation (headache, irritability, or neck stiffness) develop, inform the physician immediately. Keep the room quiet and dark, and provide an analgesic or antipyretic.

NORMAL RESULTS

- Contrast medium flowing freely through the subarachnoid space
- No obstruction or structural abnormality appearing

ABNORMAL RESULTS

- Extradural lesions suggesting possible herniated intervertebral disks or metastatic tumors
- Lesions within the subarachnoid space suggesting possible neurofibromas or meningiomas
- Lesions within the spinal cord suggesting possible ependymomas or astrocytomas
- Fluid-filled cavities in the spinal cord and widening of the cord itself suggesting possible syringomyelia

Oropharyngeal motility (swallowing test)

PURPOSE

- To diagnose hiatal hernia, diverticula, and varices
- To detect strictures, ulcers, tumors, polyps, and motility disorders

PATIENT PREPARATION

- Make sure that the consent form is signed by the child's parents or legal guardians.
- Explain that the test evaluates the function of the pharynx and esophagus.
- Maintain the child on a nothing-by-mouth status beginning at midnight before the test. (For an infant, delay feeding to ensure complete digestion of the barium.)
- The child may be given a restricted diet for 2 to 3 days before the test.
- Describe the test, who will perform it, and where it will take place.
- Describe the milk shake consistency and chalky taste of the barium preparation. Although flavored, it may be unpleasant to swallow.
- Explain to the child that he'll first receive a thick mixture, then a thin one; he must drink 12 to 14 oz (355 to 414 ml) during the examination.
- Inform the child that he'll be placed in various positions on a tilting X-ray table and that X-rays will be taken.
- Emphasize the importance of remaining still during the X-rays.
- Reassure the child about safety precautions.
- Withhold antacids, histamine-2 receptor antagonists, and proton pump inhibitors, if gastric reflux is suspected.
- Instruct the child to put on a gown without snap closures and to remove jewelry, hair clips, or other radiopaque objects. Provide assistance as needed.

PROCEDURE

- The child is placed in an upright position behind the fluoroscopic screen, and his heart, lungs, and abdomen are examined.
- The child is instructed to take one swallow of the thick barium mixture; pharyngeal action is recorded using cineradiography.

- The child is instructed to take several swallows of the thin barium mixture. Passage of the barium is examined fluoroscopically; spot films of the esophageal region are taken from lateral angles and from right and left postero-anterior angles.
- To accentuate small strictures or demonstrate dysphagia, the child may be asked to swallow a "barium marshmallow" (soft white bread soaked in barium) or barium pill.
- The child is then secured to the X-ray table and rotated to Trendelenburg's position to evaluate esophageal peristalsis or demonstrate hiatal hernia and gastric reflux.
- The child is instructed to take several swallows of barium while the esophagus is examined fluoroscopically; spot films are taken.
- After the table is rotated to a horizontal position, the child takes several swallows of barium so that the esophagogastric junction and peristalsis may be evaluated.
- Passage of the barium is fluoroscopically observed, and spot films are taken with the patient in the supine and prone positions.
- During fluoroscopic examination of the esophagus, the stomach and duodenum are also carefully studied because neoplasms in these areas may invade the esophagus and cause obstruction.

POSTPROCEDURE CARE

- Check that additional films and fluoroscopic evaluation haven't been ordered before allowing the child to resume his usual diet.
- Instruct the child to drink plenty of fluids, unless contraindicated, to help eliminate the barium.
- Give a cathartic if prescribed. Monitor bowel movements for excretion of barium and monitor GI function.
- Inform the child and his parents that stools will be chalky and light-colored for 24 to 72 hours.

NORMAL RESULTS

■ Swallowed barium bolus pouring over the base of the
tongue into the pharynx
■ Peristaltic wave propelling the bolus through the entire
length of the esophagus in about 2 seconds
■ When the wave reaches the base of the esophagus, the
cardiac sphincter opening, allowing the bolus to enter the
stomach; after passage of the bolus, the cardiac sphincter
closing
■ Bolus evenly filling and distending the lumen of the
pharynx and esophagus, and the mucosa appearing
smooth and regular

ABNORMAL RESULTS

■ Hiatal hernia, diverticula, varices; lung aspiration
■ Strictures, tumors, polyps, ulcers, and motility disorders
(definitive diagnosis requires further testing)

Positron emission tomography scan

PURPOSE

■ To detect organ dysfunction through positrons being
emitted from radioactive chemicals in the organ that are
sensed by a series of detectors positioned around the
child
■ To evaluate the heart and brain in many aspects of oncol-
ogy (most common use)
■ To help detect cerebral dysfunction caused by tumors,
seizures, head trauma, and some mental illnesses
■ To evaluate myocardial metabolism, and distinguish vi-
able from infarcted cardiac tissue

PATIENT PREPARATION

■ Make sure that the consent form is signed by the child's
parents or legal guardians.

- Note and report all allergies.
- Provide reassurance that the test is painless, other than minor discomfort if the patient receives an I.V. access insertion.
- Inform the child and his parents that he may need to fast after midnight the night before the test.
- Inform the child and his parents that he may need to abstain from caffeinated beverages for 24 hours before the test.
- Explain that food or fluids may need to be restricted for 4 hours on the day of the test.
- Stress the importance of remaining still during the study.

PROCEDURE

- The child is positioned appropriately.
- An attenuation scan, lasting about 30 minutes, is performed.
- The appropriate positron emitter is given and scanning is completed.
- A different positron emitter may be given if comparative studies are needed.

POSTPROCEDURE CARE

- Instruct the child to move slowly immediately after the procedure to avoid orthostatic hypotension.
- Encourage the child to drink liquids and urinate frequently to help flush the radioisotope from the bladder.

NORMAL RESULTS

- No areas of ischemic tissue present
- If the child receiving two tracers, flow and distribution should be matching

ABNORMAL RESULTS

■ Reduced blood flow with increased glucose use indicating ischemia
■ Reduced blood flow with decreased glucose use indicating necrotic, scarred tissue

Pulmonary function test

PURPOSE

■ To evaluate pulmonary status and function through a series of spirometric measurements
■ To assess the effectiveness of a specific therapeutic regimen

PATIENT PREPARATION

■ Make sure that the consent form is signed by the child's parents or legal guardians.
■ Note and report all allergies.
■ Withhold bronchodilators and intermittent positive-pressure breathing therapy before the pulmonary function test (PFT).
■ Explain the procedure to the child and his parents, stressing that there's no pain involved.
■ Have the child practice tasks, such as handling equipment, holding his breath, and inhaling on cue.
■ Note that results may not be accurate because the young child may have difficulty following the necessary directions.

> **ALERT** *Most children aren't able to perform the testing until about age 5 because it requires manipulating equipment, holding their breath, and exhaling on cue with directions.*

■ Instruct the child and his parents that the child should have only a light meal before the test.

- If appropriate, tell the child that he shouldn't smoke for 4 to 6 hours before the test.
- Just before the PFT, tell the child to void and loosen tight clothing, and obtain the child's height and weight.

PROCEDURE

- For tidal volume (V_T), the child breathes normally into the mouthpiece 10 times.
- For expiratory reserve volume (ERV), the child breathes normally for several breaths and then exhales as completely as possible.
- For vital capacity (VC), the child inhales as deeply as possible and exhales into the mouthpiece as completely as possible. This is repeated three times, and the largest volume is recorded.
- For inspiratory capacity (IC), the child breathes normally for several breaths and inhales as deeply as possible.
- For functional residual capacity (FRC), the child breathes normally into a spirometer. After a few breaths, the levels of gas in the spirometer and in the lungs reach equilibrium. The FRC is calculated by subtracting the spirometer volume from the original volume.
- For forced vital capacity (FVC) and forced expiratory volume (FEV), the child inhales as slowly and deeply as possible and then exhales into the mouthpiece as quickly and completely as possible. This is repeated three times, and the largest volume is recorded. The volume of air expired at 1 second (FEV_1), at 2 seconds (FEV_2), and at 3 seconds (FEV_3) during all three repetitions is recorded.
- For maximal voluntary ventilation, the child breathes into the mouthpiece as quickly and deeply as possible for 15 seconds.
- For diffusing capacity for carbon monoxide, the child inhales a gas mixture with a low level of carbon monoxide and holds his breath for 10 to 15 seconds before exhaling.

UNDERSTANDING PFT RESULTS

You may need to interpret pulmonary function test (PFT) results in your assessment of a patient's respiratory status. Use this chart as a guide to common PFTs.

Restrictive and obstructive defects

The chart mentions restrictive and obstructive defects.

- A restrictive defect is one in which a person can't inhale a normal amount of air; it may occur with chest wall deformities, neuromuscular diseases, or acute respiratory tract infections.
- An obstructive defect is one in which something obstructs the flow of air into or out of the lungs; it may occur with such disorders as asthma, chronic bronchitis, emphysema, and cystic fibrosis.

Test	Implications
Tidal volume (V_T): amount of air inhaled or exhaled during normal breathing	Decreased V_T may indicate restrictive defect and indicates need for further tests such as full chest X-rays.
Minute volume (MV): amount of air breathed per minute	Normal MV can occur in emphysema. Decreased MV may indicate other diseases such as pulmonary edema.
Inspiratory reserve volume (IRV): amount of air inhaled after normal inspiration	Abnormal IRV alone doesn't indicate respiratory dysfunction. IRV decreases during normal exercise.
Expiratory reserve volume (ERV): amount of air that can be exhaled after normal expiration	ERV varies, even in healthy people.
Vital capacity (VC): amount of air that can be exhaled after maximum inspiration	Normal or increased VC with decreased flow rates may indicate reduction in functional pulmonary tissue. Decreased VC with normal or increased flow rates may indicate respiratory effort, decreased thoracic expansion, or limited diaphragm movement.
Inspiratory capacity (IC): amount of air that can be inhaled after normal expiration	Decreased IC indicates restrictive defect.
Forced vital capacity (FVC): amount of air that can be exhaled after maximum inspiration	Decreased FVC indicates flow resistance in the respiratory system from obstructive disorders, such as chronic bronchitis, emphysema, and asthma.

	UNDERSTANDING PFT RESULTS *(continued)*	
Test	**Implications**
Forced expiratory volume (FEV): volume of air exhaled in the first (FEV_1), second (FEV_2), or third (FEV_3) FVC maneuver	Decreased FEV_1 and increased FEV_2 and FEV_3 may indicate obstructive disease. Decreased or normal FEV_1 may indicate restrictive defect.

POSTPROCEDURE CARE

■ Watch the child for respiratory distress, changes in pulse rate and blood pressure, coughing, and bronchospasm.

NORMAL RESULTS

■ Results based on age, height, weight, and sex; values expressed as a percentage (see *Understanding PFT results*)
■ V_T: 5 to 7 mg/kg of body weight
■ ERV: 25% of VC
■ IC: 75% of VC
■ FEV_1: 83% of VC after 1 second
■ FEV_2: 94% of VC after 2 seconds
■ FEV_3: 97% of VC after 3 seconds

ABNORMAL RESULTS

■ FEV_1 less than 80% suggesting obstructed pulmonary disease
■ FEV_1 to FVC ratio greater than 80% suggesting restrictive pulmonary disease
■ Decreased V_T suggesting possible restrictive disease
■ Decreased minute volume (MV) suggesting possible disorders such as pulmonary edema
■ Increased MV suggesting possible acidosis, exercise, or low compliance states
■ Reduced carbon dioxide response suggesting possible emphysema, myxedema, obesity, hypoventilation syndrome, or sleep apnea

- Residual volume greater than 35% of total lung capacity after maximal expiratory effort suggesting obstructive disease
- Decreased IC suggesting restrictive disease
- Increased FRC suggesting possible obstructive pulmonary disease
- Low total lung capacity (TLC) suggesting restrictive disease
- High TLC suggesting obstructive disease
- Decreased FVC suggesting flow resistance from obstructive or restrictive disease
- Low forced expiratory flow suggesting obstructive disease of the small and medium-sized airways
- Decreased peak expiratory flow rate suggesting upper airway obstruction
- Decreased diffusing capacity for carbon monoxide suggesting possible interstitial pulmonary disease

Skin testing, delayed-type hypersensitivity

PURPOSE

- To assess for exposure to or activation of certain diseases, most commonly tuberculosis (TB)
- To assess the status of a child's immune system during illness
- To evaluate sensitivity to environmental antigens in the child with persistent symptoms

PATIENT PREPARATION

- Make sure that the consent form is signed by the child's parents or legal guardians.
- Explain to the child and his parents that a small amount of antigenic material will be injected superficially or applied to the skin.

- Inform the child and his parents that the testing takes only a few minutes for each antigen. Reactions will be evaluated 48 to 72 hours later.
- The test may be repeated in 2 to 3 weeks if the first result is negative. The first test "reminds" the body that it was previously exposed to the antigen, and a response is noted on retesting. This is a common procedure for TB testing and is called the *two-step test.*
- Ask the child and his parents about the child's sensitivity to the test antigens, whether he has had previous skin testing, and what the outcomes of that testing were.
- Ask the child and his parents if the child has had TB or been exposed to it and if he has had the bacilli Calmette-Guerin vaccination.

PROCEDURE

- Confirm the child's identity by checking two patient identifiers.
- Inject each antigen being tested intradermally, using a separate tuberculin syringe, on the child's forearm.
- Inject the control allergy diluent on the other forearm.
- Inspect the injection sites for reactivity after 48 to 72 hours.
- Record induration and erythema in millimeters.
- Confirm a negative test result at the first concentration of antigen by using a higher concentration.
- If appropriate, store antigens in a lyophilized (freeze-dried) form at 39.2° F (4° C) and protect it from light. Reconstitute shortly before use and check expiration dates. If the child may be hypersensitive to the antigens, apply them initially in low concentrations.
- If the child's forearms aren't disease-free (for example, if he has atopic dermatitis), use other sites such as the back.

POSTPROCEDURE CARE

- Watch closely for severe local reactions that may occur at the test site, such as pain, blistering, swelling, induration,

itching, and ulceration. Scarring or hyperpigmentation
may also result.

- Observe for swelling and tenderness in lymph nodes at
  the elbow or axillary region. Check for tachycardia and
  fever, although these rarely occur. Symptoms typically
  appear in 15 to 30 minutes.

- If the child experiences hypersensitivity, inform the child
  and his parents that steroids will control the reaction;
  skin lesions may persist for 10 to 14 days.

- Advise the child to avoid scratching or otherwise disturb-
  ing the affected area.

- If signs or symptoms of anaphylactic shock develop, give
  the child epinephrine and notify the physician immediately.

NORMAL RESULTS

- Positive test result at least 5 mm of induration at the test
  site, appearing 48 hours after injection

ABNORMAL RESULTS

- Diminished delayed-type hypersensitivity (DTH) demonstrated by a positive response to fewer than two of the
  test antigens, a persistent unresponsiveness to intrader-
  mal injection of higher-strength antigens, or a generalized diminished reaction (causing less than 10 mm combined induration)

- Diminished DTH possibly resulting from Hodgkin's disease; sarcoidosis; liver disease; a congenital immunodeficiency, such as ataxia-telangiectasia, DiGeorge syndrome,
  and Wiskott-Aldrich syndrome; uremia; acute leukemia;
  viral diseases, such as influenza, infectious mononucleosis, measles, mumps, and rubella; fungal diseases, such
  as coccidioidomycosis and cryptococcosis; bacterial diseases, such as leprosy or TB; terminal cancer; and immunosuppressive or steroid therapy or viral vaccination

Ultrasonography

PURPOSE

- To measure organ size and evaluate structure
- To detect foreign bodies and differentiate between a cyst and solid tumor
- To monitor tissue response to radiation or chemotherapy

PATIENT PREPARATION

- Make sure that the consent form is signed by the child's parents or legal guardians.
- Note and report all allergies.
- Explain to the child and his parents that the procedure is painless and safe and that no radiation exposure is involved.
- Stress the importance of remaining still during scanning to prevent a distorted image.

PROCEDURE

- Assist the child into a supine position; use pillows to support the area to be examined.
- Coat the target area with a water-soluble jelly. The transducer is used to scan the area, projecting the images on the oscilloscope screen. The image on the screen is photographed for subsequent examination.
- It may be necessary to assist the child into right or left lateral positions for subsequent views.

POSTPROCEDURE CARE

- After the procedure, remove the contact jelly from the child's skin.

NORMAL RESULTS

Abdominal aorta
- Abdominal aorta descending through the retroperitoneal space, anterior to the vertebral column and slightly left of the midline
- Four of the abdominal aorta's major branches being well visualized including the celiac trunk, renal arteries, superior mesenteric artery, and common iliac arteries

Gallbladder and biliary system
- Gallbladder appearing sonolucent; appearing circular on transverse scans and pear-shaped on longitudinal scans, and its outer walls normally appearing sharp and smooth
- Cystic duct appearing serpentine and possibly indistinct; common bile duct having a linear appearance but sometimes being obscured by overlying bowel gas

Kidneys and perirenal
- Kidneys appearing between the superior iliac crests and the diaphragm, and in the center of each kidney, renal collecting systems appearing as irregular areas of higher density than surrounding tissue

Liver
- Liver demonstrating a homogeneous, low-level echo pattern, interrupted only by the different echo patterns of its vascular channels

Pancreas
- Pancreas demonstrating a coarse, uniform echo pattern (reflecting tissue density) and usually more echogenic than the adjacent liver

Pelvis
- Bladder, uterus, and ovaries appearing normal in size and shape in females
- Bladder and, possibly, the prostate gland appearing normal in size and shape in males
- No other masses visible

Spleen
- Splenic parenchyma demonstrating a homogeneous, low-level echo pattern

Thyroid
- Uniform echo pattern appearing throughout the gland

ABNORMAL RESULTS

Abdominal aorta
- Luminal diameter of the abdominal aorta indicating an aneurysm

Gallbladder and biliary system
- Mobile, echogenic areas, usually linked to an acoustic shadow, suggesting gallstones within the gallbladder lumen or biliary system
- Dilated biliary system and, usually, a dilated gallbladder suggesting obstructive jaundice

Kidneys and perirenal
- Fluid-filled circular structures that don't reflect sound waves suggesting cysts, and multiple echoes appearing as irregular shapes suggesting tumors
- Increased urine volume or residual urine postvoiding possibly indicating bladder dysfunction

Liver
- Dilated intrahepatic biliary radicles and extrahepatic ducts suggesting obstructive jaundice

Pancreas
- Alterations in the size, contour, and parenchymal texture of the pancreas suggesting possible pancreatic disease

Pelvis
- Homogeneous densities suggesting cysts and solid masses; however, solid masses (such as fibroids) appearing more dense on ultrasonography

Spleen
■ Increased echogenicity and enlarged vascular channels, especially in the hilar region, suggesting splenomegaly

Thyroid
■ Smooth-bordered, echo-free areas with enhanced sound transmission suggesting cysts
■ Solid and well-demarcated areas with identical echo patterns suggesting adenomas and carcinomas

Upper and lower GI

PURPOSE

Upper GI
■ To detect hiatal hernia, diverticula, and varices
■ To aid in the diagnosis of strictures, ulcers, tumors, regional enteritis, and malabsorption syndrome
■ To detect motility disorders

Lower GI
■ To aid in the diagnosis of inflammatory disease
■ To detect polyps, diverticula, and structural changes in the large intestine

PATIENT PREPARATION

■ Make sure that the consent form is signed by the child's parents or legal guardians.
■ Note and report all allergies.

Upper GI
■ Withhold oral medications after midnight and anticholinergics and opioids for 24 hours because these drugs affect small intestine motility.
■ Withhold antacids, histamine-2 receptor antagonists, and proton pump inhibitors if gastric reflux is suspected.

- Instruct the parents that the child is to maintain a low-residue diet for 2 or 3 days before the test and to fast after midnight before the test.
- Assist the child in removing hair clips, jewelry, and other metal items as necessary.
- Make sure that the lead apron is properly placed around the genital area.
- Describe the milk shake consistency and chalky taste of the barium preparation. Although flavored, it may be unpleasant to swallow.
- Warn the child that the abdomen may be compressed to ensure proper coating of the stomach or intestinal walls with barium or to separate overlapping bowel loops.
- Inform the child and his parents that the test may take up to 6 hours to complete.

Lower GI

- Explain that the test permits examination of the large intestine through X-rays taken after a barium enema.
- Accurate test results depend on the child's cooperation with prescribed dietary restrictions and bowel preparation.
- Common bowel preparation includes restricted intake of dairy products and maintenance of a liquid diet for 24 hours before the test. The child is encouraged to drink five 8-oz glasses of water or clear liquids 12 to 24 hours before the test.
- A polyethylene glycol and electrolyte solution (GoLYTELY) preparation isn't recommended because it leaves the bowel too wet for the barium to coat the walls of the bowel.
- The child should receive enemas until the return is clear.
- Tell the child and his parents that he shouldn't eat breakfast before the procedure; if the test is scheduled for late afternoon, he may have clear liquids.
- The child may experience cramping pains or the urge to defecate as the barium or air is introduced into the intestine. Instruct him to breathe deeply and slowly through his mouth to ease the discomfort.

■ The child must contract his anal sphincter tightly against the rectal tube.

■ Stress the importance of retaining the barium.

PROCEDURE

Upper GI

■ After securing the child in a supine position on the X-ray table, the table is tilted until the patient is erect, and the heart, lungs, and abdomen are examined fluoroscopically.

■ The child is then instructed to take several swallows of the barium suspension; its passage through the esophagus is observed.

■ Occasionally, the child is given a thick barium suspension, especially when esophageal pathology is strongly suspected.

■ During fluoroscopic examination, spot films of the esophagus are taken from lateral angles and from right and left posteroanterior angles.

■ When barium enters the stomach, the child's abdomen is palpated or compressed to ensure adequate coating of the gastric mucosa with barium.

■ To perform a double-contrast examination, the child is instructed to sip the barium through a perforated straw. As he does so, a small amount of air is also introduced into the stomach to allow detailed examination of the gastric rugae, and spot films of significant findings are taken.

■ The child is instructed to ingest the remaining barium suspension, and the filling of the stomach and emptying into the duodenum are observed fluoroscopically.

■ Two series of spot films of the stomach and duodenum are taken from posteroanterior, anteroposterior, oblique, and lateral angles, with the child erect and then in a supine position.

■ The passage of barium into the remainder of the small intestine is then observed fluoroscopically, and spot films are taken at 30- to 60-minute intervals until the barium reaches the ileocecal valve and the region around it.

- If abnormalities in the small intestine are detected, the area is palpated and compressed to help clarify the defect, and a spot film is taken.
- When barium enters the cecum, the examination is complete.

Lower GI

- After the child is in a supine position on a tilting X-ray table, spot films of the abdomen are taken.
- The child is assisted to the Sims' position; a well-lubricated rectal tube is inserted through the anus. For anal sphincter atony or severe mental or physical debilitation, a rectal tube with a retaining balloon is inserted.
- The barium is given slowly. The filling process is monitored fluoroscopically. To aid filling, the table is tilted or the child assisted to supine, prone, and lateral decubitus positions.
- As barium flow is observed, significant spot films are taken.
- The rectal tube is withdrawn and the child escorted to a toilet or given a bedpan to expel as much barium as possible.
- After evacuation, additional overhead film is taken to record mucosal pattern and evaluate the efficiency of colonic emptying.
- A double-contrast barium enema may directly follow the examination or may occur separately. If performed immediately, a thin film of barium remains in the intestine, coating the mucosa, and air is carefully injected to distend the bowel lumen.
- If a double-contrast technique is performed separately, instill a colloidal barium suspension, filling the intestine to either the splenic flexure or the middle of the transverse colon. The suspension is then aspirated, and air is forcefully injected into the intestine. If filling the intestine to the lower descending colon, forcefully inject air without first aspirating the suspension.
- The child is assisted to erect, prone, supine, and lateral decubitus positions in sequence. Filling is monitored flu-

oroscopically, and spot films are taken of significant findings.
- After films are taken, the child is escorted to a toilet or provided with a bedpan.

POSTPROCEDURE CARE

Upper GI
- Make sure additional X-rays aren't needed before allowing the child food, fluids, and oral drugs.
- Instruct the child to drink plenty of fluid (unless contraindicated) to help eliminate the barium.
- Give a cathartic or enema.
- Inform the child and his parents that his stools will be light-colored for 24 to 72 hours.
- Because barium retention in the intestine may cause obstruction or fecal impaction, notify the physician if the child doesn't pass barium within 2 to 3 days.
- Tell the child and his parents to notify the physician if the child experiences abdominal fullness or pain or a delay in a return to brown stools.
- Monitor the child's vital signs, intake and output, and bowel movements.
- Watch for abdominal distention.
- Monitor bowel sounds.

Lower GI
- Make sure that the child isn't to have further studies before allowing him to have food and fluids. Encourage him to take extra fluids because the bowel preparation and test itself can cause dehydration.
- Encourage the child to rest because the bowel preparation and test are exhausting.
- Barium retention can cause an intestinal obstruction or fecal impaction. If this happens, give a mild cathartic or enema. The child's stools will be light colored for 24 to 72 hours. Record and describe stools.

NORMAL RESULTS

Upper GI

■ After swallowing, barium suspension pouring over the base of the tongue into the pharynx and propelled by a peristaltic wave through the entire length of the esophagus in about 2 seconds

■ Bolus evenly filling and distending the lumen of the pharynx and esophagus, and the mucosa appearing smooth and regular

■ Peristaltic wave reaching the base of the esophagus, the cardiac sphincter opening, allowing the bolus to enter the stomach; closing of the cardiac sphincter following

■ Barium then entering the stomach and outlining the characteristic longitudinal folds called rugae, which are best observed using the double-contrast technique

■ When the stomach completely fills with barium, outer contour appearing smooth and regular without evidence of flattened, rigid areas suggesting intrinsic or extrinsic lesions

■ After entering the stomach, barium quickly emptying into the duodenal bulb through relaxation of the pyloric sphincter

■ Although the mucosa of the duodenal bulb appears relatively smooth, circular folds becoming apparent as barium enters the duodenal loop; these folds deepening and becoming more numerous in the jejunum

■ Barium temporarily lodging between these folds, producing a speckled pattern on the X-ray film

■ With barium entering the ileum, the circular folds becoming less prominent and, except for their broadness, resembling those in the duodenum

■ Diameter of the small intestine tapering gradually from the duodenum to the ileum

Lower GI

■ Single-contrast enema: barium uniformly filling the intestine, and colonic haustral markings appearing clear; intestinal walls collapsing as the child expels the barium,

and the mucosa having a regular, feathery appearance on the post-evacuation film
- Double-contrast enema: intestines uniformly distending with air and having a thin layer of barium, providing excellent detail of the mucosal pattern

ABNORMAL RESULTS

Upper GI
- Structural abnormalities of the esophagus suggesting possible strictures, tumors, hiatal hernia, diverticula, varices, and ulcers
- Dilation of the esophagus suggesting possible benign strictures
- Erosive changes in the esophageal mucosa suggesting possible malignant strictures
- Filling defects in the column of barium suggesting possible esophageal tumors; malignant esophageal tumors changing the mucosal contour
- Narrowing of the distal esophagus strongly suggesting achalasia (cardiospasm)
- Backflow of barium from the stomach into the esophagus suggesting gastric reflux
- Filling defects in the stomach, which usually disrupt peristalsis, suggesting malignant tumors, usually adenocarcinomas
- Outpouchings of the gastric mucosa that usually don't affect peristalsis suggesting benign tumors, such as adenomatous polyps and leiomyomas
- Evidence of partial or complete healing, characterized by radiating folds extending to the edge of the ulcer crater, suggesting benign ulcers
- Radiating folds that extend beyond the ulcer crater to the edge of the mass suggesting malignant ulcers
- Edematous changes in the mucosa of the antrum or duodenal loop, or dilation of the duodenal loop suggesting possible pancreatitis

- Edematous changes, segmentation of the barium column, and flocculation in the small intestine suggesting possible malabsorption syndrome
- Filling defects of the small intestine suggesting possible Hodgkin's disease and lymphosarcoma

Lower GI
- Adenocarcinoma or sarcoma occurring higher in the intestine
- Carcinoma, either as a localized filling defect with a sharp transition between normal and necrotic mucosa or circumferential with an "apple-core" appearance (characteristics that help distinguish carcinoma from the more diffuse lesions of inflammatory disease)
- Inflammatory disease, such as diverticulitis, ulcerative colitis, and granulomatous colitis
- Saccular adenomatous polyps, broad-based villous polyps, or structural changes in the intestine, such as intussusception, telescoping of the bowel, sigmoid volvulus, sigmoid torsion, gastroenteritis, irritable colon, and vascular injury

Child abuse awareness

If you suspect a child is being harmed, contact your local child protective services or the police. Contact the Childhelp USA National Child Abuse Hotline (1-800-4-A-CHILD) to find out where and how to file a report.

The following signs may indicate child abuse or neglect.

CHILDREN

- Show sudden changes in behavior or school performance
- Haven't received help for physical or medical problems brought to the parent's attention
- Are always watchful, as if preparing for something bad to happen
- Lack adult supervision
- Are overly compliant, passive, or withdrawn
- Come to school or activities early, stay late, and don't want to go home

PARENTS

- Show little concern for the child
- Deny or blame the child for the child's problems in school or at home
- Request that teachers or caregivers use harsh physical discipline if the child misbehaves
- See the child as entirely bad, worthless, or burdensome
- Demand a level of physical or academic performance the child can't achieve
- Look primarily to the child for care, attention, and satisfaction of emotional needs

PARENTS AND CHILDREN

- Rarely look at each other
- Consider their relationship to be entirely negative
- State that they don't like each other

Child abuse signals

Here are some signs associated with specific types of child abuse and neglect. These types of abuse are typically found in combination rather than alone.

PHYSICAL ABUSE

- Has unexplained burns, bites, bruises, broken bones, black eyes
- Has fading bruises or marks after absence from school
- Cries when it's time to go home
- Shows fear at approach of adults
- Reports injury by parent or caregiver

NEGLECT

- Is frequently absent from school
- Begs or steals food or money
- Lacks needed medical or dental care, immunizations, or glasses
- Is consistently dirty and has severe body odor
- Lacks sufficient clothing for the weather

SEXUAL ABUSE

- Has difficulty walking or sitting
- Suddenly refuses to change for gym or join in physical activities
- Reports nightmares or bedwetting
- Demonstrates bizarre, sophisticated, or unusual sexual knowledge or behavior
- Becomes pregnant or contracts a venereal disease when younger than age 14

EMOTIONAL MALTREATMENT

- Shows extremes in behavior, such as overly compliant or demanding behavior, extreme passivity, or aggression
- Is inappropriately adult (parenting other children) or inappropriately infantile (frequent rocking or head banging)
- Shows delayed physical or emotional development
- Reports a lack of attachment to the parent
- Has attempted suicide

Coma scale (pediatric)

To quickly assess a child's level of consciousness and to uncover baseline changes, use the pediatric coma scale. This assessment tool grades consciousness in relation to eye opening and motor response and responses to auditory or visual stimuli. A decreased reaction score in one or more categories warns of an impending neurologic crisis. A child scoring 7 or lower is comatose and probably has severe neurologic damage.

Test	Child's reaction	Score
Best eye opening response	Open spontaneously	4
	Open to verbal command	3
	Open to pain	2
	No response	1
Best motor response	Obeys verbal command	6
	Localizes painful stimuli	5
	Flexion-withdrawal	4
	Flexion-abnormal (decorticate rigidity)	3
	Extension (decerebrate rigidity)	2
	No response	1
Best response to auditory and/or visual stimuli	*For a child older than age 2*	
	Oriented	5
	Confused	4
	Inappropriate words	3
	Incomprehensible sounds	2
	No response	1
	or	
	For a child younger than age 2	
	Smiles, listens, follows	5
	Cries, consolable	4
	Inappropriate persistent cry	3
	Agitated, restless	2
	No response	1
		Total possible score: 3 to 15

Cultural considerations in patient care

As a health care professional, you'll interact with a diverse, multicultural patient population. Each culture has its own unique set of beliefs about health and illness and dietary practices that you need to know when providing care.

Cultural group	Health and illness philosophy	Dietary practices
African Americans	■ May believe illness is related to supernatural causes, such as punishment from God or an evil spell ■ May express grief by crying, screaming, praying, singing, and reading scripture ■ May seek advice and remedies from faith or folk healers	■ May have food restrictions based on religious beliefs, such as not eating pork if Muslim ■ May view cooked greens as good for health
Arab Americans	■ Believe health is a gift from God and that one should care for self by eating right and minimizing stressors ■ If devout, may interpret illness as the will of Allah or as a test of faith and, therefore, have a fatalistic view ■ Believe in complete rest and relieving self of all responsibilities during an illness ■ May express pain freely ■ After death, may want to prepare the body by washing it and then wrapping it in a white cloth ■ Discourage postmortem examination unless required by law	■ Don't mix sweet and sour or hot and cold ■ Don't use ice in drinks; believe hot soup can help recovery ■ If Muslim, prohibited from drinking alcohol and eating pork or ham
Chinese Americans	■ Believe health is a balance of Yin and Yang and illness stems from an imbalance of these elements; health requires harmony between body, mind, and spirit ■ May use herbalists or acupuncturists before seeking medical help ■ May use good luck objects, such as jade or a rope tied around the waist ■ Family expected to take care of the patient, who assumes a passive role ■ Tend not to readily express pain; stoic by nature	■ Staples are rice, noodles, and vegetables; tend to use chopsticks ■ Choose foods to help balance the Yin (cold) and Yang (hot) ■ Drink hot liquids, especially when sick

(continued)

Cultural group	Health and illness philosophy	Dietary practices
Japanese Americans	■ Believe that health is a balance of oneself, society, and the universe ■ May believe illness is karma, resulting from behavior in present or past life ■ May believe certain food combinations cause illness ■ May not complain of symptoms until severe	■ Eat rice with most meals; may use chopsticks ■ Diet high in salt; low in sugar, fat, animal protein, and cholesterol
Latino Americans	■ May view illness as a sign of weakness, punishment for evil doing, or retribution for shameful behavior ■ May use the terms hot and cold in reference to vital elements needed to restore equilibrium to body ■ May consult with a curandero (healer) or voodoo preist (Caribbean) ■ May view pain as a necessary part of life and believe that enduring pain is a sign of strength (especially men) ■ May openly express grief, such as by praying for the dead or saying the rosary ■ May use amulets to ward off evil ■ Typically involve family members in all aspects of decision making, such as with terminal illness	■ Beans and tortillas are staples ■ Eat lots of fresh fruits and vegetables
Native Americans	■ Use herbs and roots; each tribe has its own unique medicinal practices ■ Most use modern medicine where available ■ Use Medicine Wheel, an ancient symbol ■ For some, 4 is a sacred number, associated with the four primary laws of creation: Life, Unity, Equality, and Eternity ■ May use tobacco for important religious, ceremonial, and medicinal purposes; may sprinkle it around the bed of sick people to protect and heal them ■ May believe that the spirit of a dying person can't leave the body until the family is present	■ Have balanced diet of seafood, fruits, greens, corn, rice, and garden vegetables; salt consumption is low ■ Specific dietary practices are based on location; urban dwellers commonly eat most types of meat, while rural dwellers commonly consume only lamb and goat

Development patterns

This chart shows the patterns of development and their progression and gives examples of each.

Pattern	Path of progression	Examples
Cephalocaudal	From head to toe	Head control preceding ability to walk
Proximodistal	From the trunk to the tips of the extremities	The young infant moving his arms and legs but not picking up objects with his fingers
General to specific	From simple tasks to more complex tasks (mastering simple tasks before advancing to those that are more complex)	The child progressing from crawling to walking to skipping

Development stages

- *Infancy:* Birth to age 1
- *Toddler stage:* Ages 1 to 3
- *Preschool stage:* Ages 3 to 6
- *School-age:* Ages 6 to 12
- *Adolescence:* Ages 12 to 19

Development theories

The child development theories discussed in this chart shouldn't be compared directly because they measure different aspects of development. Erik Erikson's psychosocial-based theory is the most commonly accepted model for child development, although it can't be empirically tested.

Age-group	Psychosocial theory	Cognitive theory	Psycho-sexual theory	Moral development theory
Infancy (birth to age 1)	Trust versus mistrust	Sensori-motor (birth to age 2)	Oral	Not applicable
Toddlerhood (ages 1 to 3)	Autonomy versus shame and doubt	Sensori-motor to preoperational	Anal	Preconventional
Preschool age (ages 3 to 6)	Initiative versus guilt	Preoperational (ages 2 to 7)	Phallic	Preconventional
School age (ages 6 to 12)	Industry versus inferiority	Concrete operational (ages 7 to 11)	Latency	Conventional
Adolescence (ages 12 to 19)	Identity versus role confusion	Formal operational thought (ages 11 to 15)	Genitalia	Postconventional

Dosage calculation formulas and common conversions

COMMON CALCULATIONS

$$\text{child's dose in mg} = \text{child's body surface area (BSA) in m}^2 \times \frac{\text{pediatric dose in mg}}{\text{m}^2/\text{day}}$$

$$\text{child's dose in mg} = \frac{\text{child's BSA in m}^2}{\text{average adult BSA (1.73 m}^2)} \times \text{average adult dose}$$

$$\text{mcg/ml} = \text{mg/ml} \times 1{,}000$$

$$\text{ml/minute} = \frac{\text{ml/hour}}{60}$$

$$\text{mg/minute} = \frac{\text{mg in bag}}{\text{ml in bag}} \times \text{flow rate} \div 60$$

$$\text{mcg/minute} = \frac{\text{mg in bag}}{\text{ml in bag}} \div 0.06 \times \text{flow rate}$$

$$\text{mcg/kg/minute} = \frac{\text{mcg/ml} \times \text{ml/minute}}{\text{weight in kg}}$$

COMMON CONVERSIONS

1 kg = 1,000 g	1 ml = 1,000 micro-	8 oz = 240 ml
1 g = 1,000 mg	liters	1 oz = 30 g
1 mg = 1,000 mcg	1 tsp = 5 ml	1 lb = 454 g
1″ = 2.54 cm	1 tbs = 15 ml	2.2 lb = 1 kg
1 L = 1,000 ml	2 tbs = 30 ml	

English-to-Spanish basic translations

My name is _____.	Mi nombre es _____.
I am your nurse.	Soy su enfermero(a).
Come in, please.	Entre, por favor.
What is your name?	¿Cómo se llama?
How are you feeling?	¿Cómo se siente?
How old are you?	¿Cuántos años tiene?
Do you take any medications?	¿Toma medicamentos?
Are you allergic to any medications?	¿Es usted alérgico(a) a algún medicamento?
Who is your doctor?	¿Quién es su médico?
Are you comfortable?	¿Está cómodo(a)?
Do you follow a special diet?	¿Tiene Ud. una dieta especial?

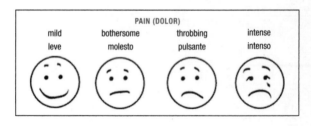

PAIN (DOLOR)

mild	bothersome	throbbing	intense
leve	molesto	pulsante	intenso

I would like to give you:	*Quisiera darle a Ud. un(a):*
■ an injection.	■ inyección.
■ an I.V. medication.	■ medicamento por vía intravenosa.
■ a liquid medication.	■ medicamento en forma líquida.
■ a medicated cream or powder.	■ medicamento en pomada o polvo.
■ a medication through your epidural catheter.	■ medicamento por el catéter epidural.
■ a medication through your rectum.	■ medicamento por el recto.
■ a medication through your _____ tube.	■ medicamento por su _____ tubo.
■ some pill(s).	■ píldoras.
■ a suppository.	■ supositorio.

Food Guide Pyramid

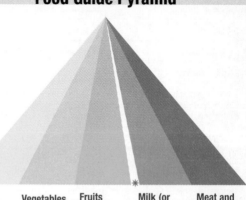

Grains
- An ounce equivalent is:
  - 1 piece of bread
  - ½ cup of cooked cereal such as oatmeal
  - ½ cup of rice or pasta
  - 1 cup cold cereal.
- 4- to 8-year-olds need 4- to 5 oz equivalents per day.
- 9- to 13-year-old girls need 5 oz equivalents per day.
- 9- to 13-year-old boys need 6 oz equivalents per day.

Vegetables
- 4- to 8-year-olds need 1½ cups per day.
- 9- to 13-year-old girls need 2 cups per day.
- 9- to 13-year-old boys need 2½ cups per day.

Fruits
- 4- to 8-year-olds need 1 to 1½ cups per day.
- 9- to 13-year-olds need 1½ cups per day.

✳ Fats
- 2- to 3-year-olds need 30% to 35% of total daily calories to come from fat.
- 4- to 18-year-olds need 25% to 35% of total daily calories to come from fat.
- Most fat should come from fish, nuts, and vegetable oils.

Milk (or other calcium-rich foods, such as yogurt, cheese, or calcium-fortified orange juice)
- 4- to 8-year-olds need 1 to 2 cups per day (or other calcium-rich foods).
- 9- to 13-year-olds need 3 cups per day (or other calcium-rich foods).

Meat and beans
- An ounce equivalent is:
  - 1 oz of meat, poultry, or fish
  - 1/4 cup dry beans cooked
  - 1 egg
  - 1 tablespoon of peanut butter
  - small handful of nuts or seeds.
- 4- to 13-year-olds need 5½ oz equivalents per day.

Adapted from U.S. Department of Agriculture, Center for Nutrition Policy and Promotion, April 2005. Available at *www.mypyramid.gov*.

Infant reflexes

Reflex	How to elicit	Age at disappearance
Trunk incurvature	When a finger is run laterally down the neonate's spine, the trunk flexes and the pelvis swings toward the stimulated side.	2 months
Tonic neck (fencing position)	When the neonate's head is turned while he's lying supine, the extremities on the same side extend outward while those on the opposite side flex.	2 to 3 months
Grasping	When a finger is placed in each of the neonate's hands, his fingers grasp tightly enough to be pulled to a sitting position.	3 to 4 months
Rooting	When the cheek is stroked, the neonate turns his head in the direction of the stroke.	3 to 4 months
Moro (startle reflex)	When lifted above the crib and suddenly lowered (or in response to a loud noise), the arms and legs symmetrically extend and then abduct while the fingers spread to form a "C."	4 to 6 months
Sucking	Sucking motion begins when a nipple is placed in the neonate's mouth.	6 months
Babinski's	When the sole on the side of the small toe is stroked, the neonate's toes fan upward.	2 years
Stepping	When held upright with the feet touching a flat surface, the neonate exhibits dancing or stepping movements.	Variable

I.M. injection sites

When selecting the best site for a child's I.M. injection, consider his age, weight, and muscle development; the amount of subcutaneous fat over the injection site; the type of drug you're administering; and the drug's absorption rate. These guidelines may assist you in making a selection.

VASTUS LATERALIS

Appropriate age
- Infants
- Toddlers

Needle size and length
- Infants under 4 months: 23G to 25G, ⅝" needle
- Infants over 4 months and toddlers: 22G to 25G, 1" needle

Recommended maximum amount
- Give 1 ml or less to infants.
- Give 2 ml or less to toddlers.

Special considerations
- The vastus lateralis is a large, well-developed muscle with few major blood vessels or nerves.
- The rectus femoris muscle should be avoided when using this injection site

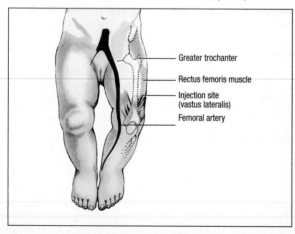

Greater trochanter

Rectus femoris muscle

Injection site (vastus lateralis)

Femoral artery

VENTROGLUTEAL

Appropriate age
- Infants
- Toddlers
- Preschool age and older children
- Adolescents

Needle size and length
- 23G to 25G, ⅝″ needle for infants less than 4 months
- 22G to 25G, 1″ needle for all other age-groups

Recommended maximum amount
- Give 1 ml or less to infants.
- Give 2 ml or less to toddlers.
- Give 3 ml or less to preschool age and older children.
- Give 5 ml or less to adolescents.

Special considerations
- This site is less painful than the vastus lateralis.
- This site is also relatively free from major nerves and blood vessels.

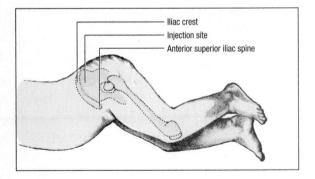

Iliac crest
Injection site
Anterior superior iliac spine

DORSOGLUTEAL

Appropriate age
- Children older than age 2

Needle size and length
- 20G to 25G, ½″ to 1½″ needle

Recommended maximum amount
- Give 1.5 ml or less to children ages 2 to 6.
- Give 2 ml or less to children over age 6.

Special considerations
- This site isn't recommended for children who haven't been walking for at least 1 year.
- Injury to the sciatic nerve is possible when using this site.

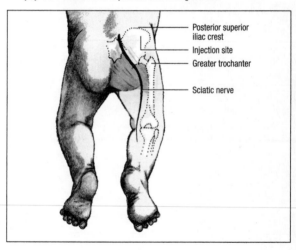

Posterior superior iliac crest
Injection site
Greater trochanter
Sciatic nerve

DELTOID

Appropriate age
- Toddlers
- Preschool age and older children
- Adolescents

Needle size and length
- 22G to 25G, ⅝″ to 1″ needle in all age-groups

Recommended maximum amount
- Give 1 ml or less in toddlers and preschool age and older children.
- Give 1 to 1½ ml in adolescents.

Special considerations
- This site is associated with less pain than the vastus lateralis site.
- Because blood flows faster in the deltoid muscle than in other muscle sites, drug absorption is faster.
- Injury to the radial nerve is possible when using this site.

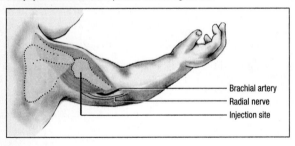

Brachial artery
Radial nerve
Injection site

Immunization schedule

This schedule shows the recommended ages for routine administration of childhood vaccines, as approved for 2005 by the Centers for Disease Control and Prevention.

Vaccine	Birth	1 month	2 months	4 months	6 months	12 months
Hepatitis B (HepB)	HepB	HepB		†HepB		HepB #3
Diphtheria, tetanus, pertussis (DTaP)			DTaP	DTaP	DTaP	
Haemophilus influenzae type b (Hib)			Hib	Hib	Hib*	Hib
Inactivated poliovirus (IPV)			IPV	IPV		IPV
Measles, mumps, rubella (MMR)						MMR
Varicella						Varicella
Meningococcal						
Pneumococcal (PCV)			PCV	PCV	PCV	PCV
Influenza						Influenza (yearly)
Hepatitis A						HepA series

Key:

Range of recommended ages

Assessment at age 11-12 years

Catch-up immunization

	15 months	18 months	24 months	4-6 years	11-12 years	13-14 years	15 years	16-18 years
				HepB series				
	DTaP			DTaP	Td		Td	
				IPV				
				MMR		MMR #2		
					Varicella			
	Vaccines within broken line are for selected populations			MCV	MCV		MCV	
				MCV			MCV	
			PCV					
					PPV			
				Influenza (yearly)				
				Hepatitis A series				

†4-month dose not needed if monovalent HepB used

*6-month dose not needed if PRP-OMP is administered at age 2 and 4 months

Immunization schedule (catch-up)

The next two charts show schedules and minimum intervals between doses for children who have delayed immunizations.

FOR CHILDREN AGES 4 MONTHS TO 6 YEARS

Vaccine	Minimum age for dose 1	Minimum interval between doses
		Dose 1 to dose 2
DTaP	6 wk	4 wk
IPV	6 wk	4 wk
HepB	Birth	4 wk
MMR	12 mo	4 wk
Varicella	12 mo	—
Hib	6 wk	■ 4 wk (if first dose given at < 12 mo) ■ 8 wk (as final dose if first dose given at 12 to 14 mo) ■ No further doses needed (if first dose given at ≥ 15 mo)
PCV	6 wk	■ 4 wk (if first dose given at < 12 mo and current age is < 24 mo) ■ 8 wk (as final dose if first dose given at ≥ 12 mo or current age is 24 to 59 mo) ■ No further doses needed (for healthy children if first dose given at age ≥ 24 mo)

FOR CHILDREN AGES 7 TO 18 YEARS

Vaccine	Minimum interval between doses	
	Dose 1 to dose 2	*Dose 2 to dose 3*
Td	4 wk	6 mo
IPV	4 wk	4 wk
HepB	4 wk	8 wk (and 16 wk after first dose)
MMR	4 wk	—
Varicella	4 wk	—

Dose 2 to dose 3	Dose 3 to dose 4	Dose 4 to dose 5
4 wk	6 mo	6 mo
4 wk	4 wk	—
8 wk (and 16 wk after first dose)	—	—
—	—	—
—	—	—
▪ 4 wk (if current age is < 12 mo) ▪ 8 wk (as final dose if current age is ≥ 12 mo and second dose at age < 15 mo) ▪ No further doses needed (if first dose given at ≥ 15 mo)	▪ 8 wk (as final dose; only necessary for children ages 12 mo to 5 yr who received 3 doses before age 12 mo)	—
▪ 4 wk (if current age < 12 mo) ▪ 8 wk (as final dose if current age ≥ 12 mo) ▪ No further doses needed (for healthy children if first dose given at age ≥ 24 mo)	▪ 8 wk (as final dose; only necessary for children ages 12 mo to 5 yr who received 3 doses before age 12 mo)	—

Dose 3 to booster dose

▪ 6 mo (if first dose given at < 12 mo and current age is < 11 yr)
▪ 5 yr (if first dose given at ≥ 12 mo, third dose given at < 7 yr, and current age is ≥ 11 yr)

▪ Children who received all OPV or IPV, 4th dose not needed if 3rd dose given ≥ 4 years
▪ IPV not recommended for those age ≥ 18 years.

—

—

—

Insulin injection sites in children

Use these illustrations to instruct the child and his parents about the injection sites for insulin administration that are recommended by the American Diabetes Association.

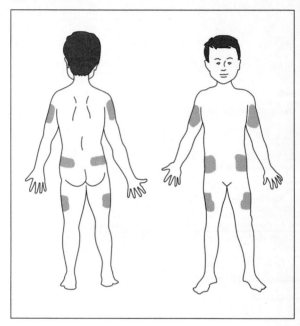

I.V. insertion sites in infants

This illustration shows the preferred sites for inserting venous access devices in infants. If a scalp vein is used, hair may be shaved around the area to enable better visualization of the vein and monitoring of the site after insertion. (Be sure to prepare the parents for this possibility and save the hair for them.)

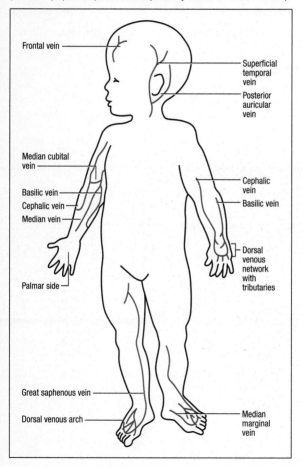

Laboratory findings in children

COMPREHENSIVE METABOLIC PANEL

Test	Conventional units	SI units
Alanine aminotransferase	< 1 yr: 5 to 28 units/L > 1 yr: 820 units/L	< 1 yr: 5 to 28 units/L > 1 yr: 820 units/L
Albumin	3.5 to 5 g/dl	35 to 50 g/L

Alkaline phosphatase	2 to 10 yr: 100 to 300 units/L
	11 to 18 yr:
	  Male: 50 to 375 units/ L;
	  Female: 30 to 300 units/L
		2 to 10 yr: 100 to 300 units/L
		11 to 18 yr:
		  Male: 50 to 375 units/ L;
		  Female: 30 to 300 units/L

Aspartate aminotransferase	< 1 yr: 15 to 60 units/L > 1 yr: ≤ 20 units/L	< 1 yr: 15 to 60 units/L > 1 yr: ≤ 20 units/L
Bilirubin, total	< 10 mg/dl	< 171 µmol/L
Blood urea nitrogen	5 to 20 mg/dl	2 to 7 mmol/L
Calcium, ionized	4.48 to 4.92 mg/dl	1.12 to 1.23 mmol/L
Calcium, total	8 to 10.5 mg/dl	2 to 2.6 mmol/L
Carbon dioxide	22 to 26 mEq/L	22 to 26 mmol/L
Chloride	94 to 106 mEq/L	94 to 106 mmol/L
Creatinine	0.3 to 0.7 mg/dl	27 to 62 µmol/L
Glucose	60 to 105 mg/dl	3.3 to 5.8 mmol/L
Potassium	3.5 to 5 mEq/L	3.5 to 5 mmol/L
Protein, total	6.5 to 8.6 g/dl	65 to 86 g/L
Sodium	135 to 145 mEq/L	135 to 145 mmol/L

THYROID PANEL

Test	Conventional units	SI units
Triiodothyronine	1 to 5 yr: 105 to 269 ng/dl	1 to 5 yr: 1.62 to 4.14 nmol/L
	5 to 10 yr: 94 to 241 ng/dl	5 to 10 yr: 1.45 to 3.71 nmol/L
	10 to 15 yr: 83 to 215 ng/dl	10 to 15 yr: 1.28 to 3.31 nmol/L
Thyroid-stimulating hormone	0.7 to 6.4 micro international units/ml	0.7 to 6.4 micro international units/m
Thyroxine (T_4), free	0.7 to 1.7 ng/dl	9 to 22 pmol/L
T_4, total	1 to 5 yr: 7.3 to 15 mcg/dl	1 to 5 yr: 94 to 194 nmol/L
	5 to 10 yr: 6.4 to 13.3 mcg/dl	5 to 10 yr: 83 to 172 nmol/L
	10 to 15 yr: 5.6 to 11.7 mcg/dl	10 to 15 yr: 72 to 151 nmol/L

OTHER CHEMISTRY TESTS

Test	Conventional units	SI units
Ammonia	13 to 48 mcg/dl	9 to 34 µmol/L
Amylase	> 1 yr: 26 to 102 units/L	> 1 yr: 26 to 102 units/L
Anion gap	7 to 14 mEq/L	7 to 14 mmol/L
Bilirubin, direct	< 0.5 mg/dl	< 6.8 µmol/L
Calcium, ionized	4.48 to 4.92 mg/dl	1.12 to 1.23 mmol/L
Cortisol	a.m.: 8 to 18 mcg/dl	225 to 505 nmol/L
	p.m.: 16 to 36 mcg/dl	450 to 1010 nmol/L
C-reactive protein	< 0.8 mg/dl	< 8 mg/L
Ferritin	7 to 144 ng/ml	7 to 144 mcg/L
Folate	1.8 to 9 ng/ml	4 to 20 nmol/L
γ-glutamyl-transferase	0 to 23 units/L	0 to 23 units/L
Glycosylated hemoglobin (HbA$_{1c}$)	3.9% to 7.7%	0.039 to 0.077
Iron	53 to 119 mcg/dl	9.5 to 27 µmol/L
Iron-binding capacity	250 to 400 mcg/dl	45 to 72 µmol/L
Magnesium	1.5 to 2.0 mEq/L	0.75 to 1 mmol/L
Osmolality	285 to 295 mOsm/kg	285 to 295 mOsm/kg
Phosphate	1 yr: 3.8 to 6.2 mg/dl	1 yr: 1.23 to 2 mmol/L
	2 to 5 yr: 3.5 to 6.8 mg/dl	2 to 5 yr: 1.03 to 2.2 mmol/L
Uric acid	2 to 7 mg/dl	120 to 420 µmol/L

COMPLETE BLOOD COUNT WITH DIFFERENTIAL

Test	Conventional units	SI units
Hemoglobin	2 to 6 mo: 10.7 to 17.3 g/dl	2 to 6 mo: 107 to 173 mmol/L
	1 to 12 yr: 9.5 to 14.1 g/dl	1 to 12 yr: 95 to 141 mmol/L
	6 to 16 yr: 10.3 to 14.9 g/dl	6 to 16 yr: 103 to 149 mmol/L
Hematocrit	2 to 6 mo: 35% to 49%	2 to 6 mo: 0.35 to 0.49
	6 mo to 1 yr: 29% to 43%	6 mo to 1 yr: 0.29 to 0.43
	1 to 6 yr: 30% to 40%	1 to 6 yr: 0.30 to 0.40
	6 to 16 yr: 32% to 42%	6 to 16 yr: 0.32 to 0.42
Mean corpuscular hemoglobin	2 to 6 yr: 24 to 30 pg/cell	2 to 6 yr: 0.37 to 0.47 fmol/cell
	6 to 12 yr: 25 to 33 pg/cell	6 to 12 yr: 0.39 to 0.51 fmol/cell
	12 to 18 yr: 25 to 35 pg/cell	12 to 18 yr: 0.39 to 0.53 fmol/cell
Mean corpuscular hemoglobin concentration	34 g/dl	340 g/L
Mean corpuscular volume	2 to 6 yr: 82 mm^3	2 to 6 yr: 82 fL
	6 to 12 yr: 86 mm^3	6 to 12 yr: 86 fL
	12 to 18 yr: 88 mm^3	12 to 18 yr: 88 fL
Platelets	150,000 to 450,000/mm^3	150 to 450 $\times$ 10^9/L
Red blood cells (RBCs)	6 mo to 1 yr: 3.8 to 5.2 $\times$ 10^6/mm^3	6 mo. to 1 yr: 3.8 to 5.2 $\times$ 10^{12}/L
	6 to 16 yr: 4 to 5.2 $\times$ 10^6/mm^3	6 to 16 yr: 4 to 5.2 $\times$ 10^{12}/L

COMPLETE BLOOD COUNT WITH DIFFERENTIAL

Test	Conventional units	SI units
White blood cells (WBCs)	2 mo to 6 yr: 5,000 to 19,000 cells/mm^3	2 mo to 6 yr: 5 to 19 $\times$ 10^9
	6 to 18 yr: 4,800 to 10,800 cells/mm^3	6 to 18 yr: 4.8 to 10.8 $\times$ 10^9
Bands	5% to 11%	0.05 to 0.11
Basophils	0%	0
Eosinophils	0% to 3%	0 to 0.03
Lymphocytes	25% to 76%	0.25 to 0.76
Monocytes	0% to 5%	0 to 0.05
Neutrophils	54% to 62%	0.54 to 0.62

ANTIBIOTIC PEAKS AND TROUGHS

Test		Conventional units	SI units
Amikacin	Peak	20 to 30 mcg/ml	34 to 52 µmol/L
	Trough	1 to 4 mcg/ml	2 to 7 µmol/L
Chloramphenicol	Peak	15 to 25 mcg/ml	46.4 to 77 µmol/L
	Trough	5 to 15 mcg/ml	15.5 to 46.4 µmol/L
Gentamicin	Peak	4 to 8 mcg/ml	4 to 16.7 µmol/L
	Trough	1 to 2 mcg/ml	2.1 to 4.2 µmol/L
Tobramycin	Peak	4 to 8 mcg/ml	4 to 16.7 µmol/L
	Trough	1 to 2 mcg/ml	2.1 to 4.2 µmol/L
Vancomycin	Peak	25 to 40 mcg/ml	17 to 27 µmol/L
	Trough	5 to 10 mcg/ml	3.4 to 6.8 µmol/L

URINE TESTS

Test	Conventional units	SI units
Urinalysis Appearance	Clear to slightly hazy	—
Color	Straw to dark yellow	—
pH	4.5 to 8	—
Specific gravity	1.005 to 1.035	—
Glucose	None	—
Protein	None	—
RBCs	None or rare	—
WBCs	None or rare	—
Osmolality	50 to 1,200 mOsm/kg	—

LIPID LEVELS (CHILDREN AGES 2 TO 19)

Test	Conventional units	SI units
Total cholesterol	Acceptable: <170 mg/dl; Borderline: 170 to 199 mg/dl; High: ≥200 mg/dl	—
Low-density lipoprotein	Acceptable: <110 mg/dl; Borderline: 110 to 129 mg/dl; High: ≥130 mg/dl	—
High-density lipoprotein	≥35 mg/dl	—
Triglycerides	≤150 mg/dl	—

Normal blood pressure

Age	Weight (kg)	Systolic BP (mm Hg)	Diastolic BP (mm Hg)
Neonate	1	40 to 60	20 to 36
Neonate	2 to 3	50 to 70	30 to 45
1 month	4	64 to 96	30 to 62
6 months	7	60 to 118	50 to 70
1 year	10	66 to 126	41 to 91
2 to 3 years	12 to 14	74 to 124	39 to 89
4 to 5 years	16 to 18	79 to 119	45 to 85
6 to 8 years	20 to 26	80 to 124	45 to 85
10 to 12 years	32 to 42	85 to 135	55 to 88
> 14 years	> 50	90 to 140	60 to 90

Normal respiratory rates

Age	Breaths per minute
Birth to 6 months	30 to 60
6 months to 2 years	20 to 30
3 to 10 years	20 to 28
10 to 18 years	12 to 20

Normal temperature ranges

Age	Temperature	
	°F	°C
Neonate	98.6 to 99.8	37 to 37.7
3 years	98.5 to 99.5	36.9 to 37.5
10 years	97.5 to 98.6	36.4 to 37
16 years	97.6 to 98.8	36.4 to 37.1

Pain measurement in young children

For children who are old enough to speak and understand sufficiently, these useful tools can help them communicate information for measuring their pain. Here's how to use each one.

VISUAL ANALOG SCALE

A visual analog pain scale is simply a straight line with the phrase "no pain" at one end and the phrase "the most pain possible" at the other. Children who understand the concept of a continuum can mark the spot on the line that corresponds to the level of pain they feel.

No pain |————————————————————————————| The most pain possible

WONG-BAKER FACES PAIN RATING SCALE

The child age 3 and older can use the faces scale to rate his pain. When using this tool, make sure that he can see and point to each face and then describe the amount of pain each face is experiencing. If he's able, the child can read the text under the picture; otherwise, you or his parent can read it to him.

Avoid saying anything that might prompt the child to choose a certain face. Then ask the child to choose the face that shows how he's feeling right now. Record his response in your assessment notes..

| Happy because he doesn't hurt at all | Hurts just a little bit | Hurts a little more | Hurts even more | Hurts a whole lot | Hurts the most |

Reprinted with permission from Wong, D.L., et al. *Wong's Essentials of Pediatric Nursing,* 6th ed. St. Louis: Mosby–Year Book, Inc., 2001.

Pain rating using FLACC scale

The Face, Legs, Activity, Cry, Consolability (FLACC) scale uses the characteristics listed below to measure pain in infants.

The FLACC scale is a behavioral pain assessment scale for use in nonverbal patients who can't report pain. Here's how to use it: **1.** Rate the patient in each of the five measurement categories; **2.** Add the scores together; **3.** Document the total pain score.

	Score		
Category	0	1	2
Face	No particular expression or smile	Occasional grimace or frown, withdrawn, disinterested	Frequent to constant frown, clenched jaw, and quivering chin
Legs	Normal position or relaxed	Uneasy, restless, tense	Kicking or legs drawn up
Activity	Lying quietly, normal position, moves easily	Squirming, shifting back and forth, tense	Arched, rigid, or jerking
Cry	No cry (awake or asleep)	Moans or whimpers, occasional complaint	Crying steadily, screams or sobs, frequent complaints
Consolability	Content, relaxed	Reassured by occasional touching, hugging, or "talking to," distractible	Difficult to console or comfort

Adapted with permission from "The FLACC: A behavioral scale for scoring postoperative pain in young children," by S. Merkel, et al. *Pediatric Nursing*, 23(3), 1997, p. 293-297. Copyright 1997 Jannetti Co. University of Michigan Medical Center.

Sexual maturity in boys

Genital development and pubic hair growth are the first signs of sexual maturity in boys. The illustrations below show the development of the male genitalia and pubic hair in puberty.

Stage 1
No pubic hair is present

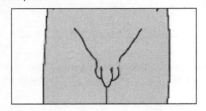

Stage 2
Downy hair develops laterally and later becomes dark; the scrotum becomes more textured, and the penis and testes may become larger.

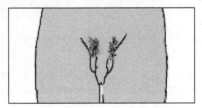

Stage 3

Pubic hair extends across the pubis; the scrotum and testes are larger; the penis elongates.

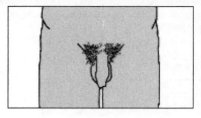

Stage 4

Pubic hair becomes more abundant and curls, and the genitalia resemble those of adults; the glans penis has become larger and broader, and the scrotum becomes darker.

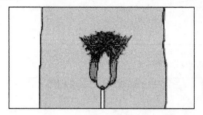

Stage 5

Pubic hair resembles an adult's in quality and pattern and the hair extends to the inner borders of the thighs; the testes and scrotum are adult in size.

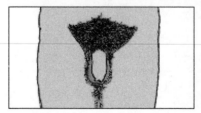

Sexual maturity in girls

Breast development and pubic hair growth are the first signs of sexual maturity in girls. These illustrations show the development of the female breast and pubic hair in puberty.

BREAST DEVELOPMENT

Stage 1
Only the *papilla* (nipple) elevates (not shown).

Stage 2
Breast buds appear; the areola is slightly widened and appears as a small mound.

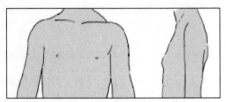

Stage 3
The entire breast enlarges; the nipple doesn't protrude.

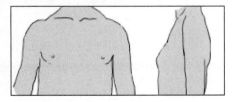

Stage 4

The breast enlarges; the nipple and the papilla protrude and appear as a secondary mound.

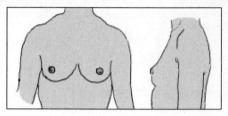

Stage 5

The adult breast has developed; the nipple protrudes and the areola no longer appears separate from the breast.

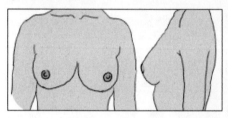

PUBIC HAIR DEVELOPMENT

Stage 1
No pubic hair is present.

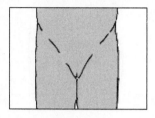

Stage 2
Pubic hair begins to appear on the labia and extends between stages 2 and 3

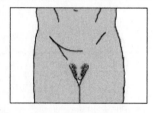

Stage 3
Pubic hair increases in quantity; it appears darker, curled, and more dense and begins to form the typical (but smaller in quantity) female triangle.

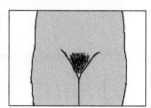

Stage 4
Pubic hair is more dense and curled; it's more adult in distribution, but less abundant than in an adult.

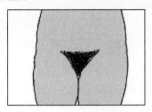

Stage 5
Pubic hair is abundant, appears in an adult female pattern, and may extend onto the medial part of the thighs

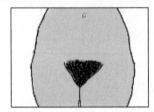

Suicide warning signs

Watch for these warning signs of impending suicide:
- withdrawal or social isolation
- signs of depression, which may include crying, fatigue, helplessness, hopelessness, poor concentration, reduced interest in daily activities, sadness, constipation, and weight loss
- farewells to friends and family
- putting affairs in order
- giving away prized possessions
- expression of covert suicide messages and death wishes
- obvious suicide messages such as, "I would be better off dead."

ANSWERING A THREAT

If a patient shows signs of impending suicide, assess the seriousness of the intent and the immediacy of the risk. Consider a patient with a chosen method who plans to commit suicide in the next 48 to 72 hours a high risk.

Tell the patient that you're concerned. Urge him to avoid self-destructive behavior until the staff has an opportunity to help him. Consult with the treatment team about psychiatric hospitalization.

Initiate the following safety precautions for those at high risk for suicide:
- Provide a safe environment.
- Remove dangerous objects, such as belts, razors, suspenders, electric cords, glass, knives, nail files, and clippers.
- Make the patient's specific restrictions clear to staff members, and plan for observation of the patient.
- Stay alert when the patient is shaving, taking medication, or using the bathroom.
- Encourage continuity of care and consistency of primary nurses.

Tooth eruption

A child's primary and secondary teeth will erupt in a predictable order, as shown in these illustrations.

PRIMARY TOOTH ERUPTION

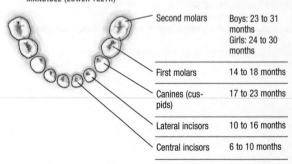

Teeth	Age of eruption
Central incisors	8 to 12 months
Lateral incisors	9 to 13 months
Canines (cuspids)	16 to 22 months
First molars	Boys: 13 to 19 months Girls: 14 to 18 months
Second molars	25 to 33 months

MAXILLA (UPPER TEETH)

MANDIBLE (LOWER TEETH)

Teeth	Age of eruption
Second molars	Boys: 23 to 31 months Girls: 24 to 30 months
First molars	14 to 18 months
Canines (cuspids)	17 to 23 months
Lateral incisors	10 to 16 months
Central incisors	6 to 10 months

SECOND TOOTH ERUPTION

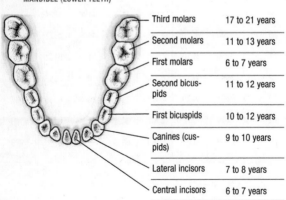

	Teeth	Age of eruption
MAXILLA (UPPER TEETH)	Central incisors	7 to 8 years
	Lateral incisors	8 to 9 years
	Canines (cuspids)	11 to 12 years
	First bicuspids	10 to 11 years
	Second bicuspids	10 to 12 years
	First molars	6 to 7 years
	Second molars	12 to 13 years
	Third molars	Variable

	Teeth	Age of eruption
MANDIBLE (LOWER TEETH)	Third molars	17 to 21 years
	Second molars	11 to 13 years
	First molars	6 to 7 years
	Second bicuspids	11 to 12 years
	First bicuspids	10 to 12 years
	Canines (cuspids)	9 to 10 years
	Lateral incisors	7 to 8 years
	Central incisors	6 to 7 years

CLINICAL TOOLS

Weight conversion

Use this table to convert from pounds and ounces to grams when weighing

Pounds	Ounces							
	0	1	2	3	4	5	6	
0	—	28	57	85	113	142	170	
1	454	484	510	539	567	595	624	
2	907	936	964	992	1021	1049	1077	
3	1361	1389	1417	1446	1474	1503	1531	
4	1814	1843	1871	1899	1928	1956	1984	
5	2268	2296	2325	2353	2381	2410	2438	
6	2722	2750	2778	2807	2835	2863	2892	
7	3175	3203	3232	3260	3289	3317	3345	
8	3629	3657	3685	3714	3742	3770	3799	
9	4082	4111	4139	4167	4196	4224	4252	
10	4536	4564	4593	4621	4649	4678	4706	
11	4990	5018	5046	5075	5103	5131	5160	
12	5443	5471	5500	5528	5557	5585	5613	
13	5897	5925	5953	5982	6010	6038	6067	
14	6350	6379	6407	6435	6464	6492	6520	
15	6804	6832	6860	6889	6917	6945	6973	

7	8	9	10	11	12	13	14	15
198	227	255	283	312	340	369	397	425
652	680	709	737	765	794	822	850	879
1106	1134	1162	1191	1219	1247	1276	1304	1332
1559	1588	1616	1644	1673	1701	1729	1758	1786
2013	2041	2070	2098	2126	2155	2183	2211	2240
2466	2495	2523	2551	2580	2608	2637	2665	2693
2920	2948	2977	3005	3033	3062	3090	3118	3147
3374	3402	3430	3459	3487	3515	3544	3572	3600
3827	3856	3884	3912	3941	3969	3997	4026	4054
4281	4309	4337	4366	4394	4423	4451	4479	4508
4734	4763	4791	4819	4848	4876	4904	4933	4961
5188	5216	5245	5273	5301	5330	5358	5386	5415
5642	5670	5698	5727	5755	5783	5812	5840	5868
6095	6123	6152	6180	6209	6237	6265	6294	6322
6549	6577	6605	6634	6662	6690	6719	6747	6776
7002	7030	7059	7087	7115	7144	7172	7201	7228

Selected references
Index

Selected references

Bowden, V.R. "Get Involved! Join a Pediatric Nursing Association Just Right for You," *Pediatric Nursing* 29(5):397-402, September-October 2003.

Bowden, V.R., and Greenberg, C.S. *Pediatric Nursing Procedures.* Philadelphia: Lippincott Williams & Wilkins, 2003.

Boynton, R.W., et al. *Manual of Ambulatory Pediatrics*, 5th ed. Philadelphia: Lippincott Williams & Wilkins, 2003.

Caputo, M., et al. "Randomized Comparison Between Normothermic and Hypothermic Cardiopulmonary Bypass in Pediatric Open-heart Surgery," *Annals of Thoracic Surgery* 80(3):982-88, September 2005.

Chiou, C., et al. "Development of the Multi-attribute Pediatric Asthma Health Outcome Measure (PAHOM)," *International Journal for Quality in Health Care* 17(1):23-30, February 2005.

Couloigner, V., et al. "Inlay Butterfly Cartilage Tympanoplasty in Children," *Otology & Neurotology* 26(2):247-51, March 2005.

Eisenbeis, J.F., and Herrmann, B.W. "Areolar Connective Tissue Grafts in Pediatric Tympanoplasty: A Pilot Study," *American Journal of Otolaryngology* 25(2):79-83, March-April 2004.

Fleitas, J. "The Power of Words: Examining the Linguistic Landscape of Pediatric Nursing," *MCN, The American Journal of Maternal/Child Nursing* 28(6):384-88, November-December 2003.

Frommelt, P.C. "Update on Pediatric Echocardiography," *Current Opinion in Pediatrics* 17(5):579- 85, October 2005.

Godshall, M. "Caring for Families of Chronically Ill Kids," *RN* 66(2):30-35, February 2003.

Hockenberry, M.J., et al. *Wong's Nursing Care of Infants and Children,* 7th ed. St. Louis: Mosby–Year Book, Inc., 2003.

Hodges, E.A. "A Primer on Early Childhood Obesity and Parental Influence," *Pediatric Nursing* 29(1):13-16, January-February 2003.

Jakubik, L.D., et al. "The ABCs of Pediatric Laboratory Interpretation: Understanding the CBC with Differential and LFTs," *Pediatric Nursing* 29(2):97-103, March-April 2003.

Kaugars, A.S., et al. "Family Influences on Pediatric Asthma," *Journal of Pediatric Psychology* 29(7):475-491, October 2004.

Limbo, R., et al. "Promoting Safety of Young Children with Guided Participation Process," *Journal of Pediatric Health Care* 17(5):245-51, September-October 2003.

Link, N. "Keeping Kids Comfortable," *Nursing2003* 33(7):22, July 2003.

Mandleco, B. *Growth and Development Handbook: Newborn Through Adolescent.* Clifton Park, N.Y.: Delmar Learning, 2004.

Miaskowski, C. "Identifying Issues in the Management of Pain in Infants and Children," *Pain Management Nursing* 4(1):1-2, March 2003.

Pillitteri, A. *Maternal and Child Health Nursing: Care of the Childbearing and Childrearing Family,* 4th ed. Philadelphia: Lippincott Williams & Wilkins, 2003.

Reed, P., et al. "Promoting the Dignity of the Child in Hospital," *Nursing Ethics* 10(1):67-76, January 2003.

Reyes, S. "Nursing Assessment of Infant Pain," *Journal of Perinatal and Neonatal Nursing* 17(4):291-303, October-November 2003.

Straight A's in Pediatric Nursing. Philadelphia: Lippincott Williams & Wilkins, 2004.

Taketomo, C.K., et al. *Pediatric Dosage Handbook,* 11th ed. Hudson, Ohio: Lexi-Comp, Inc., 2004.

Index

i refers to an illustration; t refers to a table.

---

i refers to an illustration; t refers to a table.

i refers to an illustration; t refers to a table.

i refers to an illustration; t refers to a table.

i refers to an illustration; t refers to a table.

i refers to an illustration; t refers to a table.

i refers to an illustration; t refers to a table.